W0116016

Modern System of Ophthalmology (MSO) Series

Profile and Management of
Ocular Trauma

Modern System of Ophthalmology (MSO) Series

Profile and Management of
Ocular Trauma

Editor-in-Chief

AK Khurana MS, FAICO, CTO (London)
Fellow, Moorfields Eye Hospital, London
Senior Professor and Head
Squint and Oculoplasty Services
Regional Institute of Ophthalmology
Postgraduate Institute of Medical Sciences
Rohtak, Haryana, India

Editors

Sunandan Sood MS
Professor and Head
Department of Ophthalmology
Govt Medical College and Hospital
Chandigarh, India

Mehul Shah MS, FRF, FMRF
Medical Director
Drashti Netralaya and Dahod
Tribal Community Eye Care Center
Dahod, Gujarat, India

Shreya Shah DOMS
Administrative Director
Drashti Netralaya and Dahod
Tribal Community Eye Care Center
Dahod, Gujarat, India

Aruj K Khurana DNB, FICO
Fellow, Vitreo-Retina
Narayana Nethralaya
Bengaluru, Karnataka, India

Bhawna Khurana MS, DNB, FICO
Fellow, Orbit, Oculoplasty
and Oncology
Narayana Nethralaya
Bengaluru, Karnataka, India

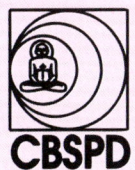

CBSPD

CBS Publishers & Distributors Pvt Ltd

New Delhi • Bengaluru • Chennai • Kochi • Kolkata • Lucknow • Mumbai
Hyderabad • Jharkhand • Nagpur • Patna • Pune • Uttarakhand

Disclaimer

Science and technology are constantly changing fields. New research and experience broaden the scope of information and knowledge. The editors have tried their best in giving information available to them while preparing the material for this book. Although, all efforts have been made to ensure optimum accuracy of the material, yet it is quite possible some errors might have been left uncorrected. The publisher, the printer and the editors will not be held responsible for any inadvertent errors, omissions or inaccuracies.

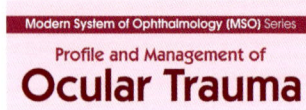

Modern System of Ophthalmology (MSO) Series

Profile and Management of
Ocular Trauma

ISBN: 978-81-239-2630-8

Copyright © AK Khurana

First Edition: 2016
Reprint 2024

All rights reserved. No part of this book may be reproduced or transmitted in any form or by any means, electronic or mechanical, including photocopying, recording, or any information storage and retrieval system without permission, in writing, from the editors and the publisher.

Published by **Satish Kumar Jain** and produced by **Varun Jain** for

CBS Publishers & Distributors Pvt Ltd

4819/XI Prahlad Street, 24 Ansari Road, Daryaganj, New Delhi 110 002, India.
Ph: 011-23289259, 23266838   Website: www.cbspd.com
                                                          e-mail: delhi@cbspd.com

Corporate Office: 204 FIE, Industrial Area, Patparganj, Delhi 110 092
Ph: 011-4934 4934   Fax: 011-4934 4935
                                        e-mail: publishing@cbspd.com; publicity@cbspd.com

Branches

• **Bengaluru:** Seema House 2975, 17th Cross, KR Road, Banasankari 2nd Stage, Bengaluru 560 070, Karnataka, India
  Ph: +91-80-26771678/79   Fax: +91-80-26771680   e-mail: bangalore@cbspd.com
• **Chennai:** 7, Subbaraya Street, Shenoy Nagar, Chennai 600 030, Tamil Nadu, India
  Ph: +91-44-26680620, 26681266   Fax: +91-44-42032115   e-mail: chennai@cbspd.com
• **Kochi:** 42/1325, 1326, Power House Road, Opp KSEB, Power House, Ernakulum Kochi 682 018, Kerala, India
  Ph: +91-484-4059061-65.67   Fax: +91-484-4059065   e-mail: kochi@cbspd.com
• **Kolkata:** 147, Hind Ceramics Compound, 1st Floor, Nilgunj Road, Belghoria, Kolkata-700056, West Bengal, India
  Ph: +033-25633055, 033-25633056   e-mail: kolkata@cbspd.com
• **Lucknow:** Basement, Khushnuma Complex, 7 Meerabai Marg (Behind Jawahar Bhawan), Lucknow-226001, UP, India
  Ph: +0522-4000032   e-mail: tiwari.lucknow@cbspd.com
• **Mumbai:** PWD Shed, Gala no 25/26, Ramchandra Bhatt Marg, Next to JJ Hospital Gate no. 2, Opp. Union Bank of India, Noorbaug, Mumbai-400009, Maharashtra, India
  Ph: 022-66661880/89   e-mail: mumbai@cbspd.com

Representatives

• Hyderabad   0-9885175004   • Jharkhand   0-9811541605   • Nagpur   0-8692091830
• Patna   0-9334159340   • Pune   0-9664372571   • Uttarakhand   0-9716462459

Printed at HT Media Ltd, Greater Noida, UP, India

to

the teachers and residents in ophthalmology for
their endeavor to dissipate and acquire knowledge
to our parents and teachers for their blessings
to our families for their understanding and encouragement
to our patients for letting us learn

Foreword

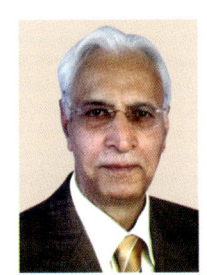

Incidence of ocular trauma is continuously on the rise in this era of unmanned high speed traffic, rapid industrialization, increasing accidents and assaults. Management of ocular trauma is a challenging task to be accomplished combinedly by a team of specialists in disorders of anterior segment, posterior segment, orbit and oculoplasty, and neuroophthalmology. At times even services of the faciomaxillary surgeon and/or neurosurgeon may also be needed to manage the complex ocular trauma cases. This book, '*Profile and Management of Ocular Trauma*' provides a concise yet comprehensive coverage an insight on this complex topic.

It is indeed a pleasure for me to write the foreword to this volume, one of the eleven books in the series Modern System of Ophthalmology (MSO) by Prof AK Khurana. A concise and comprehensive series, like MSO, was much needed for the residents in ophthalmology.

The editorial team of this volume comprises ophthalmologists dedicated to the cause. The book includes chapters on different aspects of ocular trauma by experts in different subspecialties in ophthalmology. The Editor-in-Chief has ensured that text is in a lucid and easy to comprehend style and is supplemented with abundant high quality clinical photographs, line diagrams, tables and flow charts.

I have known Dr Khurana as a keen learner since his residency period. Over the years he has established himself as a prolific writer and highly sought after author, whose books are received with great enthusiasm by the students. I am sure, like his other books, this volume of Modern System of Ophthalmology will also be useful and popular amongst residents, teachers and practitioners in ophthalmology. I congratulate and wish the entire editorial team and contributors all success for their endeavor in the form of a wonderful volume on '*Profile and Management of Ocular Trauma*'.

Prof VK Dada
Padamshree
MBBS, DOMS, MS, FAMS
Formerly Chief, Dr RP Centre for Ophthalmic Sciences, AIIMS,
Senior Consultant Sir Ganga Ram Hospital and Centre for Sight
New Delhi, India

Preface

Modern System of Ophthalmology (MSO) series comprises separate volumes on different subspecialties of ophthalmology. Each volume is planned with a very specific aim to cater to the needs of postgraduate students in ophthalmology.

Salient Features of MSO Series
- Each volume is edited by different editors, yet the layout and organization has been kept similar.
- Editors of different volumes are masters in their subspeciality with an uncanny knack of picking up the right perspectives.
- Text matter is designed to meet the needs of residents in ophthalmology with a comprehensive coverage in a concise manner. Text is complete and up-to-date with recent advances incorporated.
- Text is organized in such a way that the students can easily understand, retain and reproduce it. Various levels of headings, subheadings, bold face and italics given in the text will be helpful for a quick revision of the subject.

Profile and Management of Ocular Trauma. In this era of high-speed traffic and rapid industrialization, the incidence of injuries is increasing in general. Like any other part of the body, eyes are also not exempted from injuries; in spite of the fact that they are well protected by the lids, projected margins of the orbit, the nose and a cushion of fat from behind. It is a matter of great concern that ocular injuries have become a major cause of ocular morbidity and mortality. Further, there is a clear male predominance and that too in the younger and most productive years of their lives causing financial difficulties to the affected family and even forcing many to change their professional careers. Over the years, the diagnostic, therapeutic and surgical management of eye injuries have witnessed an exponential growth. Presently ocular trauma has emerged as an important subspeciality of ophthalmology. Consequently, a number of good books is available on this subject, however, still there is paucity of books which can provide tailor-made material for the needs of residents in ophthalmology. An effort has been made in this volume to provide information on profile and management of ocular injuries, keeping in view the requirements of trainee ophthalmologists, in a more easily understood from.

Text matter of this volume has been arranged in four sections:

Section I: Ocular Injuries: General Considerations, introduces the subject with a chapter each on 'Ocular Trauma: Classification and Terminologies'; 'Evaluation and Assessment', and 'Emergency Management of Ocular Injuries'.

Section II: Mechanical Injuries, comprehensively covers the different aspects of blunt and penetrating/ perforating ocular injuries.

Section III: Non-mechanical Injuries, includes a chapter each on 'Chemical Injuries', 'Radiational Injuries', and 'Thermal, Electrical and Barometric Injuries'.

Section IV: Prevention, Rehabilitation and Medicolegal Aspects of Ocular Injuries, comprehensively covers these aspects in the present day context.

Editorial team of this volume comprises ophthalmologists dedicated to the cause. The Editors, Prof S. Sood, Dr Mehul Shah and Dr Aruj K Khurana are devoted to the management of posterior segment ocular trauma. Dr Shreya Shah and Dr Bhawna Khurana are devoted to management of anterior segment, eyelid, ocular adnexa and orbital trauma.

Acknowledgement needs to be made to the selfless contributors of chapters for this volume and all others who have made this volume a reality. My sincere thanks are due to all of them. I want to express my gratitude to Prof CS Dhull, Head RIO, PGIMS, and Prof OP Kalra, Vice-Chancellor, UHS, Rohtak, for providing an atmosphere conducive to such academic activities. It is my pleasure to acknowledge the role of personalities behind my editorial team especially Dr Naresh Yadav, Head Vitreo-Retina Services, and Dr Roshmi Gupta and Dr Hadi, from Orbit and Oculoplasty services, Narayana Nethralaya, Bengaluru, for grooming Dr Aruj K Khurana and Dr Bhawna Khurana, respectively.

The affection and moral support, in addition to editorial help, rendered by my daughter. Dr Arushi, MD, University of Connecticut, USA, and my wife Dr Indu Khurana, Senior Professor, Department of Physiology, PGIMS, Rohtak made my task untiring. My special thanks are due to dear friends, Dr Bhujang Shetty, Dr Rohit Shetty, Major General DP Vatas, Prof PS Sandhu, Prof GS Bajwa, Prof Atul Kumar, Prof VP Gupta, Prof Vishnu Gupta, Prof BP Guliani, Prof MR Dogra, Prof Jagat Ram, Prof SM Bhati, and Prof KP Chaudhri, for their guidance and encouragement. I acknowledge with humble thanks, the respect, affection and cooperation received from faculty members of RIO, PGIMS, Rohtak, namely Dr SV Singh, Dr JP Chugh, Dr VK Dhull, Dr RS Chauhan, Dr Manisha Rathi, Dr Neebha Passi, Dr Manisha Nada, Dr Urmil Chawla, Dr Ashok Rathi, Dr Sumit Sachdeva, Dr Jitender Phogat and Dr Reena Gupta. I also acknowledge the enormous help received from Dr Shweta Goel and other residents of RIO, PGIMS, Rohtak.

The enthusiastic cooperation received from Mr SK Jain, Managing Director, Mr YN Arjuna, Senior Vice President—Publishing, Editorial and Publicity, and Mrs Ritu Chawla, Manager—Production, CBS Publishers & Distributors, New Delhi, needs special acknowledgement. Mr Sanju, graphic artist, and Mr Tarun Rajput, DTP operator, need special mention because of their efforts to provide considerable beauty to this volume.

In spite of the best efforts, a venture like this is unlikely to be error-free. Constructive criticism and suggestions from the readers are invited for further improvement in this volume.

AK Khurana
Editor-in-Chief

Editorial Board

Editor-in-Chief

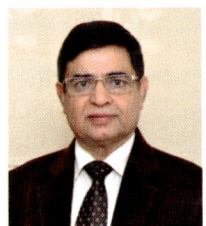

AK Khurana MS, FAICO, CTO (London)
Fellow, Moorfields Eye Hospital, London
Senior Professor and Head
Squint and Oculoplasty Services
Regional Institute of Ophthalmology
Postgraduate Institute of Medical Sciences
Rohtak, Haryana, India

Editors

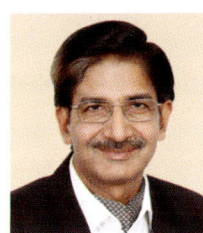

Sunandan Sood MS
Professor and Head
Department of Ophthalmology
Govt Medical College and
Hospital, Chandigarh, India

Mehul Shah MS, FRF, FMRF
Medical Director
Drashti Netralaya and Dahod
Tribal Community Eye Care Center
Dahod, Gujarat, India

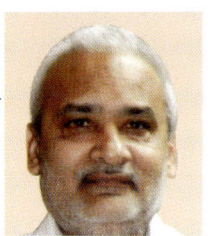

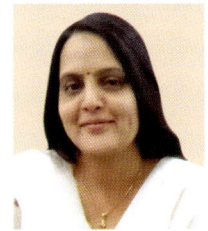

Shreya Shah DOMS
Administrative Director
Drashti Netralaya and Dahod
Tribal Community Eye Care Center
Dahod, Gujarat, India

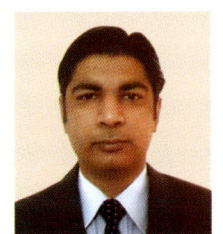

Aruj K Khurana DNB, FICO
Fellow, Vitreo-Retina
Narayana Nethralaya
Bengaluru, Karnataka, India

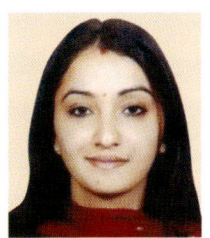

Bhawna Khurana MS, DNB, FICO
Fellow, Orbit, Oculoplasty
and Oncology
Narayana Nethralaya
Bengaluru, Karnataka, India

List of Contributors

AK Khurana MS, FAICO, CTO (London)
Senior Professor and Head
Squint and Oculoplasty Services
Regional Institute of Ophthalmology
PGIMS, Rohtak, Haryana, India

Mehul Shah MS, FMRF
Medical Director
Drashti Netralaya
Dahod, Gujarat

Aruj K Khurana DNB, FICO
Fellow, Vitreo-Retina
Narayana Nethralaya, Bengaluru

Atul Kumar MD
Prof and Head, Vitreo-Retina Services
Dr RP Centre for Ophthalmic Sciences
AIIMS, New Delhi

Naresh Yadav DOMS, FMRF
Head, Vitreo-Retina Services
Narayana Nethralaya, Bengaluru

Roshmi Gupta MS, FRCS
Head, Ophthalmicplastics, Orbital
Surgery and Ocular Oncology
Narayana Nethralaya-1, Bengaluru

Hadi-Khazaei MS, FRCS
Head, Oribt, Oculopathy and Oncology
Narayana Nethralaya-2, Bengaluru

Sudesh K Arya MD
Professor of Ophthalmology
GMCH, Chandigarh

Indu Khurana MD
Sr Professor, Physiology
PGIMS, Rohtak, Haryana

Subina Narang MS
Assoc. Prof, Ophthalmology
GMCH, Chandigarh

Arushi Khurana MD
Chief Resident, Dept. of Internal Medicine
University of Connecticut
Hartfort, USA

Anubha Bhatti MS
Sr Resident, Deptt of Ophthalmology
GMCH, Chandigarh

Panchmi Gupta MS
Sr Resident, Deptt of Ophthalmology
NDMC Hospital, New Delhi

Sunandan Sood MS
Professor and Head
Department of Ophthalmology
GMCH, Chandigarh

Shreya Shah DOMS
Administrative Director
Drashti Netralaya
Dahod, Gujarat

Bhawna Khurana MS, DNB, FICO
Fellow, Orbit, Oculoplasty and Oncology
Narayana Nethralaya
Bengaluru, Karnataka

VP Gupta MD, DNB
Prof and Head
Department of Ophthalmology
UCMS, New Delhi

SK Dhatarwal MD
Sr Prof and Head
Dept of Forensic Medicine
PGIMS, Rohtak, Haryana

Manisha Nada MS
Prof. RIO PGIMS, Rohtak

Parul Chawla Gupta MS
Assistant Prof, Advanced Eye Center
PGIMER, Chandigarh

Sumeet Khanduja MD
Assistant Prof,
RIO PGIMS, Rohtak

Prateek Topiwala MS
Sr Resident, Deptt of Ophthalmology
GMCH, Chandigarh

Shweta Goel MS (St)
Resident, RIO
PGIMS, Rohtak, Haryana

Nishita Beke MS
Resident, Deptt of Ophthalmology
GMCH, Chandigarh

Anuj Sharma MS
Resident, Deptt of Ophthalmology
GMCH, Chandigarh

Surbhi Sharma
Resident, Deptt of Ophthalmology
GMCH, Chandigarh

Contents

Section III. Non-mechanical Injuries

Section IV: Prevention, Rehabilitation and Medicolegal Aspects of Ocular Injuries

OCULAR TRAUMA: CLASSIFICATION AND TERMINOLOGIES

INTRODUCTION
- Pattern of ocular injuries
- Ocular trauma and blindness
- Grouping of ocular injuries

MECHANICAL INJURIES
Ocular trauma: Terminologies, classification, and scoring
- Birmingham eye trauma terminology

- Ocular trauma classification systems
- Ocular trauma score

NON-MECHANICAL INJURIES
- Chemical injuries
- Thermal injuries
- Electrical injuries
- Radiational injuries
- Barometric injuries

INTRODUCTION

PATTERN OF OCULAR INJURIES

Pattern of ocular injuries tends to vary from one location to another and is affected by the activities of residents in a given location. Many eye injuries are related to sports, agriculture, occupation, exposure to hazards and are caused by a variety of objects used in different settings. In addition, in this era of high-speed traffic and rapid industrialization, the incidence of injuries involving the eye is also increasing. Despite the fact that the eyes represent only 0.27% of the total body surface area and 4% of the face, these are the third most common organs affected by injuries after the hands and feet. In general, trauma is an important cause of ocular morbidity.

OCULAR TRAUMA AND BLINDNESS

Ocular trauma is an avoidable cause of blindness and visual impairment. Worldwide there are approximately 1.6 million people blind from eye injuries, 2.3 million bilaterally visually impaired and 19 million with unilateral visual loss. As a matter of fact, ocular trauma is the commonest

cause of unilateral blindness. Younger age and male gender are the most common subjects of ocular trauma. Various studies have reported that approximately one-half of patients who present to an eye emergency department are cases of ocular trauma.

GROUPING OF OCULAR INJURIES

Grouping of ocular injuries, in general, can be done comprehensively as below (Fig. 1.1):
I. Isolated ocular injuries
- Mechanical injuries
- Non-mechanical injuries.
II. Ocular injuries associated with other injuries
III. Etiological grouping

MECHANICAL INJURIES

Incidence of mechanical injuries is increasing in general in this era of high-speed traffic and industrialization, like any other part of the body, eyes are also not exempted from these injuries; in spite of the fact that they are well protected by the lids, projected margins of the orbit, the nose and a cushion of fat from behind.

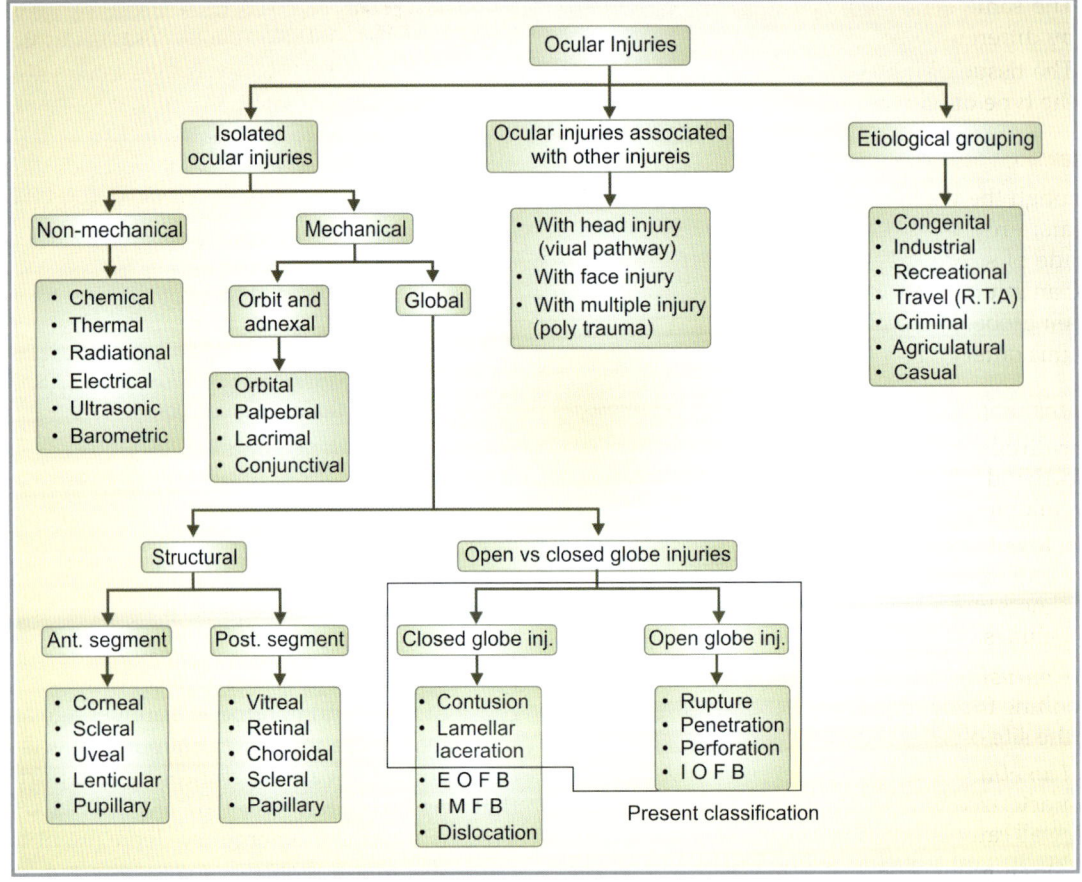

Fig. 1.1 *Comprehensive grouping of ocular injuries*

Mechanical ocular injuries can be discussed under following headings:
- Extraocular foreign bodies
- Blunt trauma
- Open globe injuries
- Sympathetic ophthalmitis

OCULAR TRAUMA: TERMINOLOGY, CLASSIFICATION AND SCORING

BIRMINGHAM EYE TRAUMA TERMINOLOGY

For individuals to communicate and understand each other, one requires a language which is both universally recognized and accepted. In a similar manner, to prevent misinterpretation of facts relating to eye injuries ophthalmologists require terms with unambiguous definitions. In many series and reports, different terms were being used interchangeably for the same ocular injury. This prevented ophthalmologists from establishing a set protocol to manage ocular trauma.

The Birmingham Eye Trauma Terminology (BETT) laid down the terminology of mechanical ocular injuries to overcome this ambiguity. Kuhn and coworkers based on their experience came up with this terminology to categorize eye injuries. This terminology, i.e. BETT was endorsed by various professional associations, such as the American Academy of Ophthalmology, International Society of Ocular Trauma and World Eye Injury Registry amongst others. The Birmingham Eye Trauma Terminology considers certain basic criteria which are looked for in an ideal terminology system.
- Includes all types of ocular injuries.
- Each type of injury is clearly defined.

- The same ocular injury cannot be described by different terms.
- The tissue of injury is mentioned along with the type of injury.

Eyewall

Though the wall of the eyeball comprises three coats; only the integrity of the external shell made of sclera and cornea needs to be broken for an injury to convert from closed globe to an open globe. Hence, the term eyewall is limited to this outer coat of the eye (sclera and cornea).

Terminologies for mechanical globe injuries

Terminologies for mechanical globe injuries modified from Birmingham Eye Trauma Terminology (Fig. 1.2) are as below:

I. **Closed globe injury** is the one in which eyewall (sclera and cornea) does not have a full thickness wound but there is intraocular damage. It includes contusion and lamellar laceration.

1. *Contusion* refers to the closed globe injury resulting from blunt trauma. Damage may occur at the site of impact or at a distant site.

2. *Lamellar laceration* is a closed globe injury characterized by a partial thickness wound of the eyewall caused by a sharp object or blunt trauma.

II. **Open globe injury** is associated with a full thickness wound of the sclera or cornea or both. It includes rupture and laceration of eyewall.

1. *Rupture refers* to a full thickness wound of eyewall caused by the impact of blunt trauma. The wound occurs due to markedly raised intraocular pressure by an inside out injury mechanism.

2. *Laceration* refers to a full thickness wound of eyewall caused by a sharp object. The wound occurs at the impact site by an outside in mechanism. It includes penetrating and perforating injuries.

i. *Penetrating injury* refers to a single laceration of eyewall caused by a sharp object which traverses the coats only once.

ii. *Perforating injury* refers to two full thickness lacerations (one entry and one exit) of the eyeball caused by a sharp object or missile. The two wounds must have been caused by the sameagent (earlier known as double perforation)

iii. *Intraocular, foreign body injury* is technically a penetrating injury associated with retained intraocular foreign body. However, it is grouped separately because of different clinical implications.

OCULAR TRAUMA CLASSIFICATION SYSTEMS

A standardization of ocular trauma classification was carried out by a group of 13 ophthalmologists, who reviewed the trauma classification systems in ophthalmology and reports on the characteristics and outcomes of eye injuries. They came up with a classification system with standardized

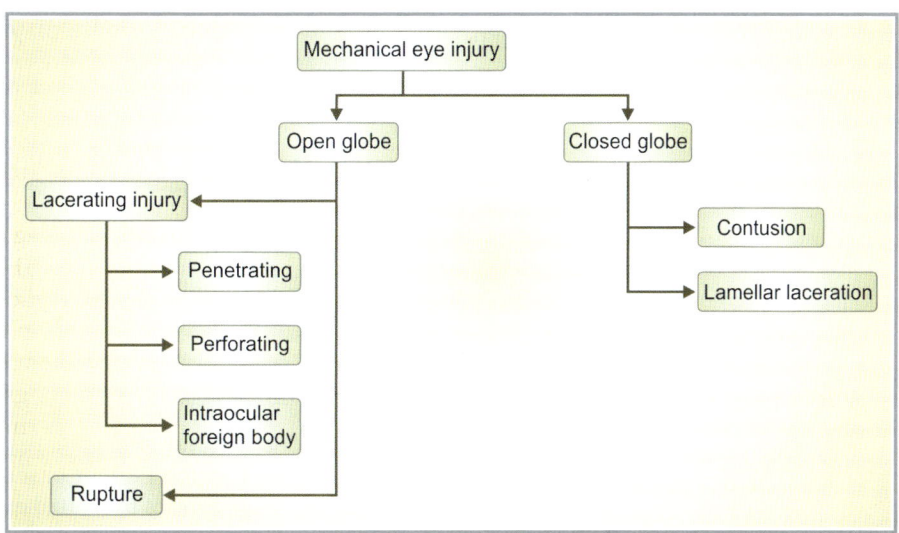

Fig. 1.2 *Birmingham eye trauma terminology*

nomenclature and prognostic indicators that need to be evaluated upon initial presentation.

The classification takes into account four variables—type, grade, zone and presence or absence of RAPD. These variables can be discerned at the initial examination or at the time of primary repair, forceful evaluation should never be attempted, lest the intraocular contents prolapse out.

System for classifying open globe injuries

Type of injury
a. Rupture
b. Penetrating
c. Intraocular foreign body
d. Perforating
e. Mixed

Grade (visual acuity at presentation)
  i. ≥ 20/40
 ii. 20/50 to 20/100
iii. 19/100 to 5/200
 iv. 4/200 to PL+
  v. Absence of light perception

Pupillary response
a. Relative afferent pupillary defect (RAPD) present in the injured eye
b. No RAPD in the injured eye

Zone (Fig. 1.3)
1. Cornea and limbus
2. Limbus to 5 mm posterior into the sclera
3. Posterior to 5 mm from the limbus

(The posterior most opening in the eyeball is considered.)

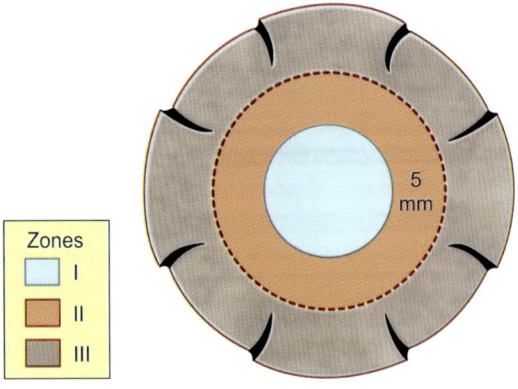

Zones
☐ I
☐ II
☐ III

Fig. 1.3 *Zones of the eyeball as per the ocular trauma classification*

System for classifying closed globe injuries

Type
1. Contusion
2. Lamellar laceration
3. Superficial corneal foreign body
4. Mixed

Grade (visual acuity at presentation)
  i. ≥ 20/40
 ii. 20/50 to 20/100
iii. 19/100 to 5/200
 iv. 4/200 to PL+
  v. Absence of light perception

Pupillary response
a. RAPD present in the injured eye
b. No RAPD in the injured eye

Zone
1. *External*, limited to bulbar conjunctiva, sclera and cornea.
2. *Anterior segment* includes structures of anterior segment along with pars plicata and the lens apparatus.
3. *Posterior segment* incluldes all internal structures posterior to posterior lens capsule.

(The posterior most structure showing evidence of structural alteration is taken into consideration.)

OCULAR TRAUMA SCORE

The patient's perspective in the scenario of ocular trauma should be borne in mind. Their leading questions "How much is the damage?" or "How much chance is there of recovery?" although cannot be determined in a single value; however, a probable idea or prognostication can be given from the ocular trauma score (OTS).

The OTS is able to tell with an accuracy of 77% the final visual outcome of the patient ± within one visual category. It helps allay the patient anxiety and helps them deal with the economic and rehabilitation issues and guides the ophthalmologist in triage and patient counselling.

Calculation of OTS

The OTS is a simple tool and is calculated as below:

Step 1. Identify the value of the raw points which can be attributed to the patient based on your assessment. At the time of the initial evaluation, ascertain the visual acuity of the patient at presentation and arrive at a tissue diagnosis (Table 1.1).

Table 1.1 *Raw points attributed to various variables in the OTS*

Variable	Raw points
A. Initial vision	
• No light perception	60
• Light perception/hand movements	70
• 1/200–19/200	80
• 20/200–20/50	90
• ≥ 20/40	100
B. Rupture	−23
C. Endophthalmitis	−17
D. Perforating injury	−14
E. Retinal detachment	−11
F. Afferent pupillary defect	−10

Step 2. Calculate the algebraic sum of the raw points (Table 1.2). Assign a raw point value for the initial visual acuity from Row 'A' of Table 1.1; subtract the appropriate row point for each diagnosis from Rows 'B' – 'F'. (For example, a patient with an initial visual acuity of 1/200, scleral, rupture and retinal detachment would receive an OTS score of 80–23–11 = 46). Higher the OTS, the better is the prognosis.

Step 3. Conversion of the sum into OTS and calculating the likelihood of final vision at 6 months. To provide an estimate of the patient's probability of attaining a specific visual acuity range at a six-month follow-up, locate the row in Table 1.2 which corresponds to the patient's OTS (As in the example above, the patient having an OTS of 46 would have a category score of 2). Table 1.2 shows the estimated probability of all potential visual outcomes after six months.

Clinical implications

It is imperative to arrive at a proper diagnosis when dealing with a patient of ocular trauma.
- *BETT terminology* helps us to define and determine the nature of injury.
- *Ocular trauma classification* guides us to label its type, grade, zone of involvement and the presence or absence of RAPD.

- *Ocular trauma score* gives an approximate idea regarding the retrieval of final visual acuity at six months follow-up of the patient thereby helping the ophthalmologist in proper patient guidance and counselling.

NON-MECHANICAL INJURIES

This group includes all ocular injuries other than caused by mechanical trauma. That include:

1. **Chemical injuries:** Chemical injuries are by no means uncommon and can be caused by chemical solution, powder or gases. These vary in severity from a trivial and transient irritation of little significance to complete and sudden loss of vision. Chemical injuries have been covered in detail in Chapter 13.

2. **Radiational injuries** can be caused by ultraviolet, infrared or ionizing radiations. These have been described in Chapter 14.

3. **Thermal injuries** are usually caused by fire, or hot fluids. The main brunt of such injuries lies on the lids. Conjunctiva and cornea may be affected in severe cases. Thermal injuries are covered in Chapter 15.

4. **Electrical injuries** are caused due to passage of electric current from the area of eye and can involve each part of the eyeball. These are covered in Chapter 15.

5. **Barometric injuries** are caused due to atmospheric pressure changes and are described in Chapter 15.

BIBLIOGRAPHY

1. Kuhn F, Morris R, Witherspoon CD, Heimann K, Jeffers JB, Treister G. A standardized classification of ocular trauma. Ophthalmology. 1996; 103(2):240–243.

2. Kuhn F, Maisiak R, Mann L, Mester V, Morris R, Witherspoon CD. The Ocular Trauma Score (OTS). Ophthalmol Clin North Am 2002; 15:163–165.

Table 1.2 *Likelihood of final visual outcome at six months*

Sum of raw points	OTS	NLP	LP/HM	1/200–19/200	20/200–20/50	≥ 20/40
0–44	1	74 %	15 %	7 %	3 %	1 %
45–65	2	27 %	26 %	18 %	15 %	15 %
66–80	3	2 %	11 %	15 %	31 %	41 %
81–91	4	1 %	2 %	3 %	22 %	73 %
92–100	5	0 %	1 %	1 %	5 %	94 %

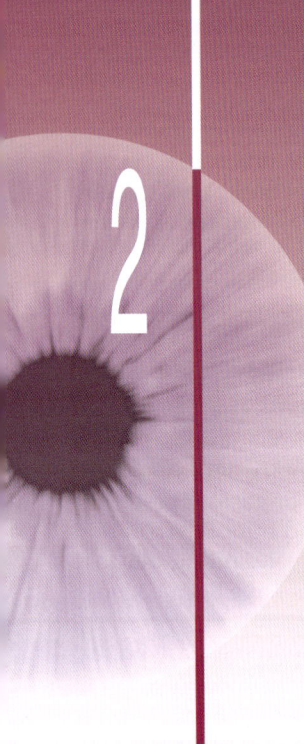

2

TRAUMATIC EYE: EVALUATION AND ASSESSMENT

INTRODUCTION

A proper evaluation of the traumatized eye is absolutely essential for appropriate and effective management of the injury. Classification of the injury and calculation of the ocular trauma score are essential aspects which should be brought into practice. It should be remembered that in case of ocular trauma, the ophthalmologist is treating the patient and not only the eye, pay attention to any systemic features, social bearing of the ocular injury and ultimately to the visual rehabilitation of the patient. Scheme of approach to a patient with ocular trauma described below is summarized in Fig. 2.1.

Initial approach. Patients usually present to the ocular emergency in a state of panic or frenzy. The sudden threat to vision can be emotionally damning. This places upon the treating ophthalmologist an added responsibility of counselling not only the patient but also their family members. It is always advisable to maintain a confident and humane approach.

Systemic evaluation. Prior to taking history and performing a thorough examination of the eye, it is important for the attending ophthalmologist to evaluate the systemic condition of the patient. Ocular trauma can be compounded by life-threatening injuries as in cases of polytrauma commonly observed in road traffic accidents. If a systemic injury is found, its treatment will obviously take precedence over the ocular management. In these cases, the emergency team stabilizes the patient before calling in for an expert ophthalmic opinion. Even in cases presenting directly to the ophthalmologist, it is always better to be suspicious of occult injury to other organ systems.

Initial triage should consist of systemic evaluation of vitals, gross mental status and obvious fractures or soft tissue injuries. The patient should be referred to a trauma facility, if at any point of the examination, the following are found:
- Unstable vital parameters
- Altered mental status or an unresponsive patient
- Serious bony or soft tissue injury

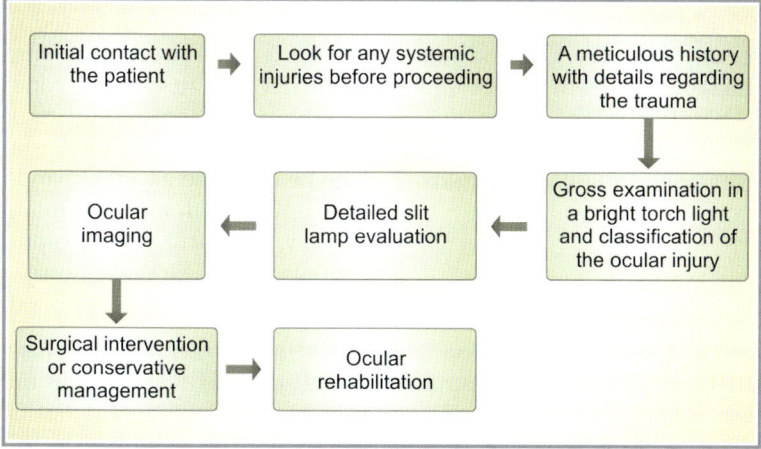

Fig. 2.1 *Scheme of approach to a patient with ocular trauma*

Once it is established that the systemic status is stable, the surgeon can turn attention to the ocular evaluation.

CLINICAL WORKUP

HISTORY

The importance of a well-taken history, at the time of initial presentation, cannot be over-emphasized. Not only does this give the ophthalmologist a chance to build a rapport and earn the trust of the patient but a well-documented history is also necessary for legal proceedings. The history will guide the ophthalmologist towards the examination.

It is best to allow the patient to tell his or her version of the incident without much of an interruption. Leading questions can be asked in between to bring the patients back on track, if they ever get diverted off course. The history should highlight the following important points:

Events leading up to the injury. It is of utmost importance to elucidate the minutest detail of activity which the patient was performing at the time of sustaining the injury, e.g. whether the activity was related to sports, bow and arrow and bursting of crackers during Diwali/Dusshera festivals, a laborer crushing stones while using a chisel and hammer, industrial or agricultural pursuits, involved in roadside accidents and finally an assault with the use of some kind of armament.

Detailed description of the mechanism of trauma to note whether:
- A high-velocity or a low-velocity trauma, and
- Injury with a blunt or a sharp object

Time of the injury and time elapsed between the insult and initial presentation should be documented:
- As it decides management. A fresh open corneal wound would be dealt with urgently and more aggressively than a self-sealed corneal laceration in a quiet eye which is a week old.
- Important for medicolegal purposes.

Rural or an urban setting should be noted. The incidence of infection in cases of trauma in rural settings is higher and so is the risk of endophthalmitis.

Chemical nature of the insulting object should be noted
- If an intraocular foreign body is suspected its nature and chemical composition must be known (iron, copper or steel)
- Any chemical agent, such as an alkali or acid, may further complicate the mechanical injury.

Prior ocular history should specifically include:
- Any history of previous ocular surgery or trauma
- Use of any ocular medications, and
- Prior vision of the injured eye and the un-injured eye.

Generalized medical history of any chronic systemic illness or use of any drugs or medications should be documented. It is important to note any drug allergies and status of tetanus immunization. If an open globe injury is suspected, general anaesthesia would be required and the patient should be asked about the time he last consumed solids and liquids.

OCULAR EXAMINATION

External inspection in diffuse illumination

Prior to examining the patient on the slit-lamp, a gross evaluation of the ocular condition can be made out with the help of a diffuse illumination of a pen torch.

- *Forehead and the periorbital tissues* should be inspected under bright illumination. Evaluate for the presence of any laceration, abrasion, periorbital edema and ecchymosis.
- *Look for exophthalmos,* enophthalmos or any foreign body, such as a stone present in the margins of the laceration.
- *Orbital walls* should be palpated to look for evidence of any bony discontinuity.
- *Crepitus and infraorbital hypoesthesia* may indicate an orbital fracture.

Inspection of globe

Attention should now be given to the ocular structures per se. The eyelids may be parted with the help of an eye speculum or a lid retractor in individuals wherein the periorbital edema makes examination difficult. Inspect the globes for:

- Prolapse of intraocular contents
- Protruding foreign bodies, and
- Any sign of occult open globe injury (hemorrhagic chemosis, pupillary peaking).

Note. It should be kept in mind that no pressure is given on the globe lest the intraocular contents prolapse out. In cases of highly swollen lids or an uncooperative patient, the examination of the globe can be deferred till imaging is done or can be carried out under sedation.

Visual function assessment

Visual acuity. The presenting visual acuity is a crucial prognostic indicator in determining the outcome of injury. The visual acuity is measured separately for each eye. It should be preferably recorded on a standardized chart (ETDRS or Snellen). If the patients are immobilized or on a stretcher, due to systemic comorbidities, visual acuity can be assessed by asking the patient to count fingers at a specific distance. Poor vision can be recorded as either hand motions or light perception with a documentation of projection of rays. The test of light perception and projection of rays should be carried out with the brightest possible light (indirect ophthalmoscope).

Relative afferent pupillary defect. The presence or absence of RAPD is an indicator of gross visual dys function. The test is performed as a swinging flash-light test with a bright light source. Apparent dilation of the pupil of the eye in which light is shown points towards the presence of RAPD. It indicates an optic nerve or a severe retinal damage with a poor prognosis.

Afferent pupillary defect can also be elucidated in cases where-in the iris is injured and the pupil is not reacting. In this case rather than visualizing the direct pupillary response in each eye, only the response in the normal reacting pupil is observed. RAPD is said to be present when the pupil of the fellow eye dilates when light is moved to the injured eye.

Visual field assessment. Rapid assessment of the peripheral visual field can be carried out in the emergency setting using the confrontation test. It can give additional information about retinal or optic nerve damage.

Ocular motility assessment

- If *injury to the cranial nerves* or bony orbital margin is suspected, ocular motility must be evaluated.
- *A case of blow-out fracture* with an entrapped inferior rectus muscle can be made out at this stage and treatment modified accordingly.
- However, it is not always possible to examine for motility as the patient's periorbital oedema or lack of cooperation may mask the findings.

Examination of conjunctiva

Foreign bodies or precipitates of chemicals may be lodged within the conjunctical fornices. The lids should be everted and fornices examined.

Double eversion of the upper lid with a Desmarres retractor is needed to look for hidden foreign bodies in the superior fornix.

Presence of hemorrhagic chemosis should make one suspect of an underlying breach in the eyewall.

Subconjunctival hemorrhage, the posterior extent of which cannot be reached, raises the possibility of a fracture of the base of the skull.

Lacerations of the conjunctiva may be difficult to make out initially. Manipulation with a cotton swab following anaesthetic instillation can clearly delineate the edge of the laceration. A thorough search for an underlying scleral wound should be made in these cases.

Examination of cornea

Epithelial defects. Patients usually present with pain and photophobia. A drop of a topical anesthetic helps to allay their discomfort and allows for a thorough examination at the slit-lamp. Fluorescein staining and documentation of the size of the epithelial defect is of prime importance. Look for abrasion, opacification and ulcerations.

Superficial corneal foreign body. The depth of penetration of the foreign body should be evaluated on the slit-lamp. If the entire thickness of the cornea is breached, the injury gets classified as an open globe injury. The foreign body in this case is best removed in the operation theatre. For smaller foreign bodies which are more superficial, removal on a slit-lamp with a hypodermic needle is sufficient.

Corneal wounds should be analysed whether they are full thickness or partial thickness. This can be carried out with the help of a Seidel's test. Leakage of aqueous from a full thickness breach would dilute the fluorescein dye forming a green stream (positive Seidel's test).

Examination of sclera

- A detailed examination of the sclera should be carried out to look for any breach in the eyewall. This is not always easy as the associated subconjunctival hemorrhage may prevent adequate visualization.

- If a defect in the continuity of the scleral wall is suspected and adequate visualization is not possible, a surgical exploration should be planned.

Examination of anterior chamber

Contents of anterior chamber should be analysed for the presence of any aqueous cells or flare. Traumatic iritis following the insult can lead to inflammation in the anterior chamber. RBCs may also be found in the anterior chamber with damage to the iris. Look for any retained foreign body, hyphema or hypopyon.

Depth of the anterior chamber must be noted:
Deep anterior chamber may be a sign of:
- Posterior dislocation of the lens, or
- Posterior scleral rupture, or
- Iridodialysis.

Shallow anterior chamber may be a sign of:
- Anterior dislocation of the lens, or
- Corneoscleral perforation, or
- Suprachoroidal haemorrhage, or
- Serous choroidal detachment.

Examination of iris

- *Iris is one of the most common sites of damage* in both open and closed globe injuries. A slit-lamp evaluation should be carried out to look for sphincter tears, iridodialysis, iridodonesis and full thickness iris defects.
- *In case of corneoscleral wounds,* the iris may be prolapsed to block the site of perforation. In old injuries, the iris tissue may get incarcerated in the wound leading to an adherent leucoma.

Examination of crystalline lens

- A note should be made of phacodonesis, dislocation, subluxation or zonular dehiscence.
- Blunt trauma can lead to a break in the posterior capsule forming a rosette-shaped concussion cataract at the posterior subcapsular region.
- Look for the integrity of the anterior capsule. A tear in the capsule would result in anterior subcapsular opacification or in leak of cortical material into the anterior chamber and further inflammation.
- Intralenticular foreign bodies must be looked for.

Intraocular pressure measurement

- Measurement of intraocular pressure should be carried out in all cases of trauma; provided an open globe injury has been ruled out.

- Following a contusion, the intraocular pressure may rise acutely, especially if inflammation and blood is present.

- An abnormally low IOP would point towards an occult open globe injury but can also be seen with ciliary body detachment.

Examination of posterior segment

- *An indepth analysis of the posterior segment* of the eye should be carried out after ruling out globe rupture before the media clarity is compromised.

- *90D slit-lamp examination* should be attempted in case the media permits or else *20D indirect ophthalmoscopy* be carried out (without indentation at this stage) in order to rule out retained intraocular foreign body, vitreous hemorrhage, retinal break (infero-temporally —direct injury) or retinal dialysis (supero-nasally—counter-coup injury), choroidal ruptures, macular edema and optic nerve avulsion, etc.

- *In most cases, mydriatics* should be used to facilitate view of the retina and vitreous. It is to be borne in mind that the use of mydriatics should be properly documented so as to avoid misinterpretation of subsequent pupillary examinations. (Pupillary reflexes are also evaluated to look for evidence of neurological damage).

- *In case of open globe injuries with prolapse of uveal tissue,* it is advisable to defer the evaluation of the posterior segment to a later date after the surgical repair is completed.

ORBITAL IMAGING

It becomes necessary to bank upon imaging modalities to provide additional information whenever significant trauma is suspected to the periorbita or in cases where in view of the posterior segment is compromised (corneal decompensation, traumatic hyphema). In cases of open globe injury, some form of an imaging investigation should be ordered to look for a retained intraocular foreign body.

PLAIN RADIOGRAPHY

- With the advent of CT scan, the dependency on plain X-ray radiography has diminished. However, if a CT scan is not available, an X-ray of the orbit can also serve as a useful tool in evaluating bony trauma (Fig. 2.2) or an intraocular foreign body (Fig. 2.3).

- In addition to the advantage of diminished exposure to radiation as compared to CT, plain X-ray orbit will save the practicing ophthalmologist from the risk of Consumer Protection Act (CPA) and must be ordered even with the slightest suspicion of retained intraocular foreign body (RIOFB).

COMPUTED TOMOGRAPHY

- *CT scan has replaced X-ray radiography* as the most commonly used and most useful investigation in patients with severe peri-orbital or ocular trauma.

- *Coronal and axial scans* provide a detailed view of the bony structure of the orbit (Fig. 2.4) as well as the ocular anatomy. The size, shape and location of a foreign body can be easily demarcated with a CT scan (Fig. 2.5).

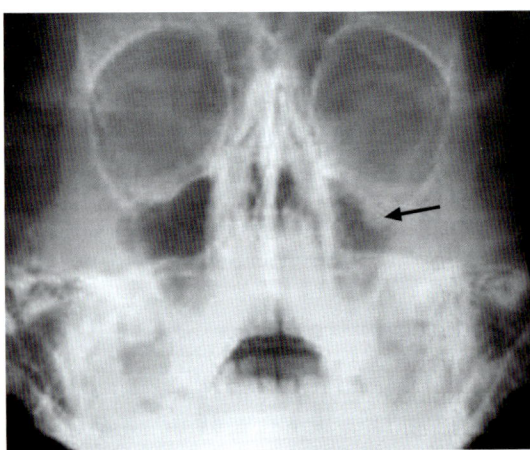

Fig. 2.2 *Plain X-ray orbit (AP view) showing herniated orbital contents (arrow) with blow-out fracture*

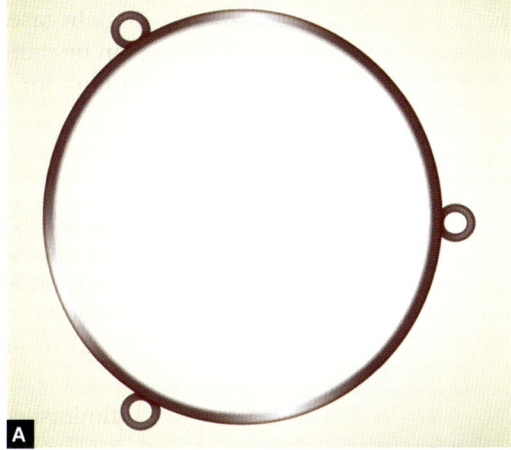

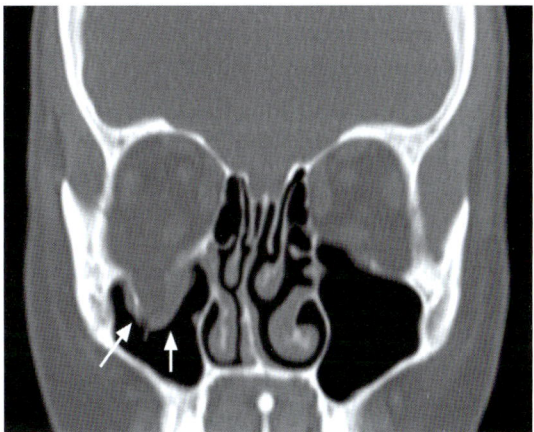

Fig. 2.4 *CT scan of orbit: Axial view depicting fracture floor of the orbit with herniation of the orbital contents*

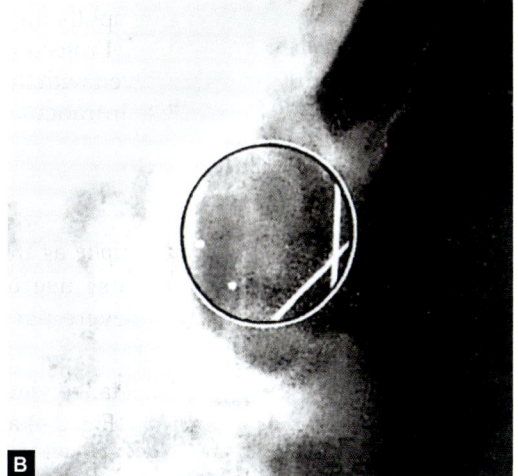

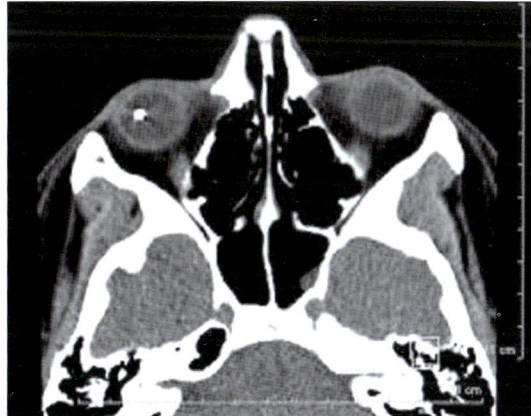

Fig. 2.3 *Limbal ring method of localizing RIOFB: (A) Limbal ring, (B) X-ray orbit lateral view with limbal ring*

Fig. 2.5 *CT scan of the orbit depicting intraocular foreign body*

- Being readily available in the emergency setting, CT scan unlike ultrasonography *can be carried out even in patients with open globe injuries.*
- *Radiologist should be advised to use thinner cuts* (1–2 mm) *so as to better delineate the ocular anatomy.*
- *Common CT scan findings* that are suggestive of open globe injury are:
  – Deformity of the globe
  – Intraocular foreign body
  – Intraocular air
  – Intraocular haemorrhage
- *Sensitivity and specificity of CT scan* in determining open globe injury are 56–68% and 79–100%, respectively.

ULTRASONOGRAPHY

- *Utilizes high frequency sound waves* to delineate ocular structures in real-time.
- *Ultrasonography requires a direct contact* with the lids and in cases of open globe injuries is contraindicated till the injury is repaired. In these cases, USG can be carried out in the operating room after repair with the patient under general anaesthesia.
- *B-scan ultrasonography helps to realize posterior segment pathology,* if the view of the fundus is compromised. It is useful in detecting (Fig. 2.6):
  – Retinal detachment (Fig. 2.6A),

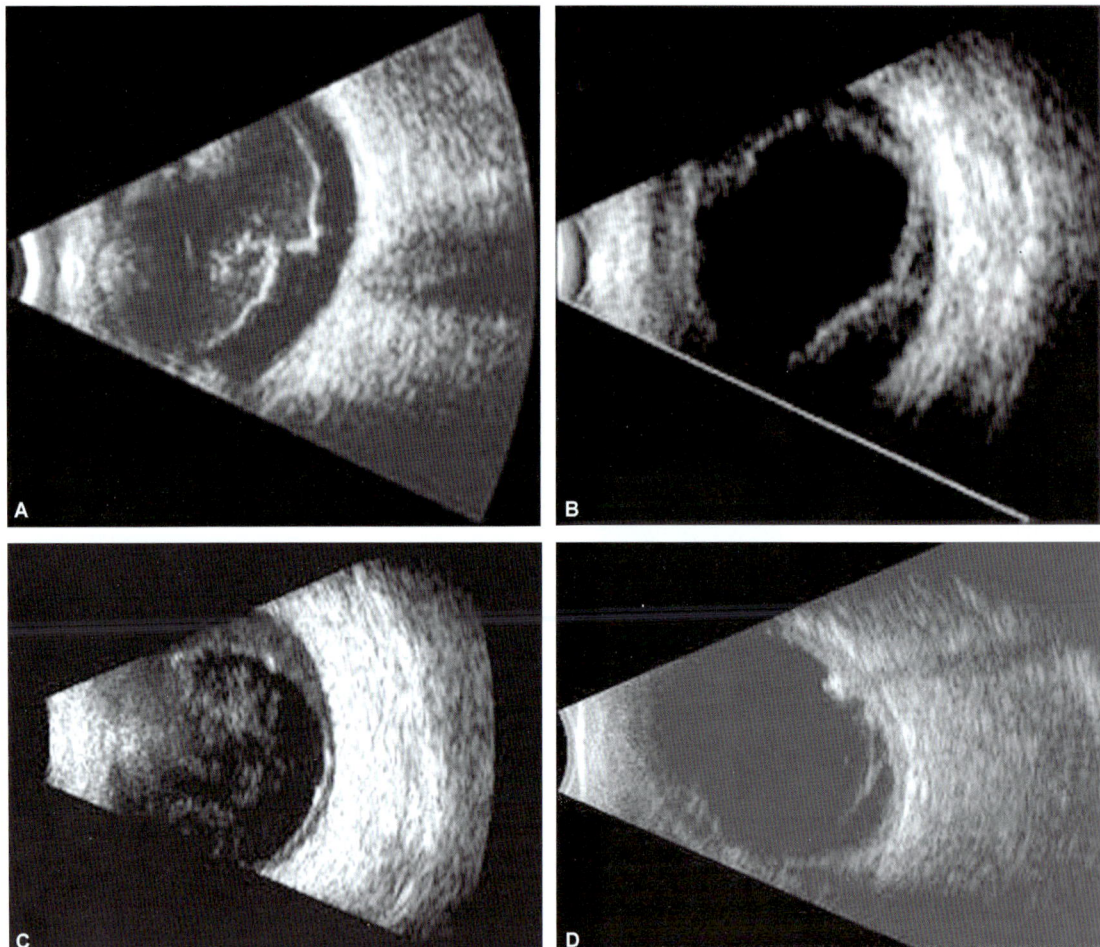

Fig. 2.6 *B scan of traumatic eyeball depicting: A. Traumatic retinal detachment; B. Choroidal detachment; C. Vitreous haemorrhage; D. Intraocular foreign body*

– Choroidal detachment (serous or haemorrhagic) (Fig. 2.6B),
– Vitreous haemorrhage (Fig. 2.6C),
– Posterior vitreous detachment
– Intraocular foreign bodies (radiolucent and radio-opaque) (Fig. 2.6D), and
– Posterior breaks in the continuity of the eyewall (perforation *vs* penetrating injury).

MAGNETIC RESONANCE IMAGING

Role of an MRI in the setting of ocular trauma is limited by its availability and longer image acquisition times. Furthermore, it cannot be used if a metallic intraocular foreign body (iron) is suspected or in patients on pacemakers.

SURGICAL EXPLORATION AND EXAMINATION UNDER ANAESTHESIA

Indications. In cases wherein significant doubt remains about the nature of injury despite imaging modalities and examination or those cases who resist examination, a surgical exploration may be necessary for accurate diagnosis.

• *General anaesthesia* should be preferred.
• *An adequate conjunctival peritomy* should be done and the scleral shell should be evaluated under high magnification for any breach. Always remember to look at weak points on the eyewall especially at the limbus, at areas of old scars and at the insertion of extraocular muscles.

- *Cornea and anterior chamber should be examined* under high magnification. The angle can be evaluated with the help of a direct gonioscope lens.
- *Ultrasonography and indirect ophthalmoscopy* can be performed to look for posterior segment pathology.

PATIENT COUNSELLING

Last but not the least patient counselling is most important sensitive part of clinical work of eye trauma. Counselling of the patient and relatives begins at the point of initial contact in the emergency environment. This begins with initial comforting of the patient and aims to allay anxiety. The counselling must be informative, truthful, accurate and should be an ongoing process till the conclusion of treatment. This is especially important in patients who would require surgical intervention. It is true that the final visual acuity remains in doubt following ocular trauma in the initial few weeks, however, a realistic opinion about the visual prognosis can be gathered from the ocular trauma score. The patient must be encouraged not to give up hope. It is important to counsel the patient for any life adjustments that may be required.

BIBLIOGRAPHY

1. Arey ML, Mootha VV, Whittemore AR, Chason DP, Blomquist PH. Computed tomography in the diagnosis of occult open-globe injuries. Ophthalmology 2007;114:1448–1452.
2. Boldt HC, Pulido JS, Blodi CF et al. Rural endophthalmitis. Ophthalmology 1989;96:1722–1726.
3. Kuhn F, Maisiak R, Mann L, Mester V, Morris R, Witherspoon CD. "The Ocular Trauma Score (OTS)". Ophthalmol Clin North Am 2002; 15:163–165.

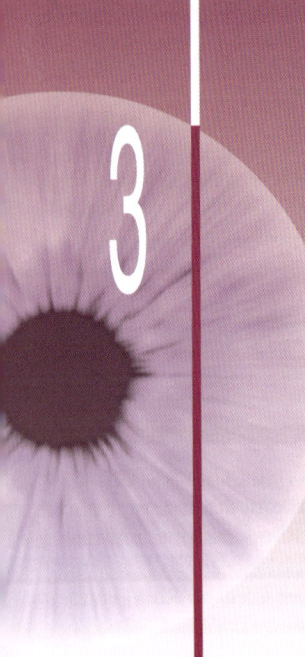

3 EMERGENCY MANAGEMENT OF OCULAR INJURIES

PRELIMINARY CONSIDERATIONS

INTRODUCTION

The approach of an ophthalmologist working in the emergency and the outpatient setting is different; in the emergency setting, the patients as well as the relatives are in a state of dismay and shock, therefore, the cordial and comforting interaction is desirable. Allaying of the patient anxiety with prompt treatment is of paramount importance and goes a long way in forming the patient–doctor bond which is quite essential in these cases as they would require motivation for undergoing repeated surgeries or long-term follow-ups. Patients in the emergency may have varied clinical presentations; this chapter aims to provide to the reader, the basic knowledge that would be required in dealing with these situations, however, for a detailed description they are referred to the relevant chapters of the book.

As mentioned previously, it is imperative to understand that management of ocular injuries in the setting of polytrauma usually takes a backseat to allow for initial evaluation of grave systemic injuries. It must, however, be noted that a prompt ophthalmological consultation of the patient should be carried out as early as the situation allows so as to formulate a treatment strategy for the same. Although it is understandable that life-threatening injuries should take priorty over ocular trauma but one should bear in mind that vision loss following ocular injuries severely dampens the quality of life of the patient.

INITIAL HISTORY AND EVALUATION

A detailed history about the nature of trauma is essential in a case of ocular injury as it guides the ophthalmologist towards the examination. A proper documentation of the records is also necessary for medicolegal purposes.

Ocular injury in many cases accompanies systemic injuries and in these patients the ophthalmologist may have limited exposure to the patient in view of life-saving interventions. A pen torch diffuse light evaluation is essential in these cases so as to have a gross idea of the nature of the ocular injury and to rule out an open globe injury. In stable and conscious patients who are co-operative for evaluation, a detailed slit-lamp examination should be performed.

In patients suffering from intracranial injuries, it must be enforced that pharmacological dilation of the pupil should not be attempted as assessment of pupillary reflexes is necessary for monitoring their systemic status. In addition, the information obtained after a fundus evaluation in this manner usually provides little or no alteration in the management strategy.

FORMULATION OF A MANAGEMENT STRATEGY

Following a thorough examination, the ophthalmologist must be in a state to formulate a plan to obtain the maximum benefit for the patient. The traditional approach focuses on a more passive role of the surgeon, taking into account a step by step approach instead of anticipating and planning ahead. This results in repeated surgeries which may have a bearing on the psychology of the patient. While forming the management strategy, the ophthalmologist must take into account the nature of the injury and anticipate complications which may occur either secondary to the trauma or during surgery. This makes the role of the ophthalmologist a more active one with fewer surgeries for the patient and an improved chance of faster visual restoration. It must be emphasized that the management strategy does not end with surgery but proper counselling of the patient should be done so that he/she is rehabilitated in the society.

ANAESTHESIA AND SPECIFIC CONSIDERATIONS FOR EMERGENCY EYE SURGERY

INDICATIONS FOR EMERGENCY EYE SURGERY

An emergency is defined as an event that has to be dealt with immediately, usually within the first hour after presentation. The commonest eye emergencies that fall into this category are chemical burns of the eye and retinal artery occlusion. Neither of these requires surgery as part of the initial management. The majority of cases presenting as emergencies can, therefore, be defined as urgent cases. Trauma is by far the commonest indication for urgent surgery. Traumatic injuries can be blunt or penetrating (open eye). The incidence is highest in young adult males and children. Trauma is often associated with industrial or motor vehicle accidents. Eye protection in the work place and car safety belts have lowered the incidence of eye trauma in many countries. Eye trauma is usually confined to one eye. Some patients may present with trauma to both eyes or with multiple injuries. There is usually enough time, however, to allow for fasting prior to surgery.

TIMING OF SURGERY

Ideally all patients should be kept fasting before undergoing general anaesthesia to minimise the risk of aspiration and subsequent lung injury. This obviously has to be weighed against the risk to the eye that delaying surgery may cause. It is essential to liase closely with the surgeon to establish the degree of urgency. Most cases involving blunt trauma can usually be delayed to allow for patient fasting. Penetrating injuries may need to be dealt with more urgently due to the risk of infection and endophthalmitis. If the patient has an open globe injury, there is also the risk of vitreous loss and retinal detachment. Even with open globe injuries, many ophthalmic surgeons are willing to delay surgery until a patient is adequately fasted prior to anaesthesia. This is especially the case where there is severe damage to the eye and surgery is not going to improve sight. This group of patients are usually admitted for bed rest and have an eyeshield covering the injured eye until they are ready for primary closure of their eye wounds. Open globe injuries in which the eye is still largely intact and the visual prognosis is good need to be dealt with more urgently. Decision need to be made on a case by case basis. The degree of urgency will depend on the size of the laceration and commensurate risk of loss of ocular contents, how dirty the wound is and the risk of infection. A fast of six hours is normally suggested in the uncomplicated patient. It is now common practice to allow patients to drink clear fluids (water, non-fizzy fruit drinks) up to two to four hours prior to the time of surgery. In patients who have had trauma or received opioids, it can take up to 24 hours for gastric emptying to take place. The most important time interval is that between the last meal and the time of the injury. If trauma occurs soon after a large meal, the patient may still have a full stomach after the standard six-hour fast. Alcohol also delays gastric emptying. If surgery is necessary in a patient with a full stomach, then a rapid sequence induction technique should be used.

How long patients should be fasted for prior to surgery with a local anaesthetic block is controversial. We feel that in the patient undergoing emergency eye anaesthesia the above principles regarding fasting should be used irrespective of the anaesthetic technique chosen.

PRE-ANAESTHETIC EVALUATION

Eye trauma requiring surgery may be associated with other injuries that may or may not require surgery. In the scenario of polytrauma, normal trauma principles must always be applied. Life-threatening problems should be dealt with before sight-threatening problems. Patients with other disease processes, such as diabetes or ischaemic heart disease, should have these optimised prior to surgery, if time allows.

LOCAL VERSUS GENERAL ANAESTHESIA

The choice of technique will depend on patient factors as well as local facilities and surgeon preferences. In many countries, extraocular, anterior segment and vitreoretinal eye surgery is routinely performed using local anaesthetic techniques. However, there are many practical reasons why a general anaesthetic is often preferable for emergency cases. Firstly, the patient must be able to lie flat, still and protect his or her own airway safely for the duration of the procedure. Thus, children, uncooperative or intoxicated patients are usually better candidates for a general anaesthetic. An uncooperative

patient with an open eye is extremely difficult to manage. Spread of local anaesthetic agents is poor in patients with eye and orbital infections.

Some procedures, such as scleral buckling for retinal detachment, can be extremely uncomfortable even with a good local anaesthetic block. In our experience, younger adults tend to tolerate surgery with a local anaesthetic technique poorly compared with elderly patients.

In open globe injuries, local anaesthetic techniques are usually avoided. Injection of local anaesthetic using peribulbar and retrobulbar techniques is associated with an increase in intraocular pressure which may lead to vitreous loss. Oculocompression after the block is also not an option, if the patient has an open globe injury. In some patients, it may be possible to operate on small open globe injuries using topical anaesthesia, sub-tenon blocks or a careful peribulbar or retrobulbar block.

SEDATION IN OCULAR INJURIES

Sedation should be used cautiously. Over sedation can convert a cooperative patient into a difficult to manage patient due to airway problems and confusion. Sedation should not be used as an alternative to a general anaesthesia in a patient with a full stomach. If a patient develops pain during surgery using a local anaesthetic technique, the patient requires analgesia and not sedation. The surgeon should supplement the block using local anaesthesia or small doses of intravenous analgesia should be given.

If sedation is to be used, then small doses of a short-acting agent, such as midazolam, should be given. Diazepam in small doses may also be an option. Propofol in small 10 mg increment doses can also be used especially prior to performing a local anaesthetic eye block. Some anaesthetists use small doses of alfentanil or fentanyl. The key to good sedation is to maintain verbal contact with the patient. Careful surgical draping is also important. Patients become claustrophobic, if their faces are draped. Use of a bar to hold up the drapes can allow a tent to be made to allow better ventilation. Oxygen should be given to the patient, especially if sedation is to be used. Patients may find a face mask or nasal oxygen cannula uncomfortable. Oxygen can be insufflated under the drapes using a breathing circuit. This also improves air circulation under the drapes.

Many of the problems associated with local techniques can be avoided with a clear explanation of the procedure to the patient prior to commencing surgery, having a comfortable operating table, and somebody to hold the patient's hand throughout. Allowing patients to empty their bladder prior to surgery also helps.

CHOICE OF DRUGS FOR GENERAL ANAESTHESIA

The choice of intravenous induction agent will depend on local availability and user familiarity. Most intravenous induction agents reduce intraocular pressure, therefore, preventing further damage to the injured eye. Ketamine possibly raises intraocular pressure although the literature is conflicting. Most textbooks state that it should be avoided in open globe injuries. If it is to be used, it is best to use it in combination with small doses of a benzodiazepine (midazolam, diazepam) to blunt its excitatory effects. The majority of problems with ketamine and intraocular pressure seem to occur when it used as a sole agent in a patient with an unprotected airway breathing spontaneously. Ideally ketamine should be used with a muscle relaxant and controlled ventilation, if intraocular pressure control is important.

All the non-depolarising muscle relaxants can be used without adverse effects on the eye so choice will depend on the availability. Suxamethonium (scoline) increases intraocular pressure, the exact mechanism of which is unclear but it is not thought to be solely due to contraction of the extraocular muscles. Suxamethonium also causes an increase in the intraocular blood volume and this may contribute to the rise in intraocular pressure.

The rise in intraocular pressure occurs after one to two minutes and wanes after six to ten minutes. The extent of the rise in intraocular pressure will depend on the other drugs used and the response to laryngoscopy and intubation. Its use in penetrating eye injury anaesthesia is controversial. The majority of eye surgeons prefer if it is not used. Adequate fasting prior to surgery will allow suxamethonium to be avoided for the majority of urgent cases. This obviously presents a dilemma in the patient with a full stomach as suxamethonium is used as part of a 'rapid sequence induction' to enable an airway to be secured quickly. In this situation, the relative risks need to be weighed, i.e. prevention of aspiration (potentially life-threatening) verses ocular damage (potentially sight-threatening). Suxamethonium-avoiding techniques include the use of large doses of vecuronium or pancuronium to speed up its onset of action as part of a modified rapid sequence induction technique. The non-depolarising neuromuscular blocker rocuronium has a rapid onset of action with a duration of 30 to 40 minutes. It can be used for a rapid sequence induction technique but can only be recommended to those who have gained experience in its use and for patients in whom airway problems are unlikely to occur. On balance, there are no case reports of ocular damage with suxamethonium use, and no good evidence that suxamethonium-avoiding techniques are any better or safer.

AIRWAY MANAGEMENT AND MODE OF VENTILATION

It is considered good practice to intubate and ventilate the patient to ensure a secure airway (the surgical field is inclose proximity) and to facilitate mild hypocarbia (this reduces intraocular pressure). The laryngeal mask airway is a popular choice for airway management for elective eye surgery in the UK. Laryngeal mask insertion avoids the presser response to laryngoscopy and intubation causing raised intraocular pressure.

ANALGESIC AND ANTI-EMETIC DRUGS IN OCULAR INJURIES

Analgesic drugs

• *Paracetamol. Children*: 90 mg/kg total per 24 hours. Avoid, if liver dysfunction peptic ulcer disease. *Acetaminophen*, orally or rectally in 4–6 divided doses dose to total of 60 mg/kg per 24 hours, if treatment for more than 48 hours. *Adults*: 1 g orally or rectally. 4 g total per 24 hours.

- *Ibuprofen. Children*: 10 mg/kg orally, 4 doses in 24 hours. Ibuprofen has the lowest side effect of the non-steroidal anti-inflammatory drugs. Avoid in renal and use with care in asthma. Not in children <7 kg.
  Adults: 400 mg orally, 4 doses maximum in 24 hours.
- *Diclofenac. Children*: 1 mg/kg orally or rectally, 3 doses in 24 hours. Cautions as for Ibuprofen.
  Adults: 150 mg total by any route in 24 hours.
- *Codeine phosphate* 0.5 mg/kg orally 6 hourly. Use with care when co-administered with other opioids.

Anti-emetic drugs

- *Droperidol.* 0.5 to 1 mg in adults, up to 3 times a day, cheap and effective but causes drowsiness, sedation, anxiety and restlessness. Risk of extrapyramidal effects.
- *Cyclizine. Children*: 1 mg/kg IV up to 3 times a day.
  Adults: 50 mg IV antihistamine and anticholinergic effect.
- *Ondansetron. Children*: 0.1 mg/kg IV 3–4 doses per 24 hours.
  Adults: 4 mg IV expensive but effective with low side effect profile. Does not protect against aspiration of gastric contents. Its use in emergency anaesthesia is, therefore, limited.

Analgesia and control of nausea and vomiting

It is possible to manage pain in the majority of patients after eye surgery with oral analgesia. Avoiding opioids, if possible, helps prevent nausea and vomiting. Regular doses of paracetamol (acetaminophen) and a non-steroidal anti-inflammatory drug (ibuprofen, diclofenac, ketoprofen) should be prescribed. Codeine phosphate can also be added. These drugs are best accepted by children, if given as an elixir (syrup).

In patients having surgery with general anaesthesia, it is a good idea to ask the surgeon to perform a local anaesthetic block before waking up the patient. If stronger analgesia is required this is best given as small intravenous doses of morphine or pethidine.

Nausea and vomiting after emergency eye anaesthesia can be a major problem in some patients. Anti-emetic prophylaxis may help prevent this. Some patients may benefit from a regular anti-emetic in the postoperative period. There is a vast number of anti-emetic drugs available. Most have a limited efficacy. Using a combination of small doses of anti-emetic drugs from different pharmacological classes may enhance efficacy and reduce side effects.

A PRACTICAL APPROACH TO EMERGENCY EYE ANAESTHESIA

- *Assess the indication for emergency anaesthesia* in discussion with the surgeon. Can surgery be deferred until normal working hours and to allow adequate fasting?
- *Carry out a full preoperative assessment* including a history and examination.
- *Are there any medical/trauma issues that need addressing first?* Decide on choice of anaesthetic technique. Provide the patient with a full explanation. Tell the patient what to expect, if a local anaesthetic technique is to be used.
- *If a general anaesthesia is chosen*, decide if the patient has a full stomach and is at risk of aspiration.
- *If the patient has a full stomach*, a rapid sequence induction technique should be used. They should be preoxygenated with 100% oxygen. Pressure on the affected eye from the mask must be avoided. The patient should then be induced with an intravenous anaesthetic agent (e.g. thiopentone 47 mg/kg) and a rapid onset muscle relaxant (suxamethonium 1–1.5 mg/kg is currently the only realistic option). While the patient is being induced, cricoid pressure should be applied by an assistant (Sellick's manoeuvre) thus occluding the oesophagus behind. The patient's trachea should be intubated after which the cricoid pressure can be removed. Note that the endotracheal tube tie should not be tight around the neck as this impedes venous drainage and raises intraocular pressure.
- *Choice of maintenance depends* on local availability, e.g. 40% O_2, 60% NO and an inhalational agent note that all inhalational agents reduce intraocular pressure.

- *Control ventilation* during the procedure aiming for low to normal end-tidal carbon dioxide. This may require the use of a longer acting muscle relaxant (e.g. vecuronium 0.1 mg/kg). A slight head up tilt helps reduce intraocular pressure.

- *At the end of the procedure, the patient should* be extubated on their side and once airway protective reflexes have returned. In patients not deemed at risk of aspiration extubation with the patient having deep and spontaneous breathing may prevent coughing. Severe coughing and straining needs to be avoided as this increases the risk of ocular haemorrhage.

- *If the patient does not have a full stomach* and is not deemed at risk of aspiration, general anaesthesia should proceed as for an elective patient. Pre-oxygenate the patient for safety and induce with an intravenous agent, give a long-acting muscle relaxant once ability to hand ventilate is established. Laryngoscopy should be performed gently. Consider spraying the vocal cords with lignocaine.

REGIONAL ANAESTHESIA FOR TRAUMATIC EYE INJURIES

Regional anaesthesia may be a reasonable alternative in those scenarios where general anaesthesia presents an unacceptable or elevated risk to either the patient systemically, or the eye in specific.

Regional anaesthesia as retrobulbar (intraconal) and peribulbar (extraconal) blocks may be performed using single-injection combinations of 2 or 4% lidocaine and .75% bupivacaine admixed with small aliquots of hyaluronidase. A prior lid block to attenuate eyelid squeezing during the orbital injection may be particularly useful in open globe trauma. In the operating room, subconjunctival irrigation of local anaesthetic via a blunt cannula may be useful in open globe trauma used as needed to supplement the initial injection. Intravenous sedation may be provided at the discretion of the anaesthetist.

Regional anaesthesia with sedation

Regional anaesthesia with sedation is a good alternative to general anaesthesia, when required.

Topical anaesthesia for traumatic eye injuries

Topical anaesthesia has gained acceptance over the past few years for cataract surgery and may be a prudent alternative in those select open globe scenarios where general or regional anaesthesia present exceptional risk.

Topical anaesthesia may consist of .4% oxybuprocaine-soaked cellulose sponges placed in the upper and lower fornices for 20 min prior to wound closure.

Topical anaesthesia and intravenous sedation may also be a reasonable alternative for less severe traumatic eye injuries.

Risks and techniques: Regional and topical anaesthesias for ophthalmic surgery are certainly not without inherent risks. A review of all monitored anaesthesia care closed malpractice claims in the American Society of anaesthesiologists Closed Claims Database revealed that one in five such legal cases derived from eye surgery.

Rethinking anaesthesia strategies for patients with traumatic eye injuries.

Unlike general anaesthesia, these techniques mandate patient cooperation. Patient movement due to cough, fluctuating levels of consciousness, rebreathing of carbon dioxide, or restlessness with prolonged duration of surgery can precipitate dire visual consequences.

EMERGENCY MANAGEMENT STRATEGIES FOR OCULAR INJURIES

Common ocular injuries encountered as emergency in day-to-day practice are open globe injuries with and without intraocular foreign bodies, closed globe injuries, chemical injuries, extraocular foreign bodies, traumatic optic neuropathy, blow-out fractures of the orbit and traumatic endophthalmitis. These are truly classified as ocular emergencies and require prompt and urgent management to safeguard vision.

ADNEXAL TRAUMA

Most patients present with injuries to the periocular structures following road traffic accidents or with a history of fall. It may range from a minor abrasion to a muscle-deep or bone-deep laceration with extensive bleeding.

- *All periocular injuries should be cleaned thoroughly* with povidone iodine or any other antiseptic agent.
- *Careful evaluation* of the lesion should be done to look for any retained foreign bodies in the wound.
- *A note should also be made of injury to the lid margin or the canaliculi* as these would require specialized treatment at the time of primary repair itself.
- *History of tetanus immunization* should be taken and wherever found to be lacking appropriate measures should be undertaken.
- *Abrasions and some superficial lacerations* require application of only an antibacterial ointment and the maintenance of proper wound hygiene.
- *Deeper laceration* would require suturing. The muscle and subcutaneous tissue should be snugly sutured with an absorbable suture (6–0 vicryl) while the overlying skin is sutured with a non-absorbable suture (5–0 silk or prolene). The skin sutures can be removed in 7–10 days as the wound healing permits.
- *Patients are instructed to maintain proper wound hygiene* and can be started on oral antibiotics and anti-inflammatory agents.

Periocular ecchymosis

- *Blunt trauma to the forehead* may result in the seepage of blood into the eyelids rendering them a purplish hue.
- *Periocular ecchymosis requires closer evaluation* as it may be the only indication of a fracture involving the base of the skull, particularly if bilateral.
- *If the site of blunt trauma is the eye* as in case of injury with a fist or a ball, a complete ocular evaluation should be carried out with full mydriasis to look at ocular injury secondary to the contusion.
- *'Raccoon eyes' or 'black eye'* requires cold compresses for resolution along with oral anti-inflammatory agents to mask the pain. Provided there is no underlying bony injury the blood usually clears away in 10–14 days.

Conjunctival injuries

Subconjunctival hemorrhage. There is usually no treatment required for subconjunctival hemorrhage following ocular trauma. An attempt should be made to trace the posterior limit of the hemorrhage, which if not reached usually points towards a fracture of the base of skull. Tear substitutes may help in providing some degree of comfort to the patient. NSAIDs should be discontinued in favour of acetaminophen which does not alter the clotting profile of the patient.

Conjunctival laceration. Lacerations of the conjunctiva can be picked up on slit-lamp examination with or without the use of fluorescein stain. The margins of the laceration tend to be rolled up due to the elastic nature of the conjunctiva. Not all lacerations require suturing and small ones can be left unsutured with pressure patching and the application of an antibacterial ointment. Most of the small lacerations tend to heal well when treated in this manner. For lacerations usually greater than 1–1.5 cm, suturing of the torn ends with 8–0 vicryl with buried knots is advocated with excellent results.

EXTRAOCULAR FOREIGN BODY

Corneal and conjunctival foreign bodies usually present with mild to moderate amount of pain with ocular discomfort.

- *Corneal abrasions and track marks* are tell tale signs of a foreign body and in all cases the conjunctival fornices should be carefully examined.
- *In cases of impacted foreign bodies,* always evaluate the depth of penetration of the object before removal.
- *Topical anaesthetic agent* in the form of 4% lignocaine or 0.5% proparacaine is administered in the cul-de-sac.
- *After appropriate anaesthesia,* the foreign body is removed with the help of a 26 G needle. While removing the foreign body gently

scrape the edge of the foreign body and approach it tangentially to avoid iatrogenic injury.

- *Iron foreign bodies may leave a small rust ring* around the site of impaction of the foreign body.
- *Following removal of the particle,* the patient must be kept under frequent follow-up till the epithelial defect heals.
- *Topical antibiotic and NSAID* should be prescribed, in cases of corneal foreign bodies, cycloplegia may help in alleviating the pain. (For details *see* Chapter 5.1)

CORNEAL INJURIES

Corneal abrasions

Presentation. Patients with corneal abrasion usually present with severe degree of pain and photophobia because of denudation of corneal nerves.

Examination. After examining and ruling out the presence of an open globe injury, application of topical proparacaine helps alleviate the symptoms and makes the patient co-operative for evaluation. Corneal abrasions can be picked up on a slit-lamp with fluorescein staining. The shape and size of the abrasion should always be clearly defined as it helps in the follow-up evaluation.

Treatment. Small corneal abrasion can be treated with the help of a bandage contact lens with frequent application of a topical antibiotic. For moderate to large abrasions, patching the eye with an antibiotic ointment is recommended. All patients with corneal abrasions should be kept under close follow-up till the epithelial defect heals. A cycloplegic agent helps to relieve the pain while a tear substitute will look after the foreign body sensation and vitamin C may help in expediting the healing process.

Corneal lacerations

Evaluation. In evaluating patients with corneal lacerations, the depth of the laceration helps to determine the treatment protocol. A Seidel's test should always be performed in cases of corneal laceration to look for occult leaks.

Treatment. Lacerations extending to the deeper stroma or lacerations with a positive Seidel's test should always be sutured with a non-absorbable 10–0 monofilament nylon sutures with micro-point spatulated needles. Superficial lacerations can be treated in the form of a corneal abrasion.

Photokeratitis

Photokeratitis, also termed as photo-ophthalmitis, is a particularly painful ocular condition arising from inadequate protection to the eyes during exposure to ultraviolet rays from natural or artificial sources.

Presentation. Typically the patient presents few hours following welding arc exposure with complaints of tearing, photophobia and ocular pain.

Evaluation. The history is very suggestive and fluorescein staining shows the presence of diffuse punctate staining under cobalt blue filter suggestive of epithelial erosions.

Treatment involves the use of a topical anti-inflammatory and copious use of artificial tears. Patients must be instructed about the occurrence of the condition and should be counselled to prevent future episodes.

Chemical injuries

Chemical burns with either acids or alkalis can prove to be devastating for the cornea, though alkali injuries are usually more severe than acid injuries.

Initial approach towards managing chemical injuries is copious irrigation; the attending ophthalmologist must consider all previous attempts at irrigation as being insufficient.

- *Irrigation helps to prevent further exposure* of the inciting agents and shortens the healing time.
- *During the process of irrigation,* the fornices should be cleared using a Desmarre's retractor.
- *Sterile saline* is the preferred agent for irrigation but no differences have been shown between saline, ringer lactate and other irrigating solutions. If none is available even tap water can be used. Irrigation should be continued to around 30 minutes.

Grading. Chemical burns can be graded using the Roperhall classification system.

- *Mild chemical burns* can be managed in the outpatient setting with the use of a topical antibiotic, copious tear substitutes, cycloplegics, topical steroids and a pressure lowering topical β-blocker. Oral anti-inflammatory agents help to reduce the pain, while vitamin C tablets accelerate the healing of the corneal epithelium. Patients must be reviewed every day till the epithelial defect heals.

- *Moderate to severe chemical burns* may require treating the patient on an in-patient basis. In severe cases, debridement of the necrotic corneal epithelium may be necessary to allow for proper re-epithelialization.

CLOSED GLOBE TRAUMA

Anterior segment trauma

Hyphema, iritis, iridodialysis

Hyphema. Layering of the RBCs in the inferior anterior chamber can occur following blunt trauma to the eyeball and may also be associated with penetrating ocular injuries. In cases of penetrating injuries, the hyphema may be drained at the time of globe repair. A slit-lamp evaluation of the hyphema is necessary for appropriate documentation. It is graded as under:

Hyphema	Suspended RBC without formation of a layered clot
1+	< 1/3 chamber hyphema
2+	1/3 – 1/2 chamber hyphema
3+	1/2 to near total hyphema
4+	Total hyphema (8-ball hyphema)

- An increase in intraocular pressure is one of the most common and dreaded complication of hyphema. The RBCs are trapped in the trabecular meshwork wherein they increase outflow resistance.

- *Outpatient management* should be considered only for adults who are compliant with a hyphema grade 2+ or less.

- *Hand-off approach.* The proper management of the condition is disputed with Romano and Phillips demonstrating a hands-off approach with excellent results. The approach consisted of using only oral steroids and hospitalization

of all patients, with no ocular manipulation in the form of tonometry or use of any eye-drops. The practice usually followed is to advise strict bed rest with head end elevation and discontinuation of any oral anticoagulants. Oral steroids are started with anti-inflammatory agent (acetaminophen should be preferred). The eye should be patched using an eyeshield. The use of cycloplegics in hyphema management is again controversial. Anti-glaucoma medications should be initiated to tide over the initial rise of IOP which is usually transient and seen in around 30% of the cases lasting for 5–7 days.

Traumatic iritis occurs secondary to blunt trauma to the anterior segment as in cases of motor vehicle accidents, firecracker injuries, battery blasts, projectile injuries. Young males tend to be affected more commonly with traumatic iritis responsible for about 20% of the cases of iritis.

- *Topical cycloplegics with a topical steroid* are beneficial in correcting this pathological entity.

- *A topical β-blocker* may be added, if increased pressures are noted.

Iridodialysis. A localized tearing away of the iris from the ciliary body can result from injuries with blunt projectiles, such as air bags, cricket-ball injuries, water-balloons, fireworks, etc. Patients with small amounts of iridodialysis need no surgical intervention and should be followed up for increased IOP. If the patient has symptoms in the form of mono-ocular diplopia or glare the iridodialysis can be repaired at a later date.

Lenticular subluxation and dislocation

Presentation. Lenticular subluxation refers to partial displacement of the lens from the patellar fossa; complete displacement is termed as dislocation. Patients can be discomforted with the sudden diminished vision that accompanies this setting due to acquired myopia, astigmatism and diplopia.

Treatment. The amount of subluxation should be noted down and the patient can be rehabilitated with refractive correction in mild cases.

- *Severe cases of subluxation* should be treated in a manner similar to dislocation with extracapsular cataract extraction and if possible an IOL fixated in the primary sitting or at a later date.
- *In cases of dislocation of the lens into the anterior chamber*, prompt surgery should be undertaken to prevent endothelial decompensation and rise of IOP.
- *Posterior dislocation* is treated by a pars plana vitrectomy, phacofragmentation and transscleral fixation of an IOL at a later stage.

Posterior segment trauma

Vitreous haemorrhage

Presentation of the patient suffering from vitreous hemorrhage following trauma is dramatic with a sudden profound deterioration in the visual acuity.

Diagnosis of vitreous haemorrhage is usually straight-forward on a slit-lamp examination with a 90 D lens. The red glow of the fundus is either very dull or absent depending upon the severity of the haemorrhage. The posterior segment evaluation should be attempted with indirect ophthalmoscopy; if not visible a B-scan ultrasonography should be carried out to look for retinal detachment, choroidal detachment, posterior vitreous detachment or globe rupture.

Treatment. Bed rest with head end elevation should be encouraged to allow for the blood to settle and provide a view of the fundus. The patient is kept under observation for a period of two months, however, early surgical intervention is advocated in cases of accompanying retinal detachment.

Preretinal haemorrhage

Presentation. Preretinal bleeds are confined to the space between the nerve-fibre layer and the internal limiting membrane of the retina. Patients present in a similar state of frenzy following marked diminished vision, particularly if the preretinal bleed rests in front of the macula.

Management. The initial management consists of only reassurance along with a complete evaluation of the fundus with indirect ophthalmoscopy. A documentation of the extent of the haemorrhage either by a diagram or better still with a fundus camera should be done so as to record the diminishing size of the haemorrhage on sequential follow-up visits.

Commotio retinae

Presentation. It is a countercoup injury to the retina following a blunt trauma to the anterior segment of the eye. The patient complains of diminished vision but the retina appears normal on initial examination. The affected area turns white and opaque some hours after the initial insult due to disorganization of the outer retinal layers.

Treatment. Usually no treatment is required and the prognosis is good. A detailed evaluation should be carried out to look for subfoveal choroidal rupture or subfoveal haemorrhages which if present carry a poorer prognosis.

OPEN GLOBE INJURY

- *When the patient is first received in the emergency setting* an effort should be made to look for an open globe injury since the management of open globe trauma differs completely from contusion injuries.
- *While evaluating cases of open globe injury* be sure not to put pressure on the globe lest the intraocular contents should prolapse out. In an uncooperative patient, if an open globe injury is confirmed or suspected never perform a forceful examination in the emergency room, in such a case, a controlled environment under sedation or general anaesthesia is preferred. In cases of open globe injury, the detail regarding the inciting insult should be explored; one should always be suspicious of a retained intraocular foreign body particularly in cases of hammer and chisel injuries.
- *Eyeball should be patched immediately* with the help of a shield to prevent chances of further injury and the patient should be instructed not to cough violently or undertake any undue stress.
- *Co-ordination with the attending anaesthesiologist* will help in early exploration and primary repair.

- *Preoperative CT scan* can be carried out not only for documentation of the injury but also to exclude any intraocular foreign body and assessment of surrounding orbital trauma. Topical medications should be avoided in any open globe injury patients.
- *Systemic antibiotic* prophylaxis should be started (iv levofloxacin 500 mg).
- *Every attempt should be carried out to salvage the eye*, however, if the trauma is too extensive and the eyeball is mutilated beyond repair despite best efforts then it can be enucleated with prior patient counselling in order to decrease the chances of development of sympathetic ophthalmia.

RETAINED INTRAOCULAR FOREIGN BODY

- *An intraocular foreign body should be suspected* in all cases of open globe injury. Small corneal wounds, iris holes or break in the anterior capsule of the lens can be clues to a retained foreign body on examination.
- *Preoperative ultrasound* can be done in patients with self-sealed lacerations, however, it should be avoided in frank open globe injuries due to the external pressure it puts on the eyeball.
- *USG B-scan and CT scan* are essential in delineating the extent and location of the foreign body.
- *MRI should be avoided* unless the non-metallic nature of the foreign body is confirmed.
- *Appropriate management strategy* should be carved out trying for primary repair and removal of the foreign body at the initial sitting.
- *Intravitreal antibiotics* should be injected in all cases. Selection of the antibiotics should include a coverage of anaerobes especially in cases of wooden foreign bodies.

TRAUMATIC ENDOPHTHALMITIS

Endophthalmitis is a known complication in open globe injury particularly in cases with retained foreign bodies, hence an emphasis is placed on prophylaxis and both intravenous and topical antibiotics should be initiated at the earliest. Post-traumatic endophthalmitis progresses rapidly and affects the prognosis of vision. The risk of endophthalmitis after penetrating injury can be reduced by prompt wound closure and early removal of intraocular foreign bodies.

TRAUMATIC OPTIC NEUROPATHY

Presentation and evaluation. A patient with traumatic optic neuropathy can be easily picked up on pen torch examination in the presence of a relative afferent pupillary defect. These individuals usually have evidences of high velocity injuries to the head and neck region and require a careful evaluation. A CT scan of the orbit should be done to look for evidence of direct injury to the optic nerve.

Management of traumatic optic neuropathy remains controversial in the absence of any randomized control trials. In indirect optic nerve injury, the favoured approach is of administration of intravenous steroids of the order of methylprednisolone 1 gram every day for 3 days followed by oral steroids, if the patient presents within 8 hours of trauma. For patients presenting later than 8 hours, a wait and watch policy can be instituted.

RETROBULBAR HAEMORRHAGE

Presentation

Retrobulbar haemorrhage following ocular trauma is a grave emergency. The patients present with severe ocular pain, diminished vision or loss of vision and diplopia which may be accompanied by nausea and vomiting.

Evaluation

The attending ophthalmologist should maintain a high index of suspicion in these cases particularly in patients on anticoagulants. Leakage of blood into the orbital space, a closed environment, gradually compresses on the ocular structures leading to an acute orbital compartment syndrome, if not treated at the earnest.

- *These patients* exhibit signs of a non-pulsating exophthalmos with resistance to retropulsion, ophthalmoplegia, increased intraocular pressure and optic disc or retinal pallor.
- *Pupillary reflex* may be absent or may show the presence of relative afferent pupillary defect (RAPD) in optic neuropathy owing to the compression on the optic nerve.

- *CT scan* can be done in the emergency setting to confirm the diagnosis and to look for any associated orbital trauma. However, it is emphasized that a radiological evaluation should not delay the prompt management of this condition.

Treatment

Treatment includes medical and surgical measures:

Medical treatment with intravenous mannitol and acetazolamide aims at reducing the intra-ocular pressure. Intravenous steroids can be administered taking into account the compressive optic neuropathy. Controversies exist in the medical management of retrobulbar haemorrhage since none of the treatment options cater to the increased intraorbital pressure. Medical treatment can only be tried in mild cases wherein no pupillary abnormalities or visual compromise is observed. These cases need to be followed up closely and, if at any time features of optic neuropathy appear, surgery should be undertaken.

Surgical treatment aims to relieve the orbital compression which is achieved by a lateral cantho-tomy and cantholysis. To perform a canthotomy, an infiltration of lignocaine and epinephrine is given in the lateral canthal region followed by incising the lateral canthal tendon with a sharp forceps. An inferior cantholysis is performed by grasping the lower lid away from the globe. A Westcott scissors is then introduced infero-laterally between the skin and the conjunctiva. Strum the tissue near the orbital rim to locate the fibrous bands of the inferior crus of the lateral canthal tendon. These fibres are then completely cut with the scissors to free the lower eyelid adequately. Mild pressure on the globe can allow for a passive egress of blood from the orbit. If sufficient decompression is not achieved by an inferior cantholysis, a superior cantholysis can be performed in a similar manner.

ORBITAL FRACTURES

Evaluation. Fractures are a relatively common result of blunt injury. While evaluating the patient of blunt trauma:

- *Bony walls* of the orbit should be palpated to look for any break in continuity.
- *Lids and periorbital skin should be palpated* to look for surgical emphysema which is indicative of an air leak from a sinus and thereby a fracture of the orbital bony cage.
- *Integrity of the globe should be evaluated* and look for extraocular movements to rule out muscle entrapment.
- *CT scan of the orbit* is necessary whenever a fracture is suspected to document the site of the break and to look for herniation of orbital contents.
- *X-ray paranasal sinuses* anterior group (maxillary sinus) may also suffice, if CT scan is not available.

Fracture of the orbital roof should be viewed with caution; it is a potentially life-threatening injury as it establishes a continuation between the cranial and the orbital cavities. A neuro-surgical consult is warranted at the earnest.

Blowout fracture of floor. An important consideration for the attending ophthalmologist is a blowout fracture of the orbital floor following concussive trauma. The diagnosis of this can be easily picked up with the clinical features of enophthalmos, pseudoptosis and reduced superior ocular movements. However, in the emergency setting with surrounding soft tissue inflammation, it may be difficult as the patient is not always co-operative for evaluation. A tear drop sign with herniation of the orbital contents should be looked for in the X-ray anterior group of paranasal sinuses. Immediate action is not usually necessary in these cases which can be managed conservatively for about 7–10 days after which a re-assessment is done to look into the magnitude of diplopia and loss of cosmesis caused by the fracture. If significant, repair of the orbital floor with release of the entrapped inferior rectus is undertaken.

Other cases of orbital fractures if the displace-ment is not significant the patients can be managed conservatively. A broad-spectrum oral antibiotic should be initiated to prevent the chances of orbital cellulitis along with an NSAID. The patients are instructed not to blow their nose and to use a cold compress for the initial 48–72 hours. A surgical intervention is usually reserved at a later date, if at all indicated.

INTRAORBITAL FOREIGN BODY

An intraorbital foreign body can be considered in high velocity periocular injuries.
- *CT scan* can be helpful in determining the site of lodging of the foreign body.
- *Foreign bodies can be either organic or inorganic.* Inorganic foreign bodies are usually inert and the injury that they cause is only limited to the initial act of the trauma.
- *Anteriorly located foreign bodies* are usually easy to remove.
- *Posteriorly located inorganic foreign bodies,* if causing no inflammation or pain, can be left in situ lest it should cause mechanical damage to the orbital contents during its surgical extraction. The same, however, cannot be said for organic foreign bodies which need to be removed as they are more likely to lead to infective complications, like orbital cellulitis, orbital abscess, meningitis and a chronically draining fistula.
- Anti-tetanus prophylaxis should be instituted for all patients.

BIBLIOGRAPHY

1. Canavan YM, O'Flaherty MJ, Archer DB, Elwood JH. A 10 year survey of injuries in northern Ireland 1967-76. Br J Ophthalmol 1980; 64:618–625.
2. Chang Y, Oh S, Chi NC. A clinical observation of ocular injuries of inpatients. J Korean OphthalmolSoc 1993; 34:257–263.
3. Dannenberg AL, Parver LM, Brechner RJ, Khoo L. Penetrating injuries in the workplace. Arch Ophthalmol 1992; 110:843–849.
4. Desai P, MacEwen CJ, Baines P, Minassian DC. Incidence of cases of ocular trauma admitted to hospital and incidence of blinding outcome. Br J Ophthalmol 1996; 80:592–596.
5. Karlson TA, Klein BEK. The incidence of acute hospital-treated eye injuries. Arch Ophthalmol 1986; 104:1473–1476.
6. Kim SS, Yoo JM. A clinical study of industrial ocular injuries. J Korean Ophthalmol Soc 1988; 29:393–403.
7. Klopfer J, Tielsch JM. Ocular trauma in the United States Eye injuries resulting in hospitalization, 1984 through 1987. Arch Ophthalmol 1992; 110:838–842.
8. Kuhn F, Morris R. A standardized classification of ocular trauma. Graefe's Arch Clin Exp Ophthalmol 1996; 614:399–403.
9. Lee KJ, Oh JH. A statistical observation of the ocular injuries. J Korean OphthalmolSoc 1990; 31:229–239.
10. Maltzman BA, Pruzon H, Mund ML. A survey of ocular trauma. Surv Ophthalmol 1976; 2:285–290.
11. Morris RE, Witherspoon CD, Helms HA Jr, Feist RM, Byrne JB Jr. Eye injury registry of Alabama (preliminary report): Demographics and prognosis of severe eye injury. South Med J 1987; 80:810–816.
12. Nash EA, Margo CE. Patterns of emergency department visits for disorders of the eye and ocular adnexa. Arch Ophthalmol 1998; 116:1222–1226.
13. Patel BC, Morgan H. Work-related penetrating eye injuries. ActaOphthalmol 1991; 69:377–381.
14. Thoradson U, Ragnarsson AT, Gudbrandsson B. Ocular trauma: Observation in 105 patients. Acta Ophthalmol 1978; 57:922–928.
15. Tielsch JM, Parver L, Shankar B. Time trends in the incidence of hospitalized ocular trauma. Arch Ophtalmol 1989; 107:519–523.
16. Tsai CC, Kau HC, Kao SC, Liu JH. A review of ocular emergencies in a Taiwanese medical center. Chung Hua I HsuehTsaChih 1998; 61:414–420.
17. Voon LW, See J, Wong TY. The epidemiology of ocular trauma in Singapore: perspective from the emergency service of a large tertiary hospital. Eye 2001; 15:75–81.

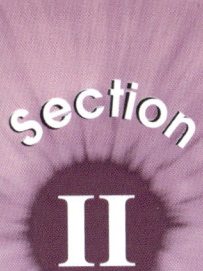

Mechanical Injuries

4

MECHANICAL OCULAR INJURIES: MODES OF TRAUMA AND MECHANISMS OF TISSUE DAMAGE

BLUNT TRAUMA
Modes of Injury
- Direct blow
- Accidental trauma

Mechanics of Blunt Trauma to Eyeball
- Direct impact on the globe
- Compression wave force
- Reflected compression wave force
- Rebound compression wave force
- Oscillatory wave force
- Indirect force

Modes of Damage
- Mechanical tearing
- Cellular damage
- Inflammatory changes
- Vascular damage
- Trophic changes
- Delayed complications

OPEN GLOBE INJURIES
Modes of Trauma
- Globe rupture
- Globe laceration

Modes of Damage
- Mechanical tearing
- Introduction of infection
- Post-traumatic iridocyclitis
- Sympathetic ophthalmitis

INTRAOCULAR FOREIGN BODY
Modes of Trauma
- Common foreign bodies

Modes of Damage
- Mechanical tearing
- Introduction of infection
- Posttraumatic iridocyclitis
- Sympathetic ophthalmitis

BLUNT TRAUMA

MODES OF INJURY

Blunt trauma may occur following:
- *Direct blow* to the eyeball by fist, a tennis or cricket or any another ball or blunt instruments, like sticks, and big stones.
- *Accidental blunt trauma* to eyeball may also occur in roadside accidents, automobile accidents, injuries by agricultural and industrial instruments/machines and fall upon the projecting blunt objects.

MECHANICS OF BLUNT TRAUMA TO EYEBALL

Blunt trauma of eyeball produces damage by different forces as described below:

1. *Direct impact on the globe.* It produces maximum damage at the point where the blow is received (Fig. 4.1A).

2. *Compression wave force.* It is transmitted through the fluid contents in all the directions and strikes the angle of anterior chamber, pushes the iris lens diaphragm posteriorly, and also strikes the retina and choroid (Fig. 4.1B). Compression of the globe by the projectile force leads to decrease in axial length and expansion of the equatorial diameter of the globle (Fig. 4.2A). This may cause considerable damage. Sometimes the compression wave may be so explosive, that maximum damage may be produced at a point distant from the actual place of impact. This is called contrecoup damage.

3. *Reflected compression wave force.* After striking the outer coats, the compression waves are reflected towards the posterior pole and may cause foveal damage (Fig. 4.1C).

4. *Rebound compression wave force.* When the projectile recoils from the cornea, the compression waves rebound back anteriorly and

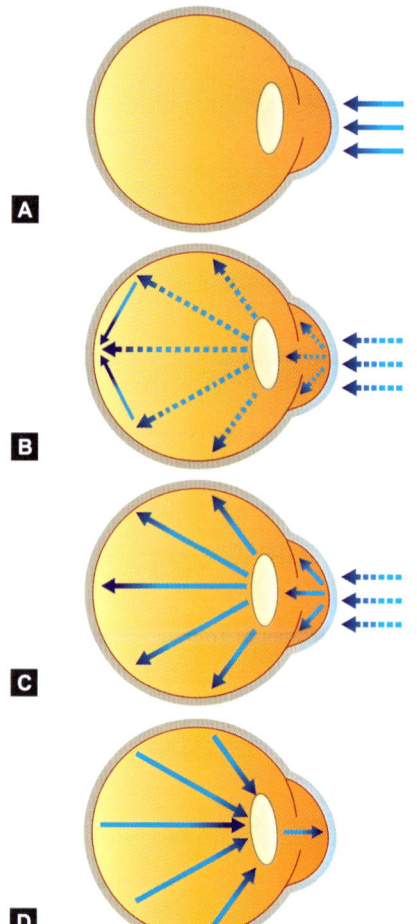

Fig. 4.1 *Mechanics of blunt trauma to eyeball: (A) Direct impact, (B) Compression wave force, (C) Reflected compression wave, (D) Rebound compression wave*

there occurs an increase in axial length and a decrease in equatorial diameter back to normal size (Fig. 4.2B). This is called *decompression phase*. Due to continued rebound forces, there occurs an increase in axial length over and above the normal length and a decrease in equatorial diameter below the normal diameter (Fig. 4.2C). This is called *overshooting phase*. This force damages the retina and choroid by forward pull and lens iris diaphragm by forward thrust from the back (Fig. 4.1D).

5. *Oscillatory wave force.* Due to compression, decompression, and overshooting, there occurs cyclical small increases and decreases in the axial length and equatorial diameter (Fig. 4.2D). This

is called *oscillatory phase*. The oscillatory wave forces also contribute to tissue damage.

6. *Indirect force.* Ocular damage may also be caused by the indirect forces from the bony walls and elastic contents of the orbit, when globe suddenly strikes against these structures.

MODES OF DAMAGE

The different forces of the blunt trauma described above may cause damage to the structures of the globe by one or more of the following modes:

I. *Mechanical tearing of the tissues of eyeball.* As described above, when blunt (non-penetrating) injury is sustained by the eye by an object moving parallel, to the visual axis, the cornea and anterior sclera is displaced backwards. This leads to a compensatory equatorial expansion. Aqueous and vitreous are relatively incompressible and transmit the force so that the ocular tissues undergo sudden expansion and possibly tearing. Mechanical tearing of tissues of eyeball may occur due to one or more mechanisms described above in the mechanics of blunt trauma (Figs 4.1 and 4.2).

Campbell, graphically has described *seven rings or circles of tissue,* anterior to the equator of globe that suddenly expand with blunt impact. These seven tissue rings are (Fig. 4.3):

1. *Ring of pupillary sphincter.* Pupillary sphincter tears.

2. *Ring of iris base.* There occurs iridodialysis, i.e. tear of iris root from ciliary body.

3. *Ring of anterior ciliary body.* There occurs angle recession or a tear in the face of the ciliary body. Rupture of the ciliary body between its longitudinal and circular fibers shows that this is the weakest portion of the ciliary body. This leads to deepening of the anterior chamber.

4. *Ring of ciliary body at its attachment to sclera.* Cyclodialysis, or a separation of the ciliary body occurs from the sclera.

5. *Ring of trabecular meshwork.* Trabecular dialysis or a tear through the trabecular meshwork.

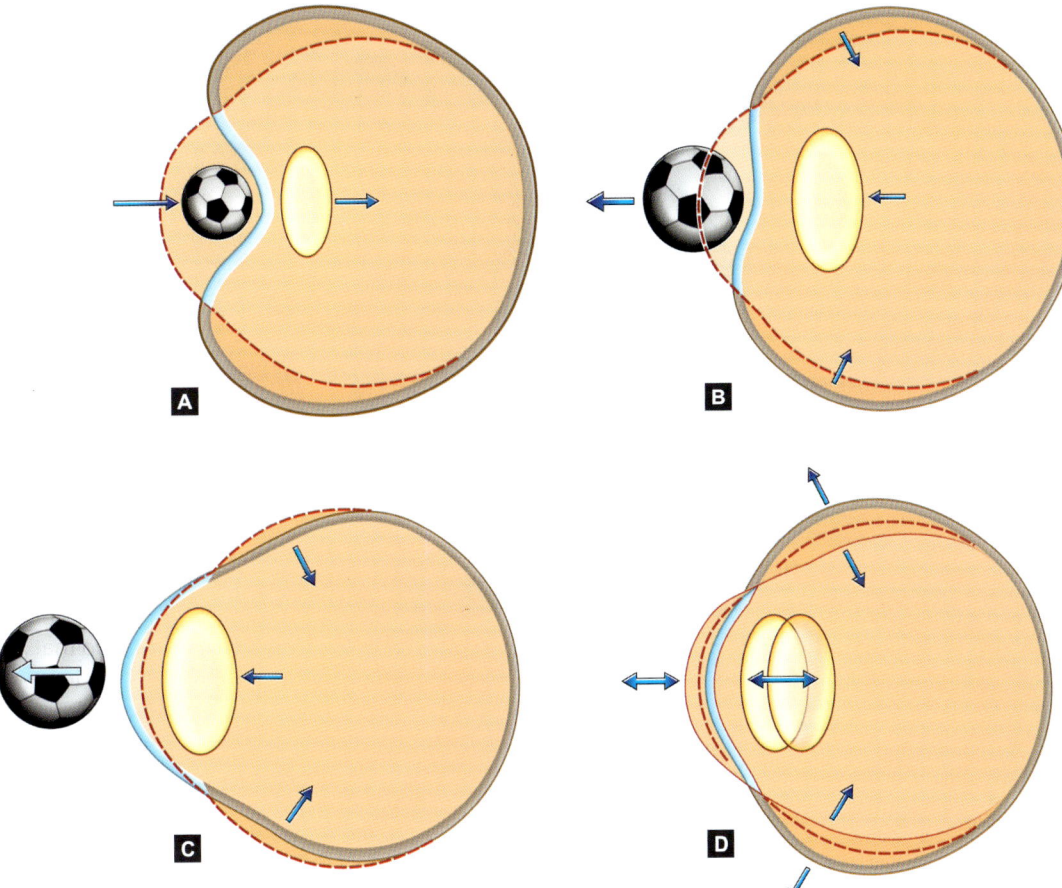

Fig. 4.2 *Phases of globe deformation by a high-speed projectile: (A) Compression phase; (B) Decompression phase, (C) Overshooting phase; (D) Oscillatory phase*

6. *Ring of lens zonules.* Tearing of the lens zonules leading to phacodonesis, iridodonesis, subluxation or total dislocation of the lens backwards.

7. *Ring of ora serrata.* Retinal dialysis at the ora or a giant retinal tear may occur.

II. *Damage to the tissue cells* sufficient to cause disruption of their physiological activity.

III. *Inflammatory changes.* Immediately following trauma, inflammatory changes are induced in ocular tissue particularly uveal tissue due to release of cytokines and prostaglandins.

IV. *Vascular damage* may occur leading to ischaemia, oedema and haemorrhages.

V. *Trophic changes* may occur due to disturbances of the nerve supply.

VI. *Delayed complications* of blunt trauma, such as secondary glaucoma, haemophthalmitis, late rosette cataract and retinal detachment.

OPEN GLOBE INJURIES

Open globe injury is defined as a full thickness wound of the eyewall (sclera or/and cornea). It includes:

1. *Globe rupture*, i.e. full thickness wound of the eyewall caused by blunt trauma.

2. *Globe laceration* refers to full thickness wound of eyewall caused by sharp objects. It includes:

i. Penetrating injury,

ii. Perforating injury, and

iii. Intraocular foreign bodies.

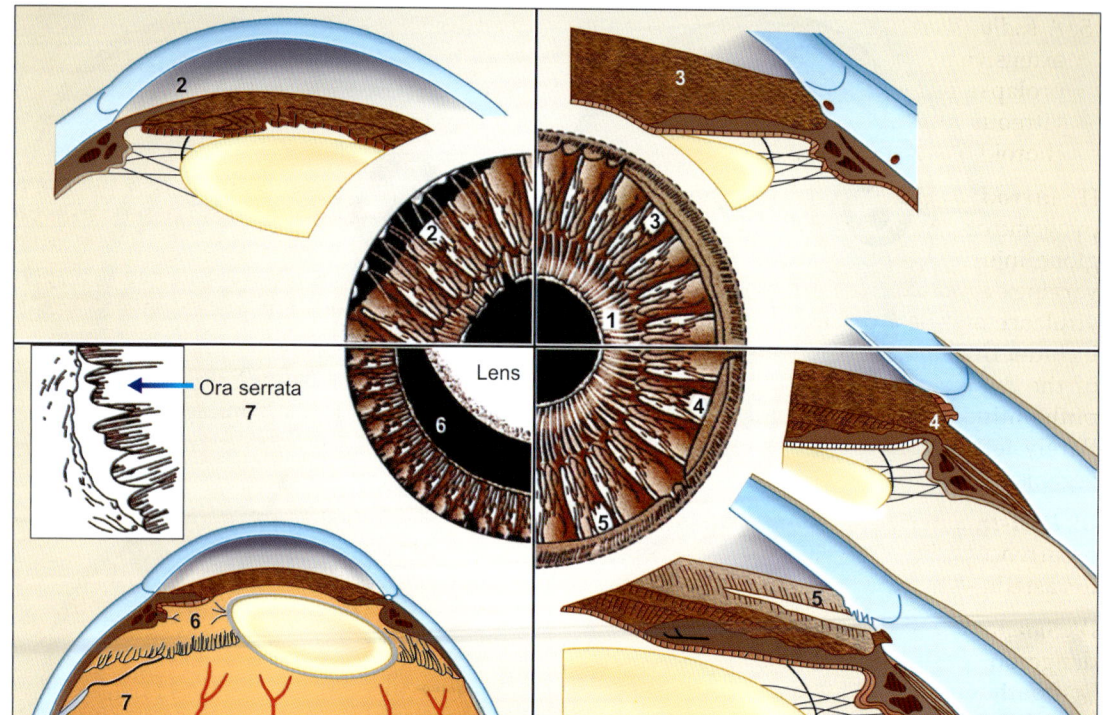

Fig. 4.3 *Campbell's seven rings or circles of tissue anterior to the equator of the globe that suddenly expand with blunt impact*

PENETRATING AND PERFORATING INJURIES

As mentioned earlier, penetrating injury is defined as a single full thickness wound of the eyewall caused by a sharp object. While perforating injury refers to two full thickness wounds (one entry and one exit) of the eyewall caused by a sharp object or missile.

These can cause severe damage to the eye and so should be treated as *serious emergencies*.

Modes of injury

1. *Trauma by sharp and pointed instruments,* like needles, knives, nails, arrows, screw drivers, pens, pencils, compasses, glass pieces and so on.
2. *Trauma by foreign bodies travelling at very high-speed,* such as bullet injuries and iron foreign bodies in lathe workers.

Modes of damage

Damage to the ocular structures may occur by following effects:

I. *Mechanical effects of the trauma* or physical changes. Mechanical effects of penetrating/ perforating trauma on the different ocular structures are as below:

1. *Wounds of the conjunctiva.* These are common and usually associated with subconjunctival haemorrhage.
2. *Wounds of the cornea.* These can be divided into uncomplicated and complicated wounds.
   i. *Uncomplicated corneal wounds.* These are not associated with prolapse of intraocular contents. Margins of such wounds swell up and lead to automatic sealing and restoration of the anterior chamber.
   ii. *Complicated corneal wounds.* These are associated with prolapse of iris, sometimes lens matter and even vitreous.
3. *Wounds of the sclera.* These are usually associated with corneal wounds.
4. *Wounds of the lens.* Small wounds in the anterior capsule may seal and lead on to traumatic cataract; which may be in the form of a localised stationary cataract, early or late rosette cataract, or complete (total) cataract. Extensive lens ruptures may be associated with vitreous loss.

5. *A badly (severely) wounded eye.* It refers to extensive corneoscleral tears associated with prolapse of the uveal tissue, lens rupture, vitreous loss and injury to the retina and choroid.

II. *Introduction of infection.* Sometimes, pyogenic organisms enter the eye during open globe injuries, multiply there and can cause varying degree of infection depending upon the virulence and host defence mechanism. These include: ring abscess of the cornea, sloughing of the cornea, purulent iridocyclitis, endophthalmitis or panophthalmitis (Chapter 9). Rarely tetanus and infection by gas forming organisms (*Clostridium welchii*) may also occur.

III. *Post-traumatic iridocyclitis.* It is of frequent occurrence and if not treated properly can cause devastating damage.

IV. *Sympathetic ophthalmitis.* It is rare but most dangerous complication of open globe injury. Sympathetic ophthalmitis refers to bilateral granulomatous panuveitis which follows open globe trauma. The injured eye is called exciting eye and the fellow involved eye is called sympathizing eye.

INTRAOCULAR FOREIGN BODIES

Modes of trauma

Penetrating injuries with foreign bodies are not infrequent. Seriousness of such injuries is compounded by the retention of intraocular foreign bodies (IOFB).

Common foreign bodies responsible for such injuries include: chips of iron and steel (90%), particles of glass, stone, lead pellets, copper percussion caps, aluminium, plastic and wood. It is important to note that during chopping a stone with an iron chisel, it is commonly a chip of the chisel and not of the stone which enters the eye.

Modes of damage

A penetrating/perforating injury with retained intraocular foreign body may damage the ocular structures by the following modes:
- Mechanical effects
- Introduction of infection

- Reaction of foreign bodies
- Post-traumatic iridocyclitis
- Sympathetic ophthalmitis

A. Mechanical effects

Mechanical effects depend upon the size, velocity and type of the foreign body. Foreign bodies greater than 2 mm in size cause extensive damage. The lesions caused also depend upon the route of entry and the site up to which a foreign body has travelled. In general these include:
- Corneal or/and scleral perforation
- Hyphema, iris hole and injury to ciliary body
- Rupture of the lens and traumatic cataract
- Vitreous haemorrhage and/or degeneration
- Choroidal perforation, haemorrhage and inflammation
- Retinal hole, haemorrhages, oedema and detachment.

B. Introduction of infection

Intraocular infection is the real danger to the eyeball. Fortunately, small flying metallic foreign bodies are usually sterile due to the heat generated on their commission. However, pieces of the wood and stones carry a great chance of infection. Unfortunately, once intraocular infection is established, it usually ends in endophthalmitis or even panophthalmitis.

C. Reactions of the foreign body

I. *Inorganic foreign body.* Depending upon its chemical nature, following four types of reactions are noted in the ocular tissues:
1. *No reaction is* produced by the inert substances which include glass, plastic, porcelain, gold, silver and platinum.
2. *Local irritative reaction* leading to encapsulation of the foreign body occurs with lead and aluminium particles.
3. *Suppurative reaction* is excited by pure copper, zinc, nickel and mercury particles.
4. *Specific reactions* are produced by iron (siderosis bulbi) and copper alloys (chalcosis).

II. *Reaction of organic foreign bodies.* The organic foreign bodies, such as wood and other vegetative materials, produce a proliferative reaction characterized by the formation of giant cell. Caterpillar hair produces ophthalmia nodosum, which is characterized by a severe granulomatous iridocyclitis with nodule formation.

D. Post-traumantic iridocyclitis

Traumatic iridocyclitis is of frequent occurrence and if not treated properly can cause devastating damage. It may occur due to:

- Direct tissue trauma,
- Lens matter, when lens is injured (phacogenic uveitis),
- Blood (hemophthalmitis),
- Irritative effects of intraocular foreign body.

E. Sympathetic ophthalmitis

Sympathetic ophthalmitis is a rare but most dangerous complication of the open-globe injury. It is a serous bilateral granulomatous panuveitis. The injured eye is called *exciting eye* and fellow normal eye which also develops uveitis is called *sympathising eye.* Sympathetic ophthalmitis has been described in detail in Chapter 8.

BIBLIOGRAPHY

1. Barr, CC. Prognostic factors in corneoscleral lacerations. Arch Ophthalmol. 1983; 101: 919–924.
2. Committee for the Classification of Retinopathy of Prematurity.An international classification of retinopathy of prematurity. Arch Ophthalmol XXXX1984YYYY; 102:1130–1134.
3. de Juan, E, Sternberg, P, Michels, R. Penetrating ocular injuries: types of injuries and visual results. Ophthalmology. 1983; 90:1318–1322.
4. Esmali, B, Elner, SG, Schork, A, Elner, VM. Visual outcome and ocular survival after penetrating trauma. Ophthalmology. 1995; 102:393–400.
5. Gilbert, CM, Soong, HK, Hirst, LW. A two-year prospective study of penetrating ocular trauma at the Wilmer Ophthalmological Institute. Ann Ophthalmol. 1987; 19:104–106.
6. Groessl, S, Nanda, SK, Mieler, WF. Assault-related penetrating ocular injury. Am J Ophthalmol. 1993; 116:26–33.
7. Hutton, WL, Fuller, DO. Factors influencing final visual results in severely injured eyes. Am J Ophthalmol. 1984; 97:715–722.
8. Kuhn, F, Morris, R, Witherspoon, D, Heimann, K, Jeffers, JB, Treister, G. A standardized classification of ocular trauma. Ophthalmology. 1996; 103:240–243.
9. Machemer, R, Aaberg, TM, Freeman, HM, Irvine, AR, Lean, JS, Michels, RM. An updated classification of retinal detachment with proliferative vitreoretinopathy. Am J Ophthalmol. 1991; 112:159–165.
10. Martin, DF, Meredith, TA, Topping, TM, Sternberg, P, Kaplan, HJ. Perforating (through and through) injuries of the globe: surgical results with vitrectomy. Arch Ophthalmol. 1991; 109:951–956.
11. Moncreiff, WF, Scheribel, KJ. Penetrating injuries of the eye: a statistical survey. Am J Ophthalmol. 1945; 28:1212–1220.
12. Snell, AC. Perforating ocular injuries. Am J Ophthalmol. 1945; 28:263–281.
13. Sternberg, P, de Juan, E, Michels, RG, Auer, C. Multivariate analysis of prognostic factors in penetrating ocular injuries. Am J Ophthalmol. 1984; 98:467–472.
14. The Retina Society Terminology Committee. The classification of retinal detachment with proliferative vitreoretinopathy. Ophthalmology 1983; 90:121–125.

ANTERIOR SEGMENT TRAUMA

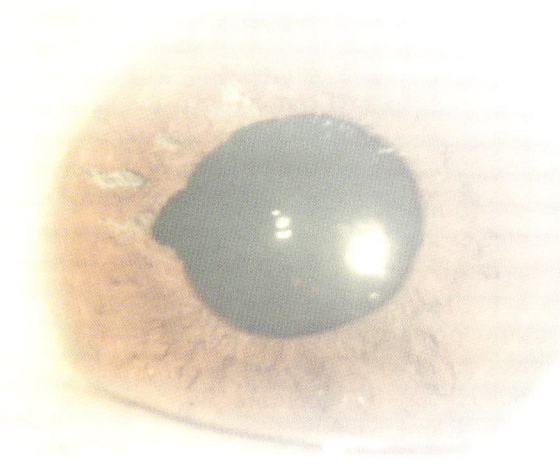

5.1 CONJUNCTIVAL AND CORNEOSCLERAL INJURIES

- Introduction
- Traumatic Conjunctival Lesions
- Traumatic Corneal Lesions
- Conjunctival and Corneal Foreign Bodies
- Corneoscleral Tears
- Summary

INTRODUCTION

In blunt as well as penetrating mechanical trauma, the anterior segment structures are second only to the lid tissue in bearing the onslaught of ocular injury. Therefore, traumatic anterior segment lesions are among the most commonly encountered injuries of the eye. The majority of the traumatic lesions are mild to moderate and are not sight-threatening, however, in some of these where the integrity of the eyeball is lost and there is superadded infection, these can prove to be devastating and detrimental to vision. In this chapter, we shall be dealing with the injuries of conjunctiva, cornea, and sclera.

Both blunt as well as penetrating traumas can involve the anterior segment structures and there can be direct as well as counter-coup forces causing variety of traumatic lesions.

TRAUMATIC CONJUNCTIVAL LESIONS

1. Subconjunctival haemorrhage

Subconjunctival haemorrhage is exceedingly common lesion, frequently alarming and worrisome to the patient that brings him to the ophthalmologist (Fig. 5.1.1). A simple haemorrhage is hardly of any consequence and best managed by reassurance since it takes 7 to 10 days to resolve spontaneously. However, one has to ensure by thorough pen-light/slit-lamp examination that it is not concealing any occult scleral rupture and is not a nidus for the entry of foreign body, particularly when the haemorrhage is severe and elevated and prolapse through palpebral fissure and is associated with subconjunctival pigmentation. Sometimes the haemorrhage is associated with trivial trauma when the causes other than trauma like systemic hypertension and Valsalva manoeuvre need to be ruled out.

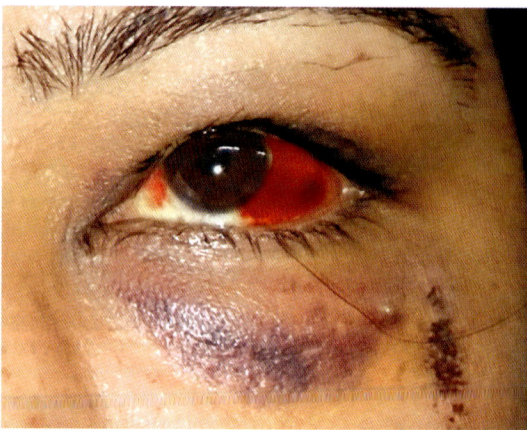

Fig. 5.1.1 *Subconjunctival haemorrhage following blunt trauma*

2. Emphysema

It is the entrapment of air in the conjunctival tissue which occurs either because of blowing of the nose, severe bout of cough and other forced exhalation or traumatic orbital bone fractures. It gives a cystic appearance of loculated air within the conjunctival stroma and on palpation crepitus is felt. Sometimes the volume of air and sudden force with which it enters is so much that it may cause exophthalmos.

Management of conjunctival emphysema is conservative and patient is cautioned to not to blow the nose and avoid sneezing by pressing the philtrum for a period of minimum of a month.

3. Conjunctival laceration

It may be either an isolated injury or part of deeper trauma and occurs mostly by injury with sharp object, such as broken glass or iron. It is commonly associated with subconjunctival haemorrhage and chemosis which may conceal underlying scleral rupture and locus of entry of foreign body (Fig. 5.1.2). It is, therefore, imperative to record complete history and

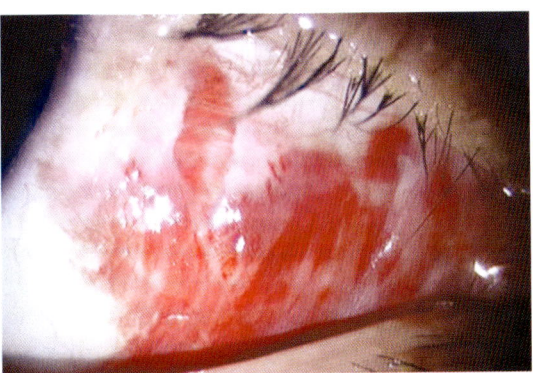

Fig. 5.1.2 *Conjunctival laceration associated with haemorrhages*

exhaustive ophthalmological examination inclusive of dilated indirect ophthalmoscopy and visualize area of the fundus corresponding to the conjunctival laceration in order to rule out scleral rupture and RIOFB. At times conjunctival laceration is not obvious as it is obscured by haemorrhage, therefore, fluorescein stain may be used to enhance the visualization of the conjuctival defect. In the absence of deeper trauma, the defects less than one centimeter may be left for spontaneous healing, however, larger defects are sutured with 8 zero absorbable polyglactin (vicryl) with buried knots avoiding the incarceration of Tenon's capsule and care is taken to not to disturb the anatomical position of caruncle and semilunar fold.

4. Conjunctival chemosis

It is the swelling of conjunctiva primarily due to the dysfunction of the vascular endothelium in response to injury and noxious stimuli. Some amount of chemosis is invariably present in most cases of ocular injury, however, its severity is not a good indicator of trauma. As already mentioned, chemosis-like haemorrhage might as well obscure deeper trauma. It is treated conservatively by putting steroid drops under the cover of antibiotics.

TRAUMATIC CORNEAL LESIONS

Out of the two refractive surfaces of the eye namely cornea and crystalline lens, the cornea is more powerful (44 D) and critical for vision. Injuries causing even minor changes in its

transparency and curvature may lead to significant changes in the visual function of the eye. Despite the fact that it is so vital a structure there are hardly any preventive measures in the form of compulsory wearing of protective glasses by the workers in the vulnerable area enforced by the law of the land. Analysis of reported data reveal that in more than 50% of all serious cases of ocular trauma, cornea is involved and vast majority are young males, in the productive years of their life.

1. Epithelial abrasion

Epithelium of the cornea has six layers of cells and the basal epithelial cells rest on the Bowman's membrane and are held in position by hemidesmosal attachments. The removal of part or all layers of the epithelium without any injury to Bowman's membrane is called as abrasion. Since the Bowman's membrane remains intact, therefore, abrasions heal completely and spontaneously without leaving behind any opacity.

Abrasions result commonly from direct tangential trauma from a foreign body, finger nail injury, branch of a tree, edge of the paper and from a contact lens.

Symptoms include pain, photophobia and watering. Since the epithelial cells of the cornea are richly supplied by the nerves, therefore, the abrasions are very painful, induce lot of photophobia because of denudation of nerve fibres and cause lacrimation. Pain and photophobia is so intense that patient does not allow proper examination which can be facilitated by local anesthetic eyedrops.

Slit-lamp examination may reveal the epithelial defects or else fluorescein stain under cobalt blue filter may enhance their visibility. Mostly the stromal infiltration and AC reaction are absent but their presence suggests superadded infection of the abrasion. Sulcus subtarsalis should be examined by lid eversion for ruling out foreign body.

Treatment. Abrasions are treated by broad spectrum antibiotic drops and ointment, short-acting cycloplegics, like 2% homatropine and bandage for 24 hrs, oral vitamin C may expedite the healing process. In the absence of infection, abrasions heal within 24 to 48 hrs. Topical steroids should be avoided. In case, the contact lens is the culprit, one should avoid contact lens and change the pair.

2. Recurrent erosions

As discussed earlier, majority of the corneal abrasions heal very fast but in about 7 to 8% of cases probably there is formation of abnormal adhesion complex in the base of epithelial defect having a weak hemidesmosomal anchorage with the Bowman's membrane. Consequently any traumatic, dystrophic disturbance can predispose to repetitive breakdown of epithelial cell layers leading to recurrent erosions.

Pathogenesis

- There is typical history of having suffered from traumatic abrasion of corneal epithelium followed by healing and then the patient reports with a sudden, very painful foreign body sensation with photophobia and lacrimation which start immediately upon awakening in the morning.
- It is being hypothesized that during sleep the lids are closed and there is absence of evaporation of tears which become hypotonic leading to the swelling of the epithelium of cornea which gets easily damaged with first blink upon awaking.

Treatment

- *Medical treatment* constitutes the application of hyperosmotic drops at night for 2 to 3 months which help in the formation of proper adhesion complex between basal epithelial cells and Bowman's membrane. Lubricating drops are applied during the daytime and oral vitamin C helps in expediting the healing process.
- If the above treatment does not help, then patient can use *extended wear contact lens*, changed every 2 weeks for 2 to 3 months.
- In case the symptoms still persist *surgical debridement* of the loose epithelium is carried out either with cotton-tipped applicator or with iris repositor under local anaesthesia followed by topical antibiotic and NSAID drops along with soft bandage contact lens.

- In case the above treatment fails another *surgical treatment* called as stromal micropuncture has been advocated in an area which is clearly defined by fluorescein staining. Partial thickness micropuncture is made with specialized 20-gauge needle having a guard to avoid full thickness penetration in a grid pattern involving the bordering normal tissue. The principle is to encourage anchorage of loose epithelium to the Bowman's membrane by normal scarring following injury to Bowman's membrane. Postoperatively topical antibiotic drops, NSAID drops should be given. Soft bandage contact lens may be helpful in case the epithelium is loose.
- Lately *superficial keratectomy by Excimer laser ablation* is also being advocated in desperate cases, however, despite this recurrence of erosion has been reported.

3. Corneal oedema

It is frequently encountered corneal pathology following blunt trauma due to the damage of Descemet's membrane and that of endothelial cell layer. Although blunt trauma of sufficient severity will cause rupture of cornea, but the one which is less severe may cause stromal, Descemet's membrane and endothelial layer damage. It is usually caused by either direct damage known as contusion injury or by counter-coup, i.e. concussion injury. The later is caused by wave of compression and decompression leading first to decrease in axial length followed by increase in equatorial diameter thereby causing damage to the layers of cornea. Two types of lesions causing corneal edema are:
- Diffuse endotheliopathy
- Descemet's membrane rupture

Diffuse endotheliopathy

Blunt injury of mild to moderate intensity usually causes diffuse endotheliopathy.

Actually, the endothelium may strike against the iris and ciliary body following impact with high-speed foreign bodies leading to rings of corneal oedema. It is postulated that rings of edema result from the transmission of foreign body impact induced hydrostatic shock waves from corneal surface to the endothelium. The rings are due to the endothelial swelling which can be visualized by specular microscopy. These lesions are transient and usually recover spontaneously without detectable abnormalities.

Descemet's membrane rupture

Blunt injury of relatively severe intensity leads to rupture of Descemet's membrane thereby breaching the endothelial cell layer. The endothelial cell pump is responsible for the maintenance of the transparency of the cornea. The breakdown of the endothelial cell pump results into acute hydrops of cornea with massive stromal oedema similar to what is seen in keratoconus and congenital glaucoma (Haab striae) following Descemet's rupture.

Although the condition is frightening leading to rapid diminution of vision, but the prognosis of retrieval of vision usually within 10–12 weeks is good. It is basically because of the fact that patients involved are young and the endothelium is healthy, thus the void created is filled by the sliding of adjacent endothelial cells leading to restoration of anatomical integrity of endothelial cells layer and revival of endothelial cell pump thereby restitution of the transparency of cornea. The condition usually does not have any effect on vision, however, healed Descemet's membrane rupture is seen as residual parallel striae or fish mouth breaks which are the sequelae of the Descemet's injury on slit-lamp examination.

Treatment of Descemet's membrane rupture is primarily reassurance of the patient and hyperosmotic topical drops and ointment. Pressure lowering drops may be added in case there is rise of IOP.

CONJUNCTIVAL AND CORNEAL FOREIGN BODIES

Conjunctival foreign bodies

These are usually associated with occupational and roadside accidents. The other common modes are while travelling on a two-wheeler without protective glasses and in labourers working with chisel and hammer.

- These foreign bodies are non-penetrating and cause irritative and foreign body sensation

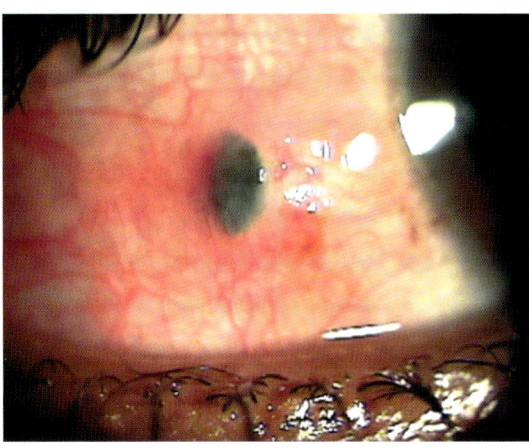

Fig. 5.1.3 *Metallic conjunctival foreign body*

only; however, stone and organic matter may cause conjunctivitis (Fig. 5.1.3).

- The suspicion of the foreign body warrants inspection of the entire globe preferably under bio-microscope. Superior fornix can be visualized by double eversion of the lid to rule out foreign body. The presence of linear epithelial defect on the cornea indicates a foreign body embedded in the sulcus subtarsalis of tarsal conjunctiva.

- Most of these foreign bodies are extruded spontaneously; however, particulate matter can be removed by irrigation with saline and by sweeping with cotton tipped applicator.

The foreign bodies which are slightly imbedded can be removed with the help of Jeweler's forceps (fine forceps) or with the bevel of 26 G needle under local anaesthesia. If the foreign body is deep, the overlying conjunctiva may have to be incised to facilitate removal. Following removal antibiotic drops and ointment should be applied.

Corneal foreign bodies
Profile

Corneal foreign bodies are the most common. Amongst the ocular foreign bodies and are second common form of ocular injury. Incidence of corneal foreign bodies varies from 17 to 40% of all ocular injuries. These are commonly seen in patients involved in activities, like welding, hammering, drilling, grinding, deriving two wheelers and in roadside and industrial accidents. Most of these are preventable provided protective glasses are used. Nature of the foreign bodies is usually metallic, organic matter or glass/plastic material.

Cornea is highly sensitive, therefore, the patients of corneal foreign body are highly symptomatic, frequently out of proportion to the severity of injury. They suffer from irritation, foreign body sensation, watering, photophobia and blurred vision.

Biomicroscopic examination is must to detect and to assess the depth of these foreign bodies (Fig. 5.1.4). One may see rust ring when it is iron in nature and stromal infiltrate in case it is there for more than 24 hrs. In the later eventuality one must suspect infective keratitis bacterial/fungal in origin particularly when the foreign body is vegetative in nature.

- In case the foreign body is transparent and suspected of glass or plastic in nature then one must examine on slit-lamp by retroillumination or sclerotic scatter otherwise these will be missed on direct illumination.
- In addition, slit-lamp examination will tell us about the depth of foreign body which is important from management point of view.

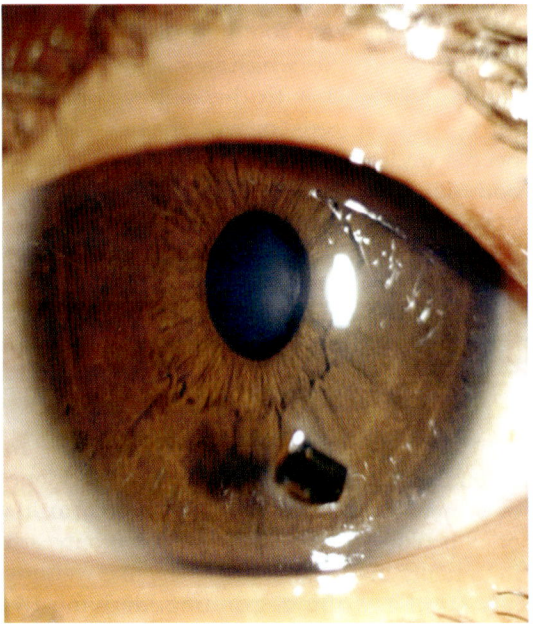

Fig. 5.1.4 *Metallic superficial corneal foreign body*

Management

Superficial foreign bodies. These foreign bodies embedded in the epithelium are easily removed in the outdoor setting under local anesthesia on a slit-lamp either with cotton-tipped applicator, foreign body spud or with 26 G needle on insulin syringe. Rust ring can be abraded with foreign body spud. The foreign bodies in anterior or mid-stroma can be removed with the help of fine-tipped tying forceps or with jeweler's forceps through the entrance wound.

Deeply embedded foreign bodies. The depth of these foreign bodies should be meticulously assessed on the slit-lamp and one should rule out perforation by performing Seidel's fluorescein test for aqueous leakage. In addition, the signs of endophthalmitis, like severe AC reaction hypopyon and vitritis, must be ruled out particularly when foreign body is few days old, although in majority of cases it is noninfectious. The removal of such foreign bodies should preferably be done in operation room setting under microscope and materials, like viscoelastics and cynoacrylate glue, should be available.

The entry wound need to be enlarged in deeply embedded foreign bodies in order to facilitate their removal.

The foreign bodies which are protruding in AC may be supported by iris repositor inside the AC via limbal incision after injecting viscoelastic in AC and then removed from outside. This manoeuvre will avoid its drop in AC or else it can be removed via AC with help of intravitreal foreign body forceps. However, magnetic foreign bodies can still be extracted from outside. Finally one must ensure that small corneal lacerations have sealed otherwise cyanoacrylate glue should be applied to make it watertight. Postoperatively, topical antibiotics, cycloplegic drops are administered and close monitoring is done daily to rule out any signs of endophthalmitis.

CORNEOSCLERAL TEARS

INTRODUCTION

Corneoscleral injury is one of the most important causes of unilateral vision loss in developing countries. It represents not only a cause of severe visual loss but also a profound psychological and economic trauma to patients and their families. These injuries are more common in the younger age groups since nearly half of patients are under 40 years of age and majority are males. Corneoscleral injuries, being a major cause of visual morbidity, therefore, urgent and appropriate measures are necessary in these cases to improve the visual outcome.

Although the terminology and classification of trauma have been dealt in Chapter 1, but before going into the details of corneoscleral injuries lets discuss these briefly. The need for a standardized terminology of the types of eye injury has led to the new widely accepted classification designed by the Ocular Trauma Group based on the "Birmingham Eye Trauma Terminology" (BETT).

CLASSIFICATION OF OPEN GLOBE INJURIES

Type
a. Rupture
b. Penetrating
c. Intraocular foreign body (IOFB)
d. Perforating
e. Mixed

Grade (visual acuity)
a. ≥ 20/40
b. 20/50 to 20/100
c. 19/100 to 5/200
d. 4/200 to light perception
e. Absence of light perception

Pupillary response
a. Positive relative afferent pupillary defect in injured eye
b. Negative relative afferent pupillary defect in injured eye

Zone
i. Cornea and limbus
ii. Limbus to 5 mm posterior into sclera
iii. Posterior to 5 mm from the limbus

EPIDEMIOLOGY

- *Incidence.* Rate of corneoscleral involvement with serious injuries is 10%.
- *Age.* Younger age group are more commonly involved. Mean age of involvement is 32 yrs.
- *Sex.* Males are five times more likely to be involved than females.
- *Place.* As per one study, the place of injury has been reported as below (Fig. 5.1.5.): 65.4% home, 13.1% roadside, 11.8% farm, 5.9% working place, and 4% school.
- *Cause* of corneoscleral injuries reported are: 33% blunt object, 13% sharp object, 12% fall, and 12% roadside accidents.

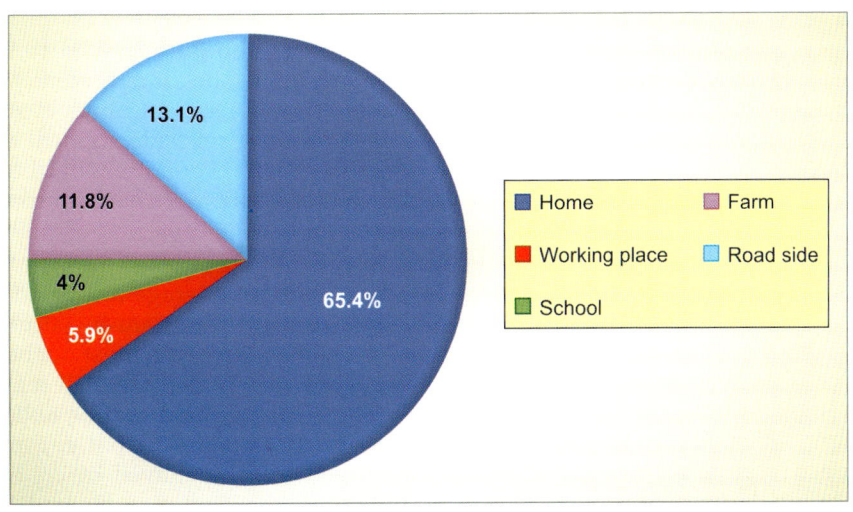

Fig. 5.1.5 *Distribution of place of injury in cases of ocular trauma*

EVALUATION OF A CASE OF CORNEOSCLERAL TEAR

History

The foremost step in the management of any corneoscleral injury repair is detailed history with regards to mode, duration, time and the object of injury. The mechanism of injury makes the examiner vigilant to identify the possibility of unsuspected or occult globe injury, such as globe perforation and posterior scleral rupture. The mode and type of injury alerts the surgeon about the possibility of concomitant microbial contamination and intraocular foreign body. Duration is important since the time elapsed between injury and presentation of the case determines the ultimate prognosis of vision. In addition, the associated life-threatening injuries need to be explored since these will take precedence over ocular injury. Nevertheless corneoscleral injuries should be addressed as early as possible in order to avoid the devastating complication, like endophthalmitis.

Ophthalmic examination

The preliminary examination may be carried out by naked eye and direct ophthalmoscope on the bedside of the patient, however, a complete and thorough ocular examination should be done preferably with slit-lamp and 90 D fundus examination whenever possible. At no point of time, pressure should be exerted on the eyeball in a suspected case of globe rupture. Best corrected visual acuity and relative afferent pupillary defect are most important prognostic factors. Signs, such as diffuse chemosis; massive subconjunctival haemorrhage; corneal laceration (partial thickness, full thickness), asymmetrical depth of anterior chamber; peaked pupil (the apex of the peak is often aligned with the meridian of the rupture), should be recorded.

Intraocular pressure measurement is contraindicated in a suspected open globe injury. However, deep anterior chamber in the presence of hypotony indicates possible posterior scleral rupture. In addition uveal show under the conjunctiva suggest scleral rupture and the one scleral rupture which may be trying to escape detection due to its posterior location should be suspected beneath the muscle insertion (thinnest sclera).

If the initial examination still fails to exclude a rupture or a hidden full thickness scleral wound, then do not hesitate to explore in the OT. Thus based on examination, the corneoscleral injury is classified as per the type, grade, zone and presence/absence of relative afferent pupillary defect.

Investigations

After assessment of the anterior segment and extent of the injury, several investigations are must in a case of corneoscleral injury.

- *X-ray orbit* both AP and lateral views to rule out presence of any foreign body and bony fractures.
- *CT scan* is the imaging modality of choice, if we are suspecting an open globe injury. Especially in cases of occult globe rupture, retained intraocular foreign bodies (RIOFBs) and orbital wall fractures.
- *MRI* is contraindicated, if we are suspecting a magnetic foreign body.
- *Cultures* should be sent from the margins of the wound, in case the wound is infected.
- *Ultrasonography* for assessment of posterior segment and any defect in the posterior layer of sclera is contraindicated till the primary repair is completed, otherwise pressure of transducer can extrude intraocular contents in an open globe injury.

MANAGEMENT

Preoperative management

The patient should be asked to stay empty stomach for 4–6 hrs. If not recently inoculated, patient should receive tetanus vaccine particularly in case of roadside accident or injury by organic matter. Patient should be started on intravenous antibiotics having broad-spectrum coverage.

Intravenous Cefazolin or Vancomycin for gram-positive coverage and third generation cephalosporin for gram-negative coverage. Open globe injury case must not be prescribed eyedrops or ointments which may permeate through open wound and be toxic to tissues. Finally the anxiety of patient and his/her relatives must be allayed by counselling and prognosis of vision may be explained on the basis of ocular trauma score (*see* Chapter 1).

Anaesthesia

General anesthesia is usually preferred, and to avoid retrobulbar/peribulbar injections which can induce or aggravate prolapse of intraocular tissues with a lot of undesirable consequences.

Goals and principles of wound repair

Goals in the management of corneoscleral injury include:
- Restoration of the integrity of the globe.
- Avoidance of further injury to ocular tissues.
- Prevention of corneal scarring and astigmatism.

Principles of wound repair are:
- *Primary aim*: Complete water-tight closure of the globe with restoration of structural integrity.
- *Secondary aim*: Restoration of normal anatomic relationships, avoidance of uveal tissue and vitreous incarceration in the wound, removal of necrotic tissue debris, removal of disrupted lens, removal of foreign bodies.

Surgical principles

Scleral wounds

Anterior scleral wounds (Fig. 5.1.6) are mostly obvious, however, posterior ones may be difficult to diagnose. Scleral ruptures can sometimes be missed since they can be hidden by the intact conjunctiva and/or large subconjunctival hematoma. In case of any doubts, globe exploration under general anaesthesia should be done. If necessary, a 360-degree peritomy is made so as to retract the conjunctiva and provide good exposure of the sclera. Special attention is given to the areas of muscle insertions as the area beneath them is one of the most common sites for a rupture.

Suturing techniques are as below:
- Full thickness scleral wounds are generally apposed with interrupted sutures with "8–0" silk or nylon. A micropoint needle with a spatulated end should be used since it is least traumatic.
- A complete 360-degree periotomy is done to ensure good exposure. The posterior extent, margins and depth of the wound should be identified. If limbus is involved, then first suturing of the limbus to reconstruct it should be done. Scleral wounds are generally closed from anterior to posterior direction.
- Also, unlike the closure of the corneal laceration, in order to prevent prolapse of intraocular contents, the sclera should be closed in a stepwise fashion the so-called "close as you go" technique. This technique involves a limited anterior dissection, exposure of a small portion of the scleral defect, and closure of the visible anterior defect prior to further posterior dissection.
- Prolapsed uveal tissue is gently reposited to avoid incarceration in the wound. If vitreous is present in the wound, then vitrectomy should be done at the scleral surface with the help of vitreous cutter. Prolapsed retinal tissue is gently reposited, if possible.
- If the scleral wound extends under an extra-ocular muscle, an assistant can retract the muscle gently using a muscle hook to aid in exposure. If more exposure is needed especially if the laceration is under the insertion of the muscle, the same may need to be temporarily disinserted so as to allow the suturing. Following the closure of the scleral defect, the muscle may be reinserted.

Corneal Wounds

Suturing techniques

As cornea forms the major refractive surface of the eye, there is a need of restoration of the optically clear, smooth surface and curvature of the cornea. The idea is to appose the edges of the laceration with properly placed sutures at landmarks, such as limbus, sharp angles of

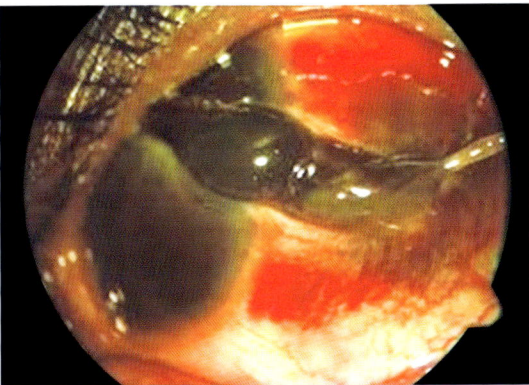

Fig. 5.1.6 *Corneoscleral laceration*

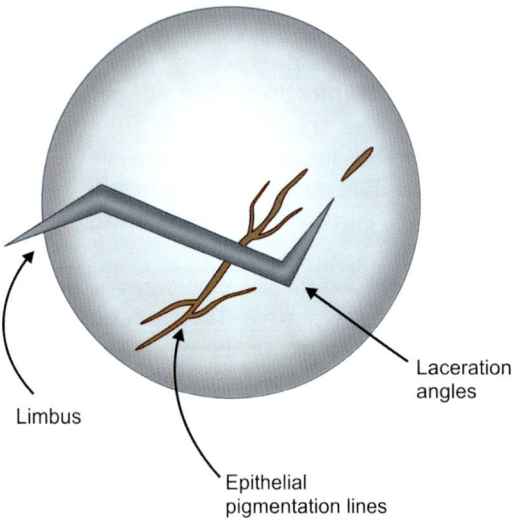

Fig. 5.1.7 *Landmarks where sutures should be applied*

laceration and pigmentation lines in epithelium (Fig. 5.1.7).

a. Basic suturing technique. Suturing with interrupted sutures with 10–0 monofilament nylon sutures and micropoint spatulated needles is the preferred method of wound apposition. Suture passes should be approximately 1.5 to 2 mm length in total, i.e. 0.75 to 1 mm on either side. The depth of the sutures should be 85–90% of full thickness, which would mean that the needle passes over the Descemet's membrane. Full thickness corneal lacerations generally have one of the following configuration:
- *Vertical/perpendicular laceration*: The distance from the wound margin to the entry site is the same as the distance from the wound margin to the exit site as shown in Fig. 5.1.8.

- *Oblique/bevelled laceration*: The distance from the anterior margin of the wound to the suture entry site is not equal to that from the same point to the suture exit site. But what matters here is the distance from the entry and exit sites to the posterior margin of the wound, which is equal as shown in Fig. 5.1.9. Sutures should be applied perpendicular to the surface of the wound to prevent slippage of the wound. Tightening of the suture will cause compression of the tissues, but if correctly done there will not be any eversion or inversion of the edges.

b. Rowsey-Hays technique of corneal suturing. The periphery of the wound is closed with long tight compression suture bites. This results in flattening of periphery and compensatory steepening of the corneal centre. The centre is then closed with short, spaced, minimally compressive suture bites to preserve the central steepening as shown in Fig. 5.1.10. This will result in flattened periphery with a spherical centre.

c. Stellate wounds. This is the most difficult problem in corneal wound repair. Techniques useful for a stellate laceration include multiple interrupted sutures, bridging sutures and purse string suture as shown in Fig. 5.1.11. The centre of a stellate laceration is difficult to appose, therefore, requires bandage contact lens application, tissue adhesive or patch grafting.

Profile of corneal wound repair

i. Corneal lacerations without incarceration. It comprises of the wound which doesn't have iris and vitreous incarceration and it doesn't extend

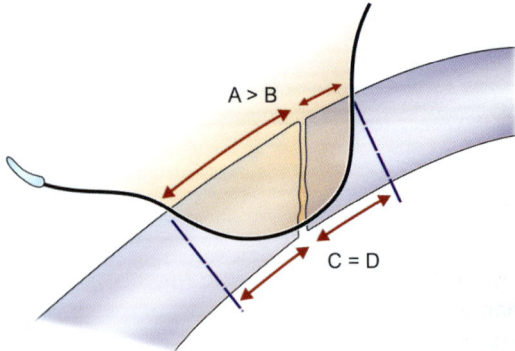

Fig. 5.1.8 *Corneal suturing technique in a vertical laceration*   Fig. 5.1.9 *Corneal suturing technique in an oblique laceration*

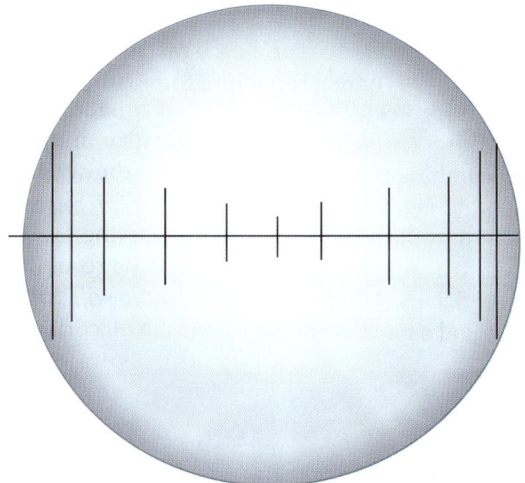

Fig. 5.1.10 *Rowsey-Hays technique of corneal suturing in a horizontal wound*

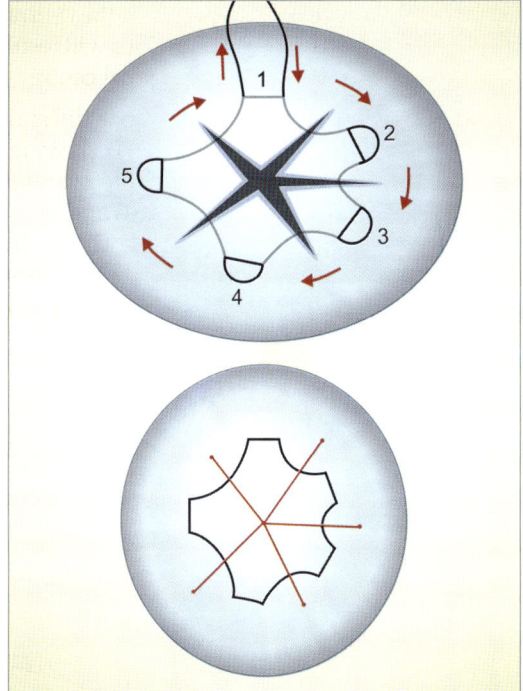

Fig. 5.1.11 *Corneal suturing technique in a stellate wound*

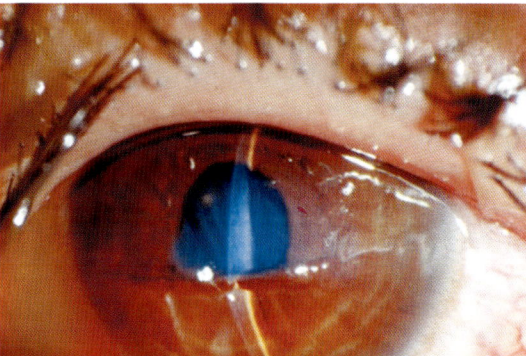

Fig. 5.1.12 *Corneal laceration without iris incarceration*

2 mm which are not self-sealing require repair in the operating room by one of the surgical technique discussed above.

ii. *Corneal laceration with iris incarceration.* Corneal wound is sutured after separating iris from the posterior surface of the wound by sweeping with help of iris repositer and recons-tructing the anterior chamber after injecting viscoelastic substance in AC. If iris prolapse is present, then the prolapsed tissue, is assessed for its viability (Fig. 5.1.13). It is important to

beyond the limbus (Fig. 5.1.12). Any wound less than 2 mm can be managed with glue with or without bandage contact lens (BCL). Glue to be used can be synthetic or natural, i.e. it can be cyanoacrylate or fibrin glue. Wounds more than

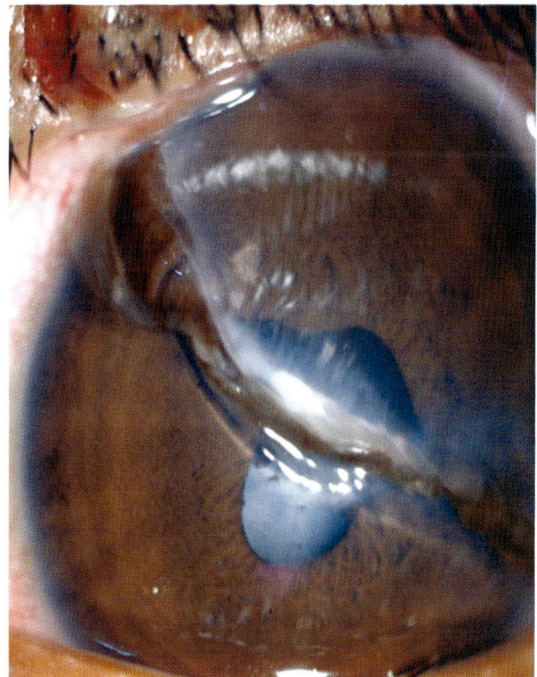

Fig. 5.1.13 *Corneal wound by glass injury with incarcerated iris tissue*

resect the prolapsed tissue, if it is more than 24 hrs old to prevent any early infection and delayed epithelial ingrowth. Viability of the iris tissue is checked and if it is not necrotic and is not contaminated by discharge and exudates, then repositioning is preferred and iridoplasty is done; whereas if iris tissue is dead, then iris is abscised.

iii. *Laceration with vitreous loss/incarceration.* Complete vitreous removal from the anterior chamber by bimanual anterior vitrectomy is must. The pupil should be circular, round without peaking. The injury with total lens extrusion and vitreous loss are bad prognosis injuries, especially those in association with intraocular haemorrhage. Such injuries should be assessed regarding the expected postoperative visual gain and if the eyes have no visual potential, then it is better to counsel the patient and his relatives regarding the poor visual prognosis before posting for primary repair.

iv. *Loss of tissue.* Tissue loss exceeding 5 mm in diameter, a corneal patch graft is usually required. A lamellar patch graft is effective and may be performed with a corneal autograft or donor sclera. These grafts are often located outside of the visual axis; therefore, graft clarity may not be essential for good postoperative vision.

Corneoscleral wounds

It is common to see corneoscleral ruptures in the superonasal area with a blunt force coming from the unprotected inferotemporal quadrant due to countercoup injury (Fig. 5.1.14). Here we need to combine the principles of corneal and scleral wound repair. Commonsense dictates that the major landmark here is the limbus which must be apposed and sutured first as shown in Fig. 5.1.15. Next continue with repair of the corneal aspect followed by the scleral aspect.

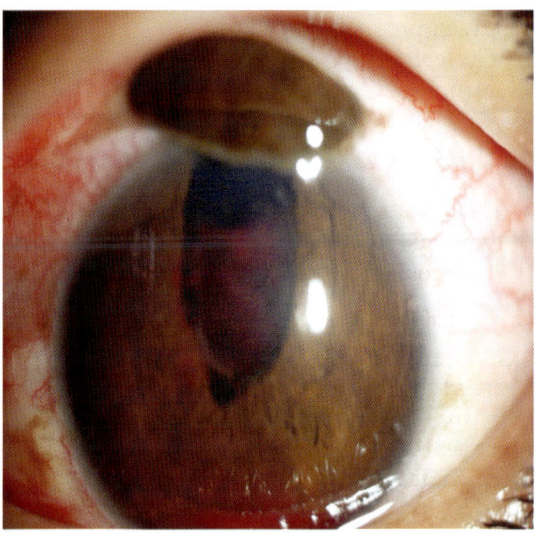

Fig. 5.1.14 *Corneal scleral tear with iris prolapse and hyphema*

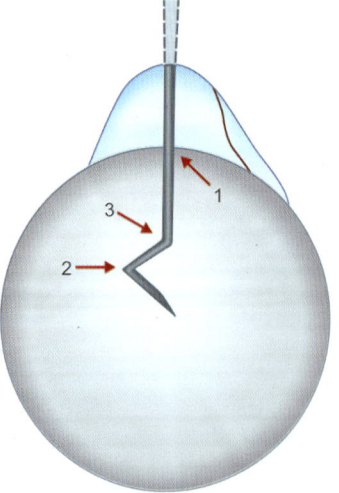
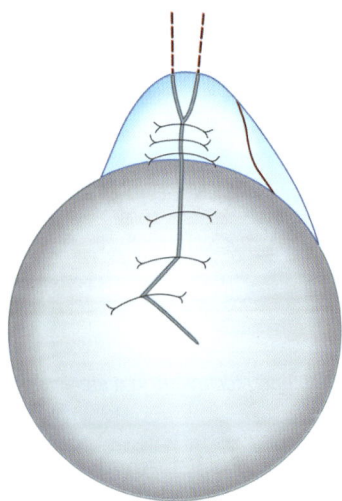

Fig. 5.1.15 *Suturing technique in a corneoscleral tear, the first suture should be applied at the limbus. Left side fig shows the anatomic landmarks identified in the corneoscleral wound. These are limbus (1) and the angles of the wound (2, 3). So first suture at (1), then corneal part and then scleral part*

Intravitreal antibiotics

Injection of 1.0 mg, vancomycin and 2.25 mg of ceftazidime intravitreally may be considered in contaminated wounds and in injuries with organic matter.

Postoperative management

- *Broad-spectrum antibiotics* topically like moxi-floxacin 0.3%. If wound seems to be infected, then fortified cefazolin 5% and tobramycin 0.3% can be added.
- *Intravenous antibiotics* are to be continued as given preoperatively.
- *Cycloplegic drugs*, like 2% homatropine/1% atropine should be given twice daily.
- *Antiglaucoma drugs* may be added, if there is rise of IOP.
- *Topical corticosteroids* are withheld and started 48 hrs later after assessing the wound in the postoperative period. In such cases, oral corticosteroids can be given immediately.

Corneal scar

Good apposition of the cut edges with deeply placed corneal sutures leaves a fine scar which gradually thins over a period of 6–9 months. Corneal scars in the pupillary axis which are significantly causing deterioration of vision can be treated by optical penetrating keratoplasty after assessing the posterior segment.

Prognosis

The main factors indicating good visual prognosis (6/18 or better) are following:
- Presenting acuity after injury of 6/60 or better,
- Wound location anterior to the pars plana,
- Wound length of 10 mm or less
- A sharp mechanism of injury.

It is seen that wounds longer than 20 mm, which extend posterior to the equator, will lead to poor final vision and subsequent enucleation in the overwhelming majority of cases.

SUMMARY

Conjunctiva and cornea are frequently injured anterior segment ocular structures. Conjunctival injuries are mostly innocuous but may conceal the presence of more serious ocular injury. Corneal injuries frequently are not isolated and are usually sight-threatening and, therefore, require timely and appropriate management.

The care of patients sustaining corneoscleral injuries calls for an approach which should be systematic and methodical. Corneoscleral lacerations are an important cause of vision loss and should be dealt diligently on an emergency basis so as to improve both structural and functional outcome. Main cause of error is non-identification of true extent of the wound so a proper examination needs to be done. The globe must be closed so that it is water-tight with the restoration of the original anatomy. Long corneal wounds are closed utilizing the Rowsey-Hays technique whereas scleral wounds extending posteriorly are closed in a stepwise fashion, proceeding posteriorly only after the anterior portion has been sutured. Timely intervention and meticulous evaluations can salvage vision in these compromised eyes.

BIBLIOGRAPHY

1. Fukuyama JI, Hayasaka S, Yamada K, Setogawa T. Causes of subconjunctival hemorrhage. Ophthalmologica 1990; 200:63–67.
2. Heier JS, Enzenauer RW, Wintermayer SF, et al. Ocular injuries and disease at a combat supported hospital in support of operation desert shield and desert storm. Arch Ophthalmol 1993; 111: 795–798.
3. Hersh SP, Zagelbeum BM. Anterior segment trauma. In: Principles and Practice of Ophthal-mology by Albert and Jakobiec. Philadelphia. 2001; 372:5201–5221.
4. McCormack P. Penetrating injury of the eye [editorial]. Br J Ophthalmol 1999; 83:1101–1102.
5. Ocular Trauma Principles and Practice-Ferenc Kuhn, Dante j Pieramici. 2002: Thieme NY 10001.
6. Scott IU, Mccabe CM, Flynn HW, et al. Local anesthesia with intravenous sedation for surgical repair of selected open globe injuries. Am J Ophthalmol 2002; 134:707–711.
7. Setlik DE, Seldomridge DL, Adelman RA, Semchyshyn TM, Afshari NA. The effectiveness of isobutyl cyanoacrylate tissue adhesive for the treatment of corneal perforations. Am J Ophthalmol. 2005; 140(5):920–921.
8. Sharma A, Kaur R, Kumar S, Gupta P, Pandav S, Patnaik B, Gupta A. Fibrin glue versus N-butyl-2-cyanoacrylate in corneal perforations. Ophthalmology 2003; 110(2):291–298.
9. Wiedemann P, Konen W, Heimann K. Recons-truction of the anterior and posterior segment of the eye after massive injury. Ger J Ophthalmol 1994; 3:1-6.

5.2 TRAUMATIC HYPHEMA AND LESIONS OF IRIS AND CILIARY BODY

- Traumatic Hyphema
- Traumatic Iris Lesions
- Traumatic Ciliary Body Lesions
- Summary

TRAUMATIC HYPHEMA

Hyphema is defined as blood in the anterior chamber. Hyphema is a common manifestation of blunt trauma to the globe. It needs thorough examination and meticulous treatment and may lead to complications, such as corneal blood staining and glaucoma, if not treated in time. Although hyphema is managed conservatively and mostly resolution of an isolated hyphema restores vision but, short-term and long-term complications may occur, which may be detrimental to vision, therefore, a systematic approach to the diagnosis and management should be followed.

EPIDEMIOLOGY

Incidence of hyphema is higher in males (male: female; 3:1) obviously because the risk of blunt trauma is higher in males than females. Hyphema is common in younger age group since 70 % are under 20 years of age. Blunt ocular trauma that results in hyphema is caused predominantly by blows (62%), projectiles (34%) and explosions (4%). Blunt trauma may be due to fist, stone, and stick injury. Sports injuries account for 60% of traumatic hyphema. Other injuries causing hyphema are violent assaults or roadside and industrial accidents.

ETIOPATHOGENESIS

In blunt ocular trauma, there are forces of compression and decompression. The compression phase causes decrease in axial length and increase in equatorial diameter of eyeball. In the decompression phase, the eyeball tends to revert back to normal diameters but it overshoots and it is in this phase that maximum damage occurs to ocular tissue by overstretching. Thus, blunt ocular trauma causes casacade of events, like stretching of limbal tissues, expansion of equatorial sclera, posterior displacement of lens/iris diaphragm and acute elevation of intraocular

pressure and consequent tearing of the anterior chamber angle (*see* Fig. 4.1, Fig. 5.2.1) resulting in rupture of vessels in the iris or ciliary bodies causing hyphema in the anterior chamber. Disruption of the major arterial circle and its branches, recurrent choroidal arteries and choroidal veins may also occur. A tear at the anterior aspect of the ciliary body is the most common site of bleeding and occurs in about 71% of cases. The blood exits from the anterior chamber via the trabecular meshwork and the Schlemm canal or the juxtacanalicular tissue.

Associated causes. Despite apparently traumatic etiology, one should rule out rubeosis iridis, vitreous hemorrhage, occult perforating injury, neoplasm (retinoblastoma, malignant melanoma and ocular metastasis).

Rebleeding. Maximum risk of rebleeding from the injured vessels occurs from three to five days after injury when clot lysis and retraction occurs. Factors that may increase the risk of rebleeding include large hyphemas, young patients and certain races, such as in African-American and Hispanic patients.

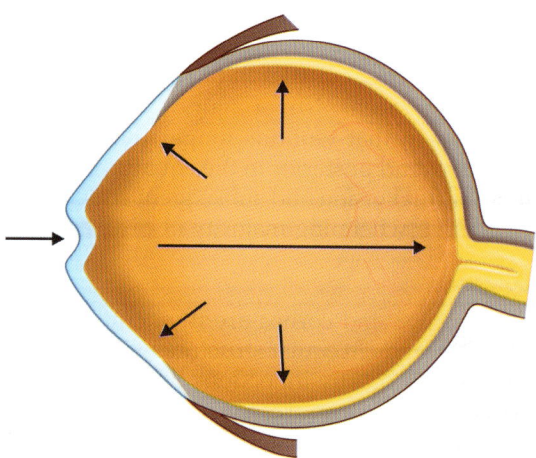

Fig. 5.2.1 *Schematic drawing showing the phase of compression in blunt ocular trauma*

CLINICAL FEATURES

Symptoms and signs

Symptoms. Symptoms of traumatic hyphema include acute pain and decreased vision. Visual recovery to 20/50 or better occurs in approximately 64% of patients with secondary haemorrhage as compared with 79.5% cases where no re-bleeding occurred.

Signs. Slit-lamp examination is done to grade the hyphema and to assess associated conjunctival, corneal and uveal tissue injuries (Fig. 5.2.2). Rebleeding is suggested by fresh blood over clotted blood in the anterior chamber. Visual acuity, hyphema size, intraocular pressure and severity of anterior uveitis have to be documented at every follow-up examination. Slit-lamp biomicroscopy, gonioscopy and fundoscopy are done for ruling out corneal blood staining, anterior chamber angle recession and signs of posterior segment trauma respectively.

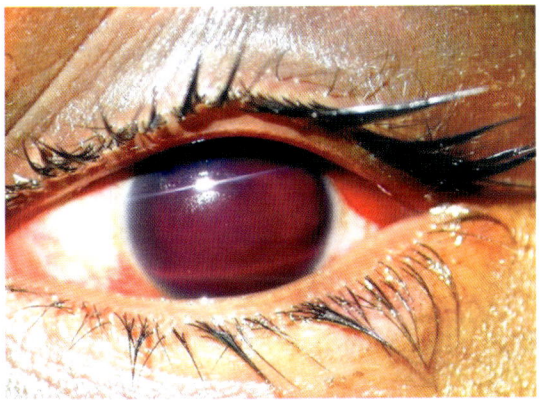

Fig. 5.2.2 *Hyphema with associated sub-conjunctival haemorrhage in a case of blunt ocular trauma*

Grading of hyphema

Table 5.2.1 describes the grading of hyphema.

Table 5.2.1 *Grading of hyphema*	
Grade	*Size of the hyphema in AC*
Microscopic	Only circulating RBCs
Grade 1	< 1/3
Grade 2	1/3 – 1/2
Grade 3	1/2 – near total
Grade 4	Total (eight ball)

Associated ocular findings

- *Corneal abrasion* may be seen after blunt trauma.
- *Corneoscleral rupture* most commonly occurs in the thinnest parts of sclera near the limbus parallel to the equator or just behind the insertion of recti perpendicular to the limbus. The site of rupture is usually superonasal in counter-coup lesions since the force of blunt trauma comes from relatively unprotected inferotemporal quadrant. Clinical signs of rupture are chemosis, subconjunctival haemorrhage, alteration in anterior chamber angle depth and hypotony (Fig 5.2.3).
- *Traumatic mydriasis* occurs in about 10% of cases secondary to sphincter muscle paresis and tears.
- *Angle recession.* There occurs a separation between longitudinal and circular muscle fibres of the ciliary muscle. Thus the ciliary body band on gonioscopy is widened. The incidence of angle recession is 6–10% of all cases of hyphema. The angle recession leads to glaucoma at a later date.
- *Traumatic iritis* is usually associated with hyphema and a vossious ring which is imprint of pigment layer of iris on the anterior surface of lens signifying compression of the pupillary margin on the anterior lens capsule may develop.

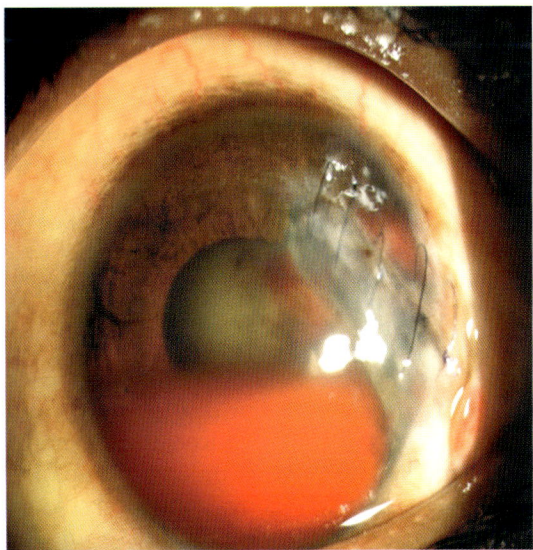

Fig. 5.2.3 *Grade II hyphema with associated repaired corneoscleral tear*

- *Cataract formation* may develop in 5–15% of cases secondary to blunt trauma. It is usually rosette-shaped nearly always in posterior subcapsular area since the capsule is thinnest there and most commonly gets ruptured in blunt trauma.
- *Posterior segment lesions*, like vitreous haemorrhage, retinal oedema, macular hole, choroidal rupture, may be seen once hyphema clears. Hence, if media permit and it is a closed globe injury, indirect ophthalmoscopy is done without indentation on presentation and on every follow-up visit with sclera indentation to look for vitreous haemorrhage and to rule out retinal dialysis, giant retinal tear, vitreous avulsion and retinal detachment.
- *Optic atrophy* may occur at a later stage as a result of direct trauma or after uncontrolled intraocular pressure rise. Such eyes suffer from irreversible loss of vision.

MANAGEMENT

Evolution of hyphema

The bleeding in anterior chamber gets arrested as a result of intraocular pressure tamponade, fibrin/platelet clot and vascular spasm. Development of clot occurs from formation of a fibrin/platelet coagulum which has been confirmed by histopathological studies. The total hyphenate once clotted may get bilobed in anterior and posterior chambers taking the shape of figure of eight and within 4–7 days maximum clot integrity is acquired. The anterior chamber is fibrinolytically active. Plasminogen is converted to plasmin which breaks down fibrin to dissolve the clot. Fibrin degradation products in the anterior chamber are cleared by trabecular outflow.

Diagnosis

A careful history of type of ocular trauma should be taken. Attention should be paid to history of sickle cell anaemia, bleeding disorders, liver and kidney disease and recent anticoagulant therapy. As mentioned already, complete examination inclusive of biomicroscopy, gonioscopy, tonometry, indirect ophthalmoscopy should be performed in a case of hyphema. If the globe is intact and media are hazy, B scan ultrasonography should not be missed to assess posterior segment. It is imperative to carry out investigations, like bleeding time, clotting time, liver function tests, to rule out any bleeding disorders. Radiological investigations are ordered, only if there is suspicion of retained intraocular foreign body (RIOFB).

Treatment of hyphema

Medical treatment

1. **Hospitalization** is recommended only if hyphema is more than one-third of anterior chamber or intraocular pressure is more than 30 mm Hg or in case of bleeding disorder, such as sickle cell haemoglobinopathy. Hospitalization has advantages, such as daily monitoring; better medical compliance and one can check and detect complications, if there are any.

2. **Bed rest.** Darr and Passmore found bilateral patching to help in hyphema rebleeding. However, patching is not easy. It increases anxiety of the patients and is a tedious task for children. Nevertheless patient should be asked to avoid strenuous activity and Valsalva manoeuvre. Most authors have noted no significant difference in results between moderate activity and strict bed rest. Head elevation is advised since it enhances dependant settling of blood and permits earlier posterior segment examination.

3. **Steroids.** Topical steroids are commonly used to decrease the discomfort related to traumatic iritis. Role of systemic steroids is controversial. They are reserved for corneal scleral rupture. A prospective study of 43 adults by Spoor and colleagues found no statistically significant difference in blood resorption and rebleeding when prednisolone 40 mg per day was used as compared to controls.

4. **Cycloplegics.** Role of cycloplegics is debatable. It is said to enhance patient comfort in traumatic iritis and facilitate fundus examination. However, Gilbert and Jensen found that topical atropine 1% had no beneficial effect on rebleeding, blood resorption or final visual acuity.

5. **Antifibrinolytic agents,** such as aminocaproic acid and tranexamic acid, are used in traumatic

hyphema to reduce rebleeding. Antifibrinolytic agents are competitive inhibitor of the activating substance that converts plasminogen into proteolytic enzyme plasmin. It secondarily inhibits plasmin itself. Plasmin lyses fibrin into smaller polypeptides and accelerates clot breakdown. Therefore, its inhibition will decrease the potential for rebleeding by stabilizing the clot. Dosage of tranexamic acid in traumatic hyphema is 25 mg/kg three times a day, i.e. in adults 500 mg tranexamic acid 2–3 tablets 2–3 times daily may be prescribed. Aminocaproic acid 50 mg/kg orally every 4 hours up to 30 gm/day for a total of 5 days. Common side effects are nausea, vomiting, diarrhoea and postural hypotension. Antifibrinolytic agents are contraindicated in bleeding disorders, pregnancy, cardiac, hepatic and renal disease. In addition, their use is also debatable because of cost issues, side effects and complications. By and large their use is avoided.

Note. Aspirin and other blood thinner are contraindicated.

Surgical treatment

Indications

Currently surgical intervention is indicated, if the IOP is raised as under.

Intraocular pressure (IOP) criteria:
- IOP more than 50 mm Hg for five days
- IOP more than 35 mm Hg for seven days.
- IOP more than 25 mm Hg for five days in total or near total hyphema.

Other criteria:
- Corneal blood staining.
- Large clot for more than 10 days.
- Total hyphema for more than five days.
- Sickle cell haemoglobinopathy.

Surgical technique
- The type of surgical technique depends whether hyphema is liquid or clotted. In case it is liquid then paracentesis and anterior chamber wash is the simplest and safest method to evacuate blood and circulating RBCs. It is very easy to perform, lowers the intraocular pressure and has the advantage of repeatability as well. Injection of air or balance salt solution after drainage do not seem to offer any additional benefit.
- For clotted blood in anterior chamber, the limbal incision needs to be enlarged and it is best delivered between 4 and 7 days, i.e. the time period of maximal consolidation and retraction of the clot. The delivery of the clot may be facilitated by viscoelastic solution which will also prevent injury to corneal endothelium, iris and lens.
- An obdurate clotted hyphema can also be removed by vitereotomy probe and anterior chamber maintainer. However, this technique requires considerable expertise and experience in phakic eyes since an inadvertent use by novice can damage iris and lens. One must see that all throughout the evacuation, the portal of cutter is blocked by clot in order to avoid sudden collapse of anterior chamber and damage to intraocular structures. In the eventuality of associated vitreous in anterior chamber or traumatic cataract, it allows additional benefit of anterior segment reconstruction.

Other surgical techniques which may be employed are peripheral iridectomy in pupillary block glaucoma and trabeculectomy in angle recession glaucoma.

COMPLICATIONS

1. *Rebleeding.* Rebleeding occurs mostly 2–5 days following injury, may be caused by clot lysis and retraction. It is assumed that retraction of clot opens up the partially closed vessels leading to rebleed. Infact rebleed continues to be a matter of anxiety in a case of hyphema as it has been reported in 3.5 to 38% of patients. Rebleeding is associated with poor prognosis. In a study, 7 of 25 rebleed patients required surgery compared with 1 of 131 non-rebleed patients. Risk factors for rebleeding include race (higher rebleeding rates are seen with black or Hispanic race), younger age, aspirin intake, larger hyphemas. Aminocaproic acid is said to decrease secondary haemorrhage after traumatic hyphema.

2. *Glaucoma.* It can be both an early and late rise of intraocular pressure.

- *The early rise of intraocular pressure* is basically because of the blockage of trabecular meshwork by RBCs, fibrin/platelet aggregates and degraded cell products. The traumatic trabeculitis and inflammation further aggravate the condition. Also as already mentioned, larger hyphemas are associated with higher intraocular pressure. Medical treatment is instituted, if the intraocular pressure is more than 25 mm Hg and aggressively, if more than 35 mm Hg.

- *Late glaucoma* may develop weeks to years after hyphema due to posterior synechiae formation with iris bombe, peripheral anterior synechiae, and ghost cell glaucoma and angle recession. When gonioscopy is performed, asymmetry of the angle recess may be noticeable between the affected and the nontraumatized eye or in different quadrants of the involved eye. Widening of the ciliary body band may be present due to retrodisplacement of the iris root. Other signs include irregular and darker pigmentation in the angle, whitening of the scleral spur due to visibly fractured iris processes, or the presence of peripheral anterior synechiae. The incidence of glaucoma is directly related to the extent of angle recessed; it is approximately 4%, if less than 180° of the angle is recessed and approximately 10%, if more than 180° is recessed. The time of onset of angle recession glaucoma is variable from 1 to 40 years.

Medical treatment is initiated when the intraocular pressure exceeds the normal range. Aqueous suppressants, both topical β blockers and oral carbonic anhydrase inhibitors are the mainstay of the therapy. Much more aggressive treatment including surgical intervention is indicated in sickle cell disease, previous glaucomatous optic nerve damage or large clots with endothelial disruption.

3. *Corneal blood staining:* It occurs in less than 5% of patients with hyphema (Fig. 5.2.4) and is associated with larger hyphema, rebleeding, prolonged clot duration, elevated intraocular pressure and decompensated endothelium. Early clinical signs include yellowish granular changes on the corneal endothelium and hazy view of the posterior stroma of the cornea on

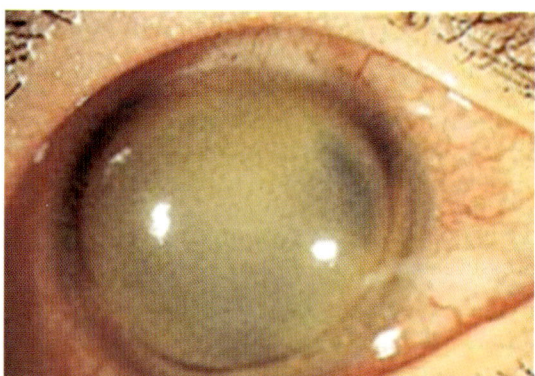

Fig. 5.2.4 *Corneal blood staining following hyphema*

higher magnification on slit-lamp examination. Blood staining resolves over several months to several years and clearing begins peripherally and posteriorly. Mostly penetrating keratoplasty is not required, however, it may be needed in children who are in amblyopic age group in order to avoid the risk of amblyopia.

4. *Posterior synechiae and peripheral anterior synechiae* are formed in hyphemas of prolonged duration of more than 9 days.

SICKLE CELL DISEASE

Although sickle cell disease is rare in Indian race, 10% of black population suffers from it. Sickle cells because of their shape and rigidity pose conspicuous problem in anterior chamber in patients of hyphema. These cells are poorly tolerated in anterior chamber and these do not egress through normal tabecular meshwork easily. Number of studies indicate that patients with sickle cell haemoglobinopathies and anterior chamber hyphema have more sickled erythrocytes in their anterior chambers than in their circulating venous blood. The sickled erythrocytes obstruct the trabecular meshwork more effectively than healthy cells, and a consequent elevation of intraocular pressure occurs even with lesser amounts of hyphema. Sickle cells are elongated and relatively of rigid characteristics that reduce their egress through normal trabecular meshwork, leading to marked elevation of intraocular pressure. This leads to more hypoxia, acidosis and hypercarbia which further increases sickling and resultant increase in intraocular pressure. Therefore, to prevent optic nerve damage and central retinal artery occlusion, intraocular pressure must be aggressively treated and monitored in these patients. The goal of treatment is to keep the intraocular pressure low without exacerbating the hypoxia. Surgery is indicated, if intraocular pressure exceeds 25 mm Hg for >24 hours.

TRAUMATIC IRIS LESIONS

It is a muscular–vascular diaphragm, fenestrated in the centre, dividing the anterior segment into anterior and posterior chambers and regulating the rays of light entering into the eye. It is thinnest at its root lying in the periphery at the site of its attachment on the anterior surface of the ciliary body. Tear of the root known as irido-dialysis is one of the most common lesions of the iris in a blunt trauma, although penetrating injuries of cornea can result in the laceration of iris or prolapsed of iris through the wound which is dealt in Chapter 5.2. In this section, lesions of the iris due to blunt trauma and their management inclusive of its reconstruction will be discussed.

ETIOPATHOGENESIS

In blunt trauma, there are forces of compression and decompression (*see* Fig. 4.1). The compression phase causes decrease in axial length and increase in equatorial diameter of eyeball. In the decompression phase, the eyeball tends to revert back to normal diameter but it overshoots and it is in this phase that maximum damage occurs to ocular tissues by overstretching. Thus, blunt ocular trauma causes casacade of events, like stretching of limbal tissue, expansion of equatorial sclera, posterior displacement of iris/lens diaphragm, acute elevation of IOP and consequent tearing of iris and ciliary body resulting into following lesions.

PROFILE OF LESIONS

Traumatic iritis

Mild to moderate blunt injury results in anterior chamber flare and cells. It is accompanied by eyeache, redness, photophobia and blurry vision. Mostly, it is controlled by topical steroids and cycloplegics and recovers in few days time.

Pigmentary changes

Release of pigment from the pigment epithelium of the iris is the rule in blunt trauma and it gets scattered all over the anterior segment. A fine dusting of pigment may be seen on the corneal endothelium in the trabecular meshwork, on the anterior surface of the lens and on the surface of iris. Most conspicuous is the imprint of the iris epithelium on the front of the anterior capsule of the lens known as Vossius ring (Fig. 5.2.5). It is usually smaller than actual size of the pupil since there is reflex miosis of pupil during trauma. It usually disappears with time, however, some residual pigment may remain permanently.

Miosis and mydriasis

Blunt trauma can cause both miosis and mydriasis depending upon the extent of injury. A mild trauma causes irritation of iris and ciliary body muscle causing miosis and spasm of accommodation whereas severe trauma will cause paralysis resulting in mydriasis and cycloplegia. It is not difficult to differentiate between traumatic mydriasis and mydriasis due to cycloplegic drugs. 2% pilocarpine will cause immediate miosis of traumatically dilated pupil whereas the constriction of pupil dilated by cycloplegic will be delayed. Traumatic miosis and mydriasis usually recovers spontaneously.

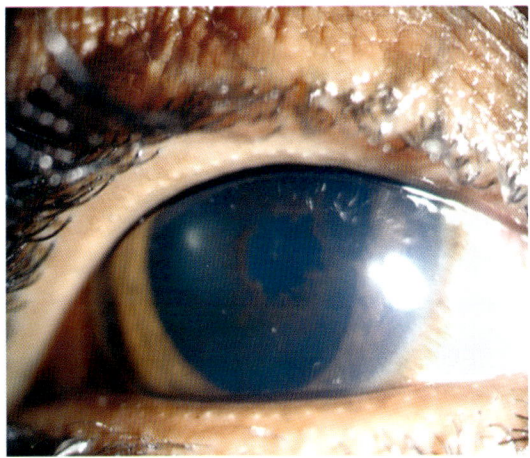

Fig. 5.2.5 *Vossius ring on the anterior surface of lens following blunt trauma*

Sphincter tears

Sphincter pupillae is located near the papillary border. The wave of concussion causes sphinteric alterations leading to single or multiple radial tears in the iris stroma appearing as small triangular defects in the pupillary border with its apex directed towards iris root (Fig. 5.2.6). Torn iris tissue leads to permanent defect since iris is devoid of healing its structure.

Sphincter lacerations

These have been reported with more severe concussive injuries, like water jets, water balloons or during phacoemulsification surgery inferiorly while sculpting anteriorly, if the critical distance between the phaco-tip and the iris is not maintained. It leads to cosmetic problem, glare and loss of sharp focus while reading the print. If the visual symptoms persist, surgical reconstruction may be considered.

Repair of sphincter laceration can be done by McCannel suture technique in a closed chamber in a pseudophakia eye. Since there is risk of damaging the crystalline lens in a normophakic patient where open sky suturing is preferred. Fig. 5.2.7 illustrates the McCannel suture technique for repairing an inferior sphincter laceration in a closed chamber in a pseudophakia eye.

Iridoschisis

It is the separation of stroma from the pigment epithelium of iris or sometimes anterior stroma

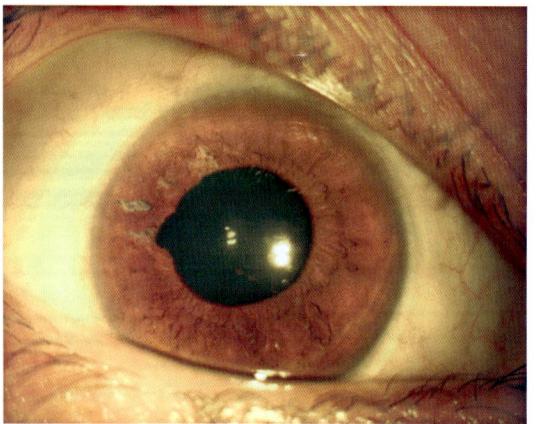

Fig. 5.2.6 *Sphincter tear following blunt trauma with a clenched fist*

may separate from posterior stroma of the iris. The detached leaf or anterior stroma may float in the anterior chamber or else the detached segment of the iris usually atrophy leaving behind thin depigmented stroma or denuded pigment epithelium.

Iridodialysis

Iris is inserted to the anterior surface of ciliary body by its root which is thinnest and weakest. During a severe concussive injury, it may get torn and iris gets separated from ciliary body and is known as iridodialysis. It results into a D-shaped pupil and in addition creates an accessory pupil of significant size at the limbus (Fig. 5.2.8). This type of injury is usually associated with hyphema which might conceal it and it becomes apparent after hyphema clears. It can be diagnosed easily on slit-lamp or seeing an alternative red glow through the iridodialysis on coaxial illumination provided the lens is clear.

Management. Small iridodialysis concealed by upper lid when asymptomatic hardly require any treatment. However, large one with good retrieval of vision and causing persistent monocular diplopia may be repaired by 10–0 double arm prolene mattress suture as depicted in Fig. 5.2.9.

Aniridia

Blunt trauma of extreme intensity may lead to complete severing of iris from its root in its entire circumstances and the iris tissue may lie like a crumbled ball in the anterior chamber and the condition is known as aniridia. This intensity of trauma is surely associated with other ocular lesions which must be recorded by thorough examination. Sometimes the posterior surface of the detached portion of the iris faces anteriorly and it is termed as *antiflexion of iris*. At other times, the whole of the iris may double back into the ciliary region and becomes invisible and known as *retroflexion of the iris*. It may mimic aniridia although it is pseudoaniridia.

- Traumatic aniridia should be differentiated from congenital aniridia which is usually bilateral, mostly associated with foveal aplasia, pendular nystagmus and glaucoma because of dysgenesis of trabecular meshwork.

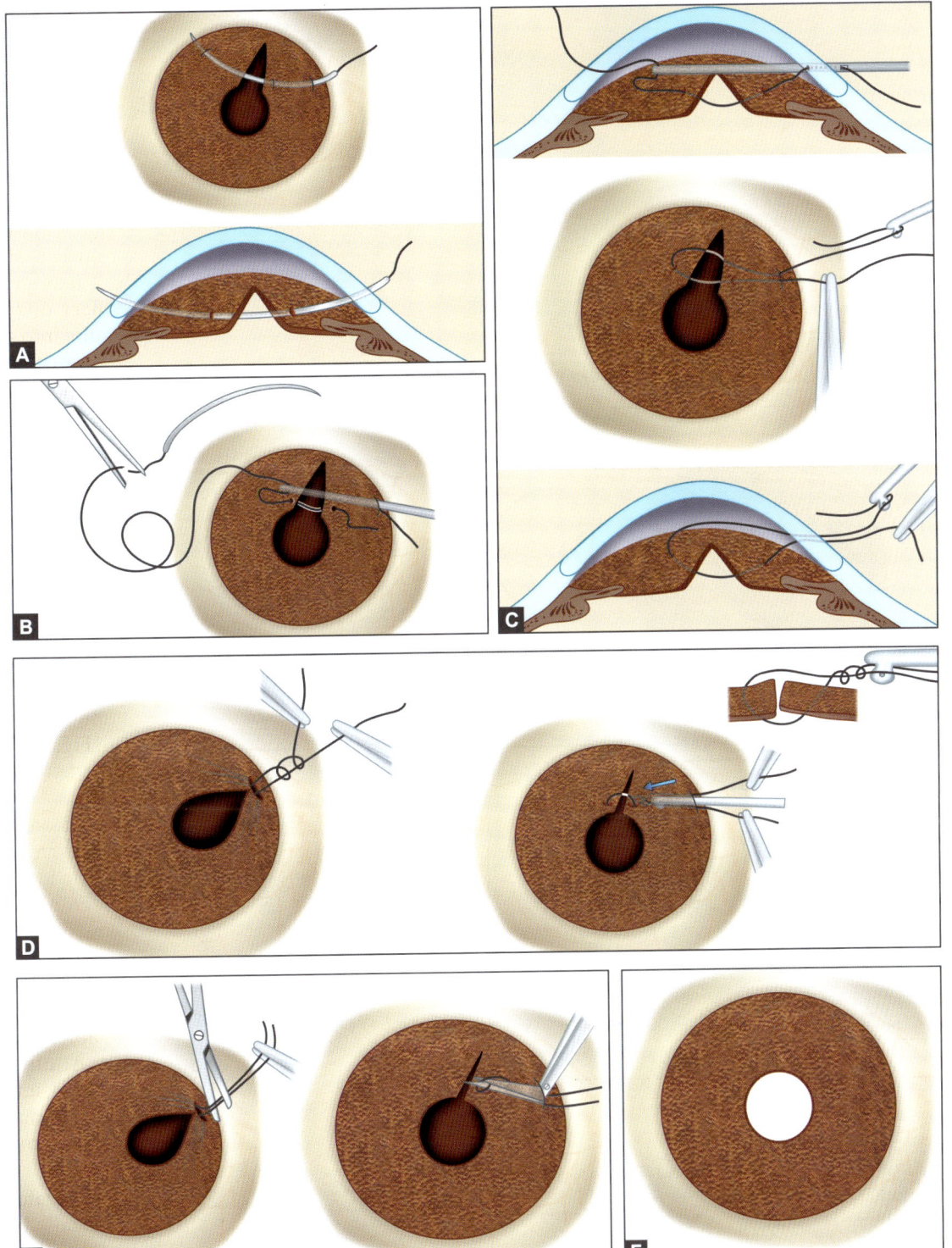

Fig. 5.2.7 *Repair of the sphincter laceration by McCannel suture from A to E*

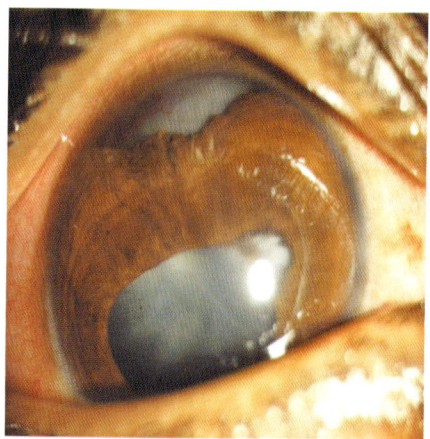

Fig. 5.2.8 *Superotemporal iridodialysis with traumatic uveitis and cataract*

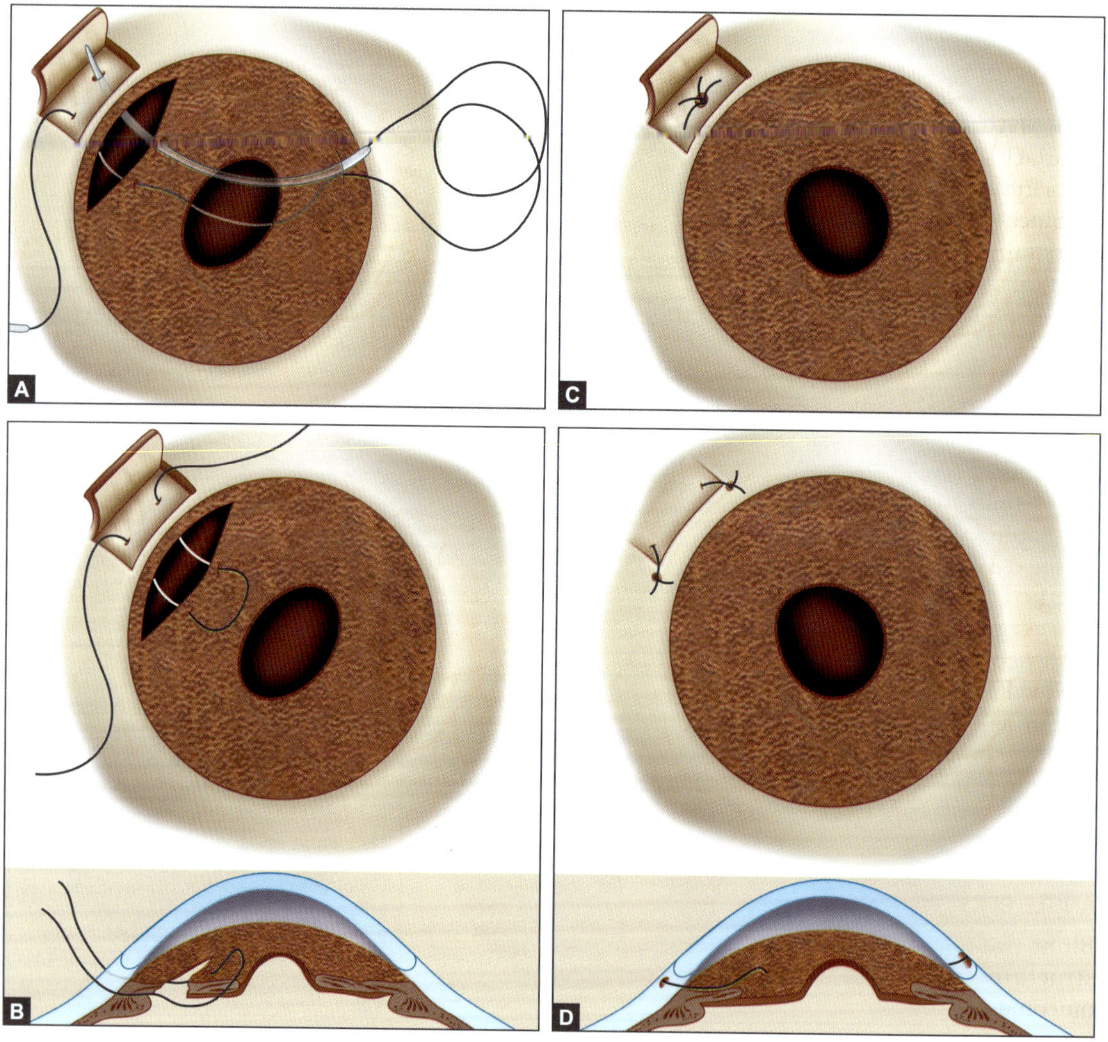

Fig. 5.2.9 *Technique of iridodialysis repair*

- Patient commonly suffers from glare and photophobia and difficulty in focusing the near print which are of serious nature and should be addressed.

Treatment. Several options are available for treatment of aniridia:

1. *Iris print contact lenses.* These are of HEMA material. These diminish glare but may also reduce visual acuity and contrast sensitivity and are good for eyes having poor visual potential.
2. *Corneal tattooing.* Since the long-term results are yet not available, therefore, corneal tattooing is best recommended for cosmesis in blind eyes. It is applied after creating lamellar corneal preparation at 50% depth of the stroma sparing the central 4 mm of corneal cap.
3. *Stained intraocular optical diaphragm.* It is either attached to capsular tension ring or as a part of intraocular lens as artificial iris diaphragm. Since these are rigid PMMA devices, these required 180° corneoscleral incision for their implantation and the capsular bag should be intact.
4. *Clear intraocular mechanical diaphragms.* These are designed particularly for severely damaged aphakic eyes requiring silicone oil tamponade in order to counter insufficiency or aqueous secretion and resultant phthisis bulbi. These are either open or closed diaphragms. The open rigid PMMA one is fixed in eyes with normal IOP and the success rate of holding back the silicone oil is 40% over a mean follow-up of 18 months. The closed (flexible) one is designed for eyes with low IOP. It is of silicone material and success rate is 50%. The closed ones are preferred, however, further modifications needs to be done.

TRAUMATIC CILIARY BODY LESIONS

ANGLE RECESSION

Blunt trauma is known to damage the angle structures and angle recession is a common outcome of contusion injury. It occurs due to tear between the longitudinal and circular fibres of ciliary body muscle, gonioscopically it is seen as widening of the ciliary body band and scleral spur band becomes distinctly white and prominent. Traumatic hyphema patients have angle recession in 70 to 100% eyes. Glaucoma is seen in about 7 to 9% of patients with angle recession. An attempt has been made to correlate the extent of angle recession and risk of glaucoma, accordingly risk is more, if angle recession exceeds 180°.

The term angle recession glaucoma is deceptive as it is not the recession of angle which leads to glaucoma but it is the collateral damage and scarring of the trabecular meshwork which is responsible for the rise of IOP. The other mechanism is extension of endothelial like layer from the cornea to angle of anterior chamber.

Patients may present with rise of IOP within 6 months to more than 10 years after injury. Gonioscopy is diagnostic and it can be performed at the time of the initial injury which may reveal the source of anterior chamber bleeding, however, it is best to wait till approximately 4 weeks post-injury. In the absence of frank hyphema, gonioscopy is essential at the time of initial examination to rule out the possibility of microhyphema.

Gonioscopic findings

Gonioscopic findings of angle trauma include torn iris processes, trabecular meshwork tears, white and distinct scleral spur, posteriorly displaced iris root and exceptionally broad ciliary body band indicating angle recession (Fig. 5.2.10). The tear into the ciliary body, which

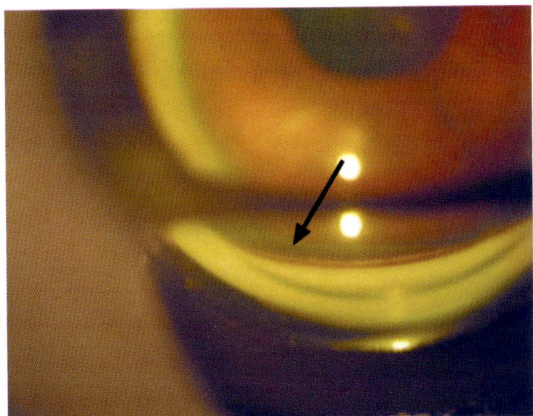

Fig. 5.2.10 *Gonioscopy picture of a patient showing traumatic angle recession measuring 3 o' clock hours in the superior angle*

splits the longitudinal and circular muscle fibres, begins to scar soon after injury. In some cases, there may be obliteration of the angle recess and peripheral anterior synechiae, which may obscure angle recession. Gonioscopy should also be performed on the normal uninjured eye for comparative analysis. Depending upon the nature of the injury, another gonioscopic finding may be excessive pigment deposition within the drainage angle. Pigment may especially be seen when there is blunt force of trauma to the eye.

Management

Since the rise of IOP can occur at any time after 6 months of injury, therefore, the patient of concussion trauma must be followed up over a period of many years to rule out glaucoma. First line of management is medical therapy by beta blockers, alpha agonists and topical and oral carbonic anhydrase inhibitors (CAI). If it fails, then filtering surgery with mitomycin C is recommended as laser therapy (ALT) yields disappointing results.

CYCLODIALYSIS

Blunt trauma of severe intensity may lead to separation of ciliary body from scleral spur. It can also be seen after anterior segment surgery. Thus, a free communication is established between anterior chamber and suprachoroidal space leading to increased fluid egress causing hypotony. Conversely in any case of hyptonous eye, cyclodialysis should be ruled out gonioscopically particularly after blunt trauma or recent surgery (Fig. 5.2.11). Cyclodialysis cleft may be small or wide. The size of cleft does not appear to have any correlation with the severity

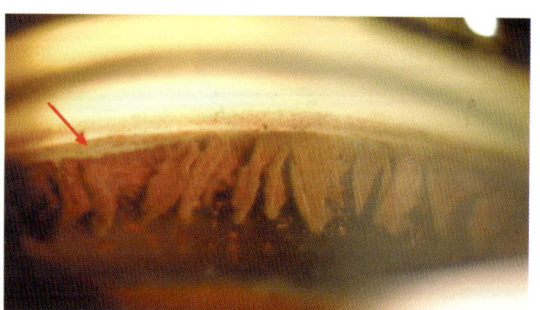

Fig. 5.2.11 *Cyclodialysis cleft as indicated by red arrow (Courtesy: Dr Parul Ichhpujani)*

of hypotony. The diagnosis of cyclodialysis cleft may be difficult in a hypotonous eye. Injection of viscoelastic in AC may aid in the diagnosis on gonioscopy.

Management

Cyclodialysis cleft may close spontaneously leading sometimes to rise of IOP to extreme levels. Laser application (Argon laser) in and around the cleft may close the cleft by inducing inflammation. If laser fails, external diathermy or cryotherapy may help in the resolution of the cyclodialysis. Finally, the ciliary body may be sutured with sclera.

SUMMARY

- *Most cases of traumatic hyphema without associated injuries resolve with restoration of normal vision.* However, in larger hyphemas with injuries to associated structures, like cornea, lens and posterior segment structures, the prognosis of vision is guarded.

- *Rebleed prevention* remains a matter of concern. Recently, the introduction of antifibrinolytic agents have shown some benefit, but their toxicity and delay in the resolution of hyphema are issues which need to be resolved.

- *Glaucoma* in early or late stage is a frequent complication, but can be controlled.

- *Corneal blood staining* is uncommon which can be avoided by maintaining intraocular pressure to normal levels.

- *Decision to use corticosteroids, cycloplegics, or nondrug interventions* (such as binocular patching, bed rest, or head elevation) should remain individualized because no solid scientific evidence supports any benefit. Since these multiple interventions, as mentioned above, are rarely used in isolation, further research to assess the additive effect of these interventions might be of value. Nevertheless, majority of hyphemas resolve, if IOP is controlled and associated uveitis is treated.

- *Damage to the iris* in most cases is without consequence; however, it may cause visually disabling symptoms requiring its surgical reconstruction.

- *Ciliary body injuries* are such that they require gonioscopy and periodic monitoring of the IOP on long-term basis so that irreversible blindness is avoided.

BIBLIOGRAPHY

1. Eye trauma by Shingleton. Mosby publications. 2010 edition.
2. Gentile RC, Pavlin CJ, Liebmann JM, et al. Diagnosis of traumatic cyclodialysis by ultrasound biomicroscopy. Ophthalmoc Surg Lasers 1996; 27:97–105.
3. Gharaibeh A, Savage HI, Scherer RW, Goldberg MF, Lindsley K. Medical interventions for traumatic hyphema (Review). Cochrane Library 2013.
4. Li Y, Zhu Y. Clinical study of medication for the treatment of traumatic hyphema. International Journal of Ophthalmology 2009; 9(10):2025–2026.
5. Pieramici DJ, Goldberg MF, Melia M, Fekrat S, BradfordCA, Faulkner A, et al. A phase III, multicenter, randomized, placebo-controlled clinical trial of topical aminocaproic acid (Caprogel) in the management of traumatic hyphema. Ophthalmology 2003; 110(11):2106–2112.
6. Vajpayee RB, Majii AB, Taherian K, Honavar SG. Frosted-iris IOL for traumatic aniridia with cataract. Ophthalmic Surg 1994; 25:730–734.
7. Walton W, Von Hagen S, Grigorian R, Zarbin M. Management of traumatic hyphema. Survey of Ophthalmology 2002; 47(4):297–334.

5.3 TRAUMATIC CATARACT

- Introduction
- Profile and pathogenesis
- Management

INTRODUCTION

Literally speaking, traumatic cataract refers lens opacification occurring as a result of traumatic lens damage caused by either mechanical injury or physical forces, such as radiation (radiation cataract), chemicals and electric current (electric cataract). However, in clinical practice, the term traumatic cataract is used for the cataract occurring due to mechanical injuries; and so only such cataracts are described in this section.

PROFILE AND PATHOGENESIS

Traumatic cataracts caused by different modes of mechanical trauma are as below.

1. CATARACT CAUSED BY CLOSED GLOBE INJURY

A blunt non-penetrating injury or concussion trauma (concussion cataract) may cause lense opacification either as an acute event or a late sequel. In some cases, blunt trauma may cause both dislocation and cataract formation.

Pathomechanism

Modes of damage. During blunt trauma, the crystalline lens may get injured by following modes:

- *Direct impact of blunt trauma* to the globe in an anterior to posterior direction causes backward displacement of the cornea and anterior sclera leading to a compensatory equatorial expansion (Fig. 4.2). The equatorial stretching may cause rupture of the lens capsule at its equator resulting in cataract formation. Equatorial globe expansion may also cause zonular disruption and resulting in subuxation of lens.

- *Contrecoup damage* to the crystalline lens may occur following a blow to the orbital area. Shock waves pass through the eyeball possibly damaging the anterior or posterior lens capsule with subsequent lens opacification.

Traumatic lesions of the lens which lead to cataract formation include:
- Mechanical damage to lens fibres
- Altered semipermeabilty of the lens capsule
- Rupture of the lens capsule

Lens concussion with intact capsule may cause cataract even several months after injury.

Lens concussion with ruptured capsule may cause a localized or generalized opacification of the lens depending upon the size of the tear. Tear in the lens capsule is associated with hydration of the lens capsule leading to rapidly developing cataract and even intumescence.

Clinical Profile

Blunt trauma may be associated with following types of lenticular opacities:

Vossius ring opacity

It is a circular ring of brown pigment seen on the anterior capsule. It occurs due to striking of the contracted pupillary margin against the crystalline lens. It is always smaller than the size of the pupil (Fig. 5.3.1).

Concussion cataract

It occurs mainly due to imbibition of aqueous and partly due to direct mechanical effects of

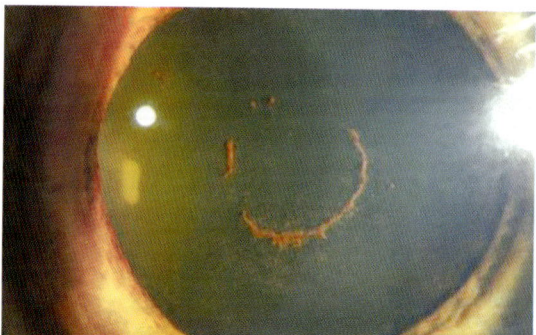

Fig. 5.3.1 *Vossius ring opacities following blunt trauma to eyeball*

the injury on lens fibres. It may assume any of the following shapes:

Localized opacities may occur due to subcapsular changes and include:

- *Disseminated subcapsular opacities* may be discrete, punctuate and scattered. These are of the most common occurrence.
- *Cobweb opacities*, which are film-like in disruption.

Early rosette cataract (punctate). It is the most typical form of concussion cataract. It appears as feathery lines of opacities along the star-shaped suture lines; usually in the posterior cortex (Fig. 5.3.2).

Late rosette cataract. It develops in the posterior cortex 1 to 2 years after the injury. Its sutural extensions are shorter and more compact than the early rosette cataract.

Traumatic zonular cataract. It may also occur in some cases, though rarely.

Diffuse (total) concussion cataract. It is of frequent occurrence and is usually associated with a capsular tear. It is characterized by total lens opacification (Fig. 5.3.3).

White soft cataract is a term suggested to denote loose cortical material found in the anterior chamber together with ruptured capsule and with fluffy opacification of the lens (Fig. 5.3.4).

Membranous cataract may occur after trauma, especially in children due to absorption of lens matter. In it, the lens, capsule and remnants of organized lens matter are fused to form a membrane of varied density (Fig. 5.3.5).

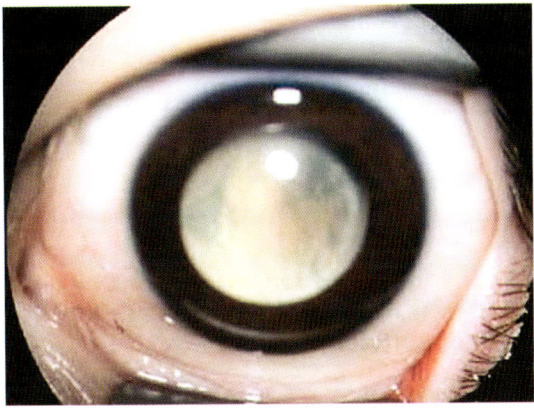

Fig. 5.3.3 *Diffuse concussion cataract*

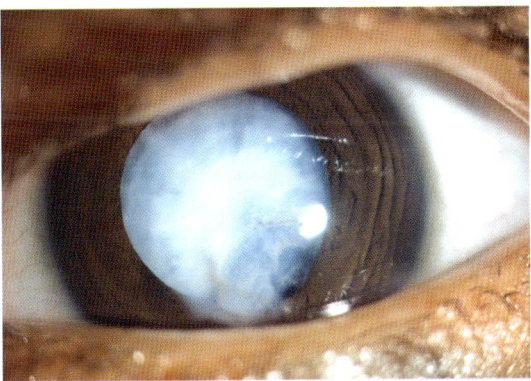

Fig. 5.3.4 *White soft traumatic cataract*

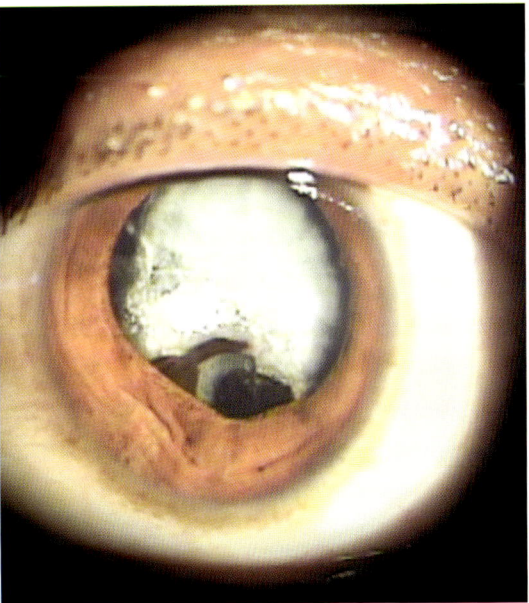

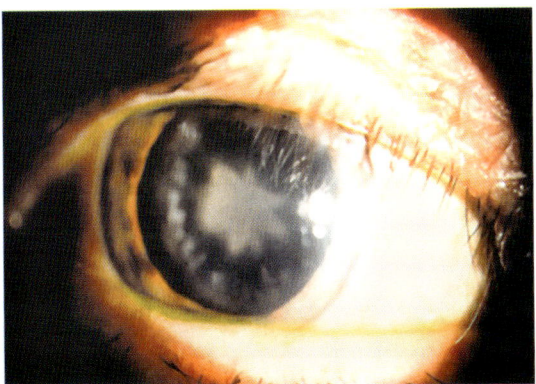

Fig. 5.3.2 *Rosette-shaped cataract following blunt trauma*

Fig. 5.3.5 *Post-traumatic membranous cataract*

Early maturation of senile cataract

Early maturation of sensile cataract may also follow the blunt trauma.

2. CATARACT CAUSED BY OPEN GLOBE INJURY

Open globe injuries include perforating and penetrating injuries. Such direct injuries to the lens may cause:

- Massive perforation of the lens capsule leading to release of free floating lens particles in the anterior chamber which becomes cataractous (Fig. 5.3.6).
- Perforating injuries of the lens often result in opacification of cortex at the site of rupture, usually progressing rapidly to complete opacification.
- A small perforation of lens capsule may occasionally heal resulting in a stationary focal cortical cataract (Fig. 5.3.7).

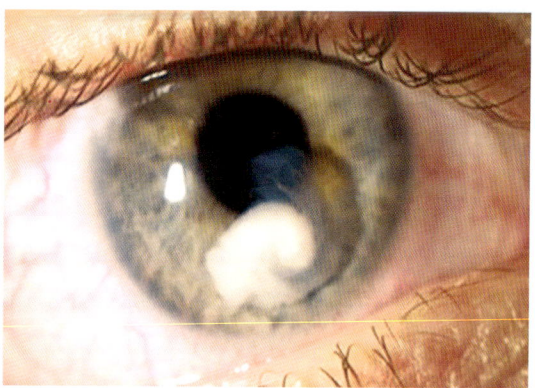

Fig. 5.3.6 *Free floating lens particle in the anterior chamber of a patient with open globe injury*

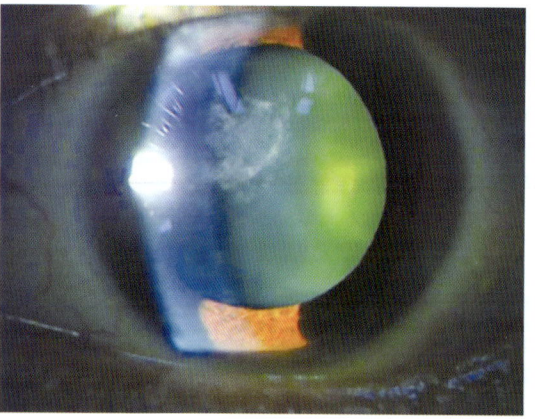

Fig. 5.3.7 *Stationary traumatic cataract*

3. CATARACT CAUSED BY INTRAOCULAR FOREIGN BODIES

The retained intraocular foreign bodies may produce cataract by following mechanisms:

i. *Direct injuries to the lens* produce effects of perforating/penetrating injury as described above.

ii. *Retained intraocular bodies* may either produce an opaque track in the lens (Fig. 5.3.8) or the lens may become completely cataractous.

iii. *Specific reactions of the foreign body* include siderosis bulbi or chalcosis.

- *Siderosis bulbi* refers to the degenerative changes produced by retained iron foreign deposits arranged radially in the anterior epithelium and lens capsule (Fig. 5.3.9). Eventually there occurs complete cortical cataract.

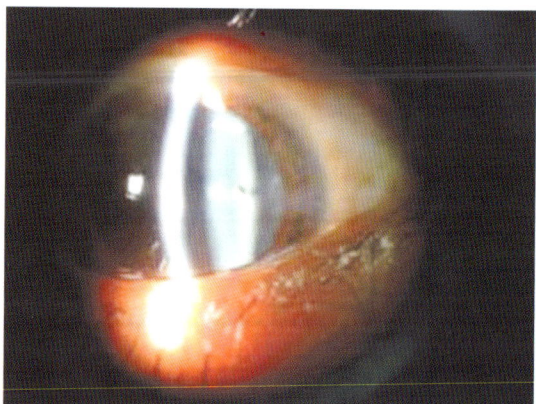

Fig. 5.3.8 *Retained intralenticular foreign body with traumatic cataract*

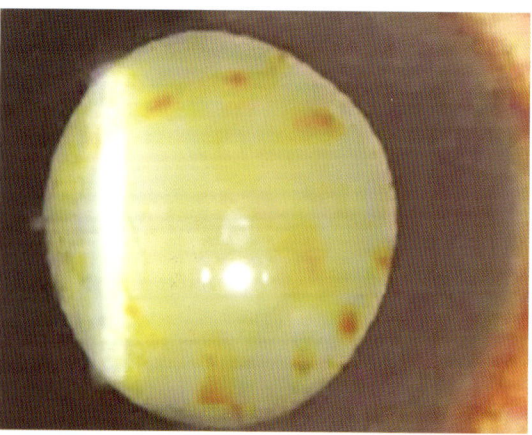

Fig. 5.3.9 *Siderotic cataract due to retained intraocular iron foreign body*

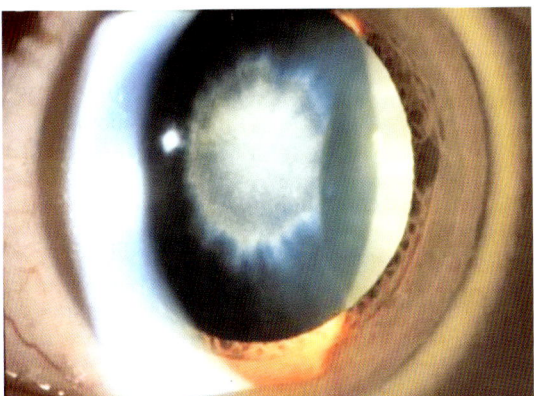

Fig. 5.3.10 *Sunflower cataract due to retained intraocular copper alloy foreign body*

- *Chalcosis* refers to the specific changes produced by a retained copper-alloy foreign body. *Sunflower cataract* is produced by deposition of copper ions under the posterior capsule. It is brilliant golden green in colour and arranged like the petals of sunflower (Fig. 5.3.10).

MANAGEMENT OF TRAUMATIC CATARACTS

ANTICIPATED RISKS AND COMPLICATIONS

Traumatic cataract, depending upon the clinical situation (severity of traumatic damage to the lens, zonules and other ocular structures), may be associated with following anticipated risks and complications.

A. Preoperatively anticipated risks and complications

1. *Calculation of IOL power* may be difficult due to irregular corneal astigmatism.
2. *Surgical procedure* may be difficult and may require vitrectomy.

B. Per-operatively anticipated risks and complications

1. *Anterior capsulorhexis* may be difficult or not possible.
2. *Posterior capsular rupture (PCR)* incidence and the incidence of associated complications may be more.
3. *Nuclear fragment loss* may occur through the PCR and/or zonular dehiscence.
4. *Vitreous loss* may occur depending upon the extent of PCR and/or zonular dehiscence.
5. *Positioning of IOL* may be difficult.

C. Anticipated postoperative risks and complications

1. *Exuberant postoperative inflammation* may be expected because of lens matter or vitreous present in the anterior chamber or injury to the iris.
2. *Prolonged postoperative increase in IOP* may be expected due to multiple factors in ocular trauma.
3. *Prolonged postoperative corneal oedema* may be expected due to associated damage to the corneal endothelium, glaucoma or hyphema.
4. *Cystoids macular oedema (CME)* may be severe and prolonged.
5. *Postoperative refractory error* due to inaccurate biometry and IOL malposition.

MANAGEMENT CONSIDERATIONS

Management considerations include:
- Preoperative considerations
- Operative considerations
- Postoperative considerations

A. Preoperative considerations

Preoperative considerations should include:
- Meticulous preoperative evaluation
- Decision and planning for surgery
- IOL consideration

Meticulous preoperative evaluation

A thorough preoperative evaluation should be carried out to:
- *Examine for RAPD* to assess for traumatic optic neuropathy
- *Corneal evaluation* for oedema, scarring, astigmatism, status of endothelium
- *Pupillary dilatation* should be assessed
- *Examination of lens* with slit-lamp to note for:
  - Signs of capsular rupture
  - Presence of a fibrotic anterior capsular plaque
  - Phacodonesis is present or absent
  - Zonular defects, when present, should be characterized preoperatively in terms of degree/clock hours of loss
  - Subluxation or dislocation of the lens
  - Vitreous prolapse is present or absent in the anterior chamber

- *Indirect ophthalmoscopy* to evaluate the posterior segment
- *B-scan ultrasonography* should be performed to evaluate the posterior segment when visualization is not possible due to opaque media. Efforts should also be made to discover any retained intraocular foreign body.
- *Biometry and keratometry* should be carried out to calculate IOL power. Many a times it may be erroneous due to difficulty obtaining axial length and keratometry measurements. Biometry of other eye should be performed to compare for accuracy.

Decision and planning for surgical management

Depending on the clinical situation, the following decision and planning should be done:

- Time of surgery
- Surgical approach

Time of surgery

The indications for removal of traumatic cataract can be acute (immediate), subacute (early) or elective (delayed).

Immediate (acute) removal of traumatic cataract is required only when there is:

- Risk of worsening of the lens-related inflammation (phacoanaphylactic uveitis)
- Loss of lens fragments in the posterior segment
- Significant risk of lens particle glaucoma from a highly disrupted lens capsule.

Early (subacute) removal of traumatic cataract is indicated during conservative management in post-traumatic period patient develops:

- Persistent inflammation
- Phacogenic uveitis
- Lens particle glaucoma

Delayed (elective) extraction of traumatic cataract should be preferred, as it permits:

- Proper management of traumatic inflammation.
- Proper decision in small traumatic cataracts which may not progress to visual axis and thus may not need extraction.
- Proper healing and stability of open globe wounds.

- More accurate measurement of IOL power calculation and planning of cataract surgery.

Surgical approaches

Once decision to operate is made, depending on the clinical situation, the surgical management of a traumatic cataract is performed using either a standard anterior limbal or posterior pars plana approach.

Anterior approach is best for a traumatic cataract unless there is complete lens dislocation or capsular rupture with significant lens material incarcerated in the vitreous. The surgeon should perform a standard phacoemulsification cataract extraction using a large capsulorhexis and initiated at the site of greatest zonular stability.

Posterior approach with vitrectomy and lensectomy is reserved for cases of posterior capsular rupture with vitreous prolapse or a posteriorly dislocated lens.

IOL considerations

- *Power of IOL,* when not possible to measure accurately, take fellow eye values. Further, plan to balance the refraction in the fellow eye to within 2 to 3 D. Always err on the myopic side.
- *Size of IOL.* Large diameter IOL (>6 mm optic size) should be preferred to minimize the symptoms, if lens decentration occurs in the future. An IOL with over all diameter 13 mm (never less than 12 mm) should be preferred.
- *IOL with PMMA haptics* should be preferred, since they are stiffer and may help to prevent capsular contraction and IOL decentration. Recommended IOLs are:
  - Foldable acrylic with PMMA haptics,
  - One piece PMMA,
  - Foldable one piece acrylic
- *Heparin surface modified and acrylic IOLs* are reported to produce minimal corneal oedema, anterior chamber reaction, formation of synechiae, and deposits on IOL.

B. Anaesthesia considerations

General anaesthesia is required in children and un-cooperative adults.

Local anaesthesia is recommended for adult patients.

- Always prefer peribulbar block anaesthesia than topical or intracameral anaesthesia.

- Avoid stressing of the zonules by overpressing the eye during local anaesthesia (i.e. avoid digital massage, Honon balloon and Super-Pinky after administration of anaesthetic solution).

C. Per-operative considerations

1. Incision considerations

In the presence of narrow non-dilating pupil, there are two different recommendations:
- *Anterior corneal* incision should be given to prevent high risk of iris prolapse with posterior corneal incision.
- *Scleral tunnel approach* should be considered, if there is increased likelyhood conversion to conventional ECCE.
- *In the presence of subluxated lens/zonular dehiscence,* follow the incision considerations given on page 74.

2. Viscoelastic considerations

- *In the presence of zonular dehiscence,* avoid hyperinflation of the anterior chamber.
- *In the presence of small pupil,* a high molecular weight viscoelastic agent is recommended to aid in pupillary dilation, synechiolysis and haemostasis. A soft shell technique should be preferred.

3. Pupil and iris considerations

Anticipated risks and complications

Anticipated risks and complications, in patients with small non-dilating pupil include:
- Difficulty during each step of surgery
- Postoperative inflammation due to excessive iris manipulation
- Iris trauma
- Peroperative and postoperative hyphema
- Postoperative glaucoma
- Temporary or permanent postoperative mydriasis

Measures to enlarge pupil size

When pharmacological dilation is of little help measures to dilate pupil include:
i. Synechiolysis with viscoelastics and use of spatula to sweep below the iris tissue. At times, cyclitic membrane along the pupillary border can be peeled off to free the pupil.

ii. Stretch pupilloplasty with the use of two y hooks, or Kugler hooks or similar instruments is a simple and effective treatment (Fig. 5.3.11). Four point pupillary dilation with the use of a microhook and Beechler's pupil dilator is also very effective (Fig. 5.3.12).

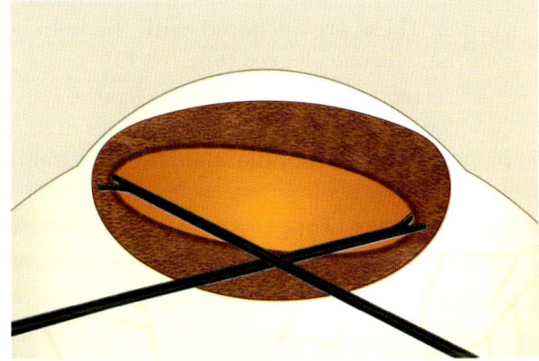

Fig. 5.3.11 *Stretch pupilloplasty using two hooks*

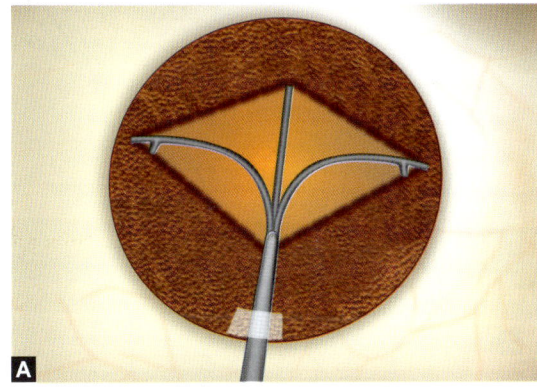

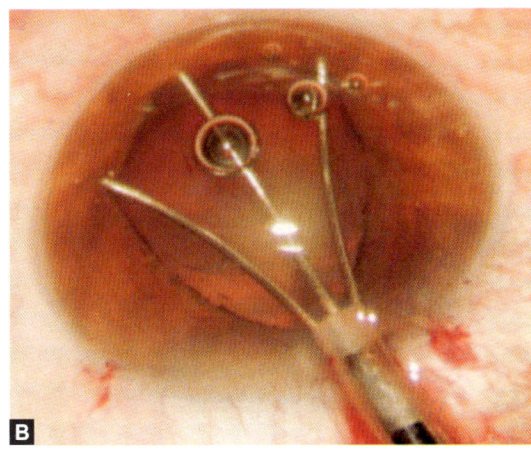

Fig. 5.3.12 *Stretch pupilloplasty using the Beehler pupil dilator: (A) Diagrammatic; (B) Clinical photograph*

iii. Use of iris retractors, and other devices has also become very popular to sustain the dilation of pharmacologically non-dilating pupil. These include:

- *Flexible iris retractors or hooks.* These are made of nylon and are applied by making four equidistant paracentesis sites in the peripheral cornea. These are anchored with the help of external silicone sleeves (Fig. 5.3.13).
- *Mackool self-retaining titanium mechanical hooks* can also be used similar to flexible iris hooks, but are much less popular than the disposable nylon hooks.
- *Malyugin ring.* This is a rectangular device made of 5–0 polypropylene which uses the scroll principle to catch the pupillary margin.
- *Hydroview iris protector ring* is a hydrogel ring, which is inserted in the anterior chamber in a dehydrated form (compressed oval). It has flanges on the edge of inner surface that capture the pupil. On hydration, it expands and thus dilates the pupil.
- *Graether pupil expander* system consists of three components: pupil expander, an inserter and an iris glide retractor expander. The pupil expander is a soft silicone ring with a circumferential groove which engages the pupillary margin and allows sustained pupillary dilation.
- *Morcher pupillary dilator* is a semicircular elastic PMMA ring which may be inserted manually or with the help of Geuder dilator injector.

iv. Surgical measures to enlarge pupil include:
- *Multiple sphincterotomies* performed at the pupillary border with the help of Vanna's scissors (Fig. 5.3.14).

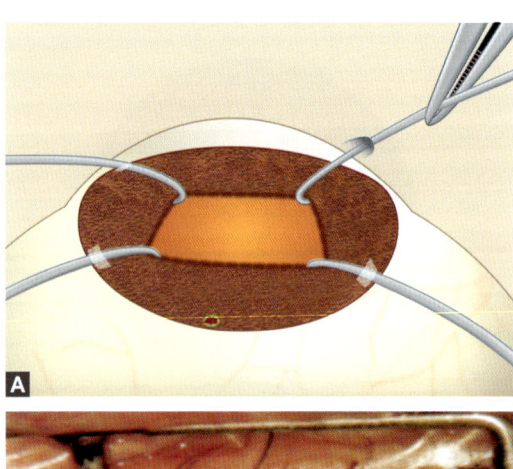

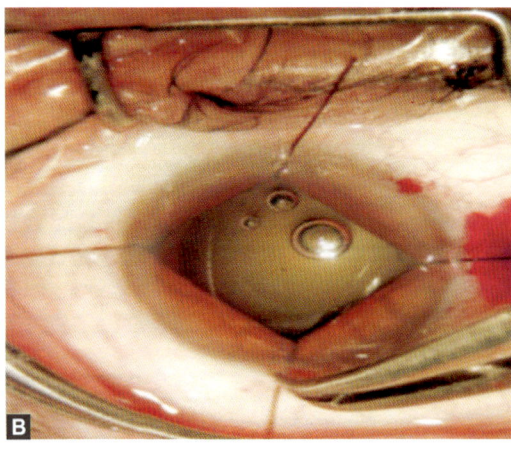

Fig. 5.3.13 *Pupil stretching using flexible nylon iris retractors equipped with adjustable silicone sleeves: (A) Diagrammatic; (B) Clinical photograph*

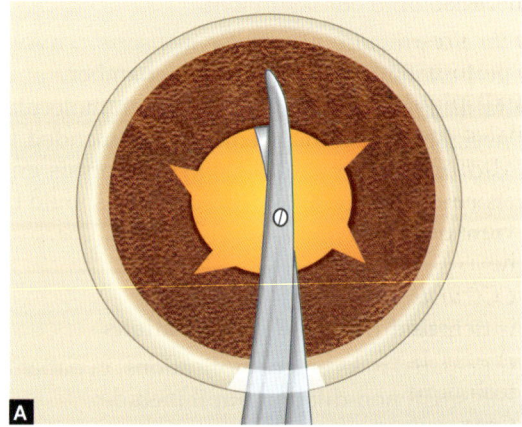

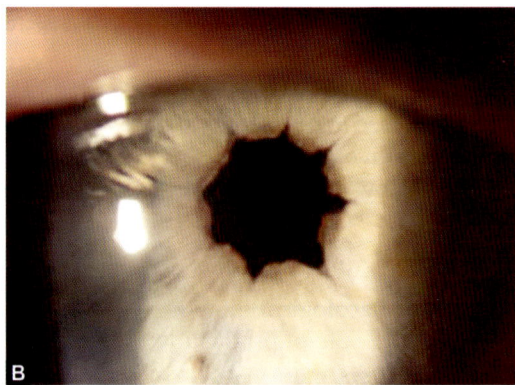

Fig. 5.3.14 *Multiple sphincterotomies performed at the pupillary border with Vanna's scissors to enlarge the pupil: (A) Diagrammatic; (B) Clinical photograph*

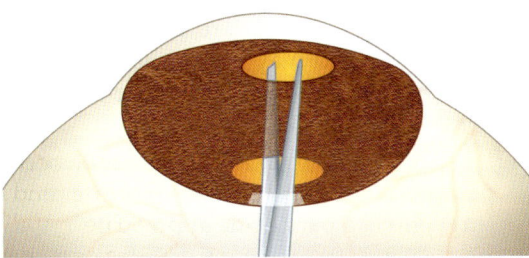

Fig. 5.3.15 *Radial iridotomy being performed through the peripheral iridectomy*

- *Radial iridotomy* made through a peripheral iridectomy either at 6 o'clock position or at 12 o'clock position results in keyhole pupil (Fig. 5.3.15). After completing the surgery, the defect can be closed using McCannel suture.

4. Considerations during capsulorhexis

Staining the capsule with trypan blue dye is recommended in all complicated and white cataracts.

In the presence of narrow of pupil. It is difficult to perform adequate sized capsulorhexis with a small pupil. Certain considerations for mid-dilated pupil include:

- *Mechanical retraction of pupil with Sinskey hook* repeatedly in different areas gives a direct view of the running margin of the capsulorhexis.
- *CCC under the iris in an air-filled anterior chamber* is practised by some surgeons. The tearing rhexis is visible through the iris in this technique.
- *Good control of capsulorhexis* is very important with a small pupil. Therefore, the technique should be performed slowly and with great ease.
- *In the presence of zonular dehiscence,* follow the considerations described on page 74.
- *In the presence of dense fibrotic subcapsular plaque,* start away from the plaque and tear completely around the plaque, if possible. Avoid tearing through the plaque.

5. Hydrodissection and hydrodelineation

Gentle but thorough cortical cleavage hydrodissection should be performed carefully so as to free the nucleus maximally and lessen the stress on the zonules during phacoemulsification.

Aggressive hydrodissection may cause a hydraulic rupture at the point of capsular compromise. Hydrodelineation may be preferred in the absence of zonular dehiscence and phacodonesis.

This technique creates a small endonucleus that can be phacoemulsified more easily.

6. Phacoemulsification, nucleus management, and cortical aspiration

In the presence of subluxation, the degree of zonular dehiscence dictates the management approach (For details *see* page 77).

In the presence of mid-dilated pupil

- *Phaco-chop* should be preferred over the nuclear fractis technique.
- *Pupillary plane* phacoemulsification should be performed after creating a deep central space.
- *Phaco parameters* recommended are low aspiration flow rates (AFR) and low vacuum rate to avoid inadvertent aspiration of the iris and posterior capsule.

Traumatic cataract without any associated complication should be managed in standard way but with more gentle and careful approach.

7. Considerations for thorough cortical clean

With narrow pupil include use of a Kuglen hook or y-hook to retract the pupil to allow direct visualization of the remaining cortical matter.

8. IOL implantation

In the capsular bag implantation of IOL, preferably foldable hydrophobic, is the recommended choice.

The use of *multifocal capsular bag IOLs* following removal of a traumatic cataract has also been explored in young patients with unilateral traumatic cataract. In comparison with standard, monofocal capsular bag IOLs, the multifocal lenses resulted in improved uncorrected near visual acuity and stereopsis, as well as decreased spectacle dependency.

Other IOL options, in case of an unsalvageable capsular bag, include ciliary sulcus fixated IOLs, trans-sclerally sutured PCIOLs, and ACIOLs. Although the ACIOLs have been advocated in special circumstances (elderly patient, good iris support, no evidence of glaucoma, no vitreous in anterior chamber), they should not be used in younger patients because of the increased risk of corneal endothelial injury and glaucoma from further angle injury.

- *Ciliary sulcus-fixated IOLs* in children following traumatic cataract removal are reported to result in visual outcomes similar to those for capsular bag IOLs but with more complications, in particular uveitis and pupillary capture.
- *Sclerally sutured PCIOLs* are also reported to produce good postoperative visual results.

9. Wound closure

Since complicated traumatic cataract patients often require additional surgical procedures, so preferably the tunnel wound should be closed with at least one suture.

D. Consideration for alternative surgical procedures

- *Combined phaco with trabeculectomy* or other glaucoma procedures need to be considered in the presence of intractable glaucoma.
- *Postponement of cataract surgery* needs to be considered in patients with uncontrolled inflammation, except in case of phacogenic uveitis.
- *ICCE* may need to be considered in markedly subluxated lens.
- *Pars plana approach* may be needed in patients with posterior capsular rupture associated with lens matter in the vitreous and in completely posteriorly dislocated lens.
- *Consider deferring surgery* in the presence of associated traumatic optic neuropathy.

E. Postoperative considerations

1. *Postoperative inflammation and CME* are likely to be more severe in patients with traumatic cataract. So, intensive topical steroid and NSAID therapy and frequent follow-up examination are recommended.

2. *Postoperative glaucoma* due to debris, (blood, pigment and inflammatory cells) is more likely to occur, and so needs to be monitored and managed efficiently.

3. *Malpositions of IOL* are frequent postoperatively and may need repositioning in patients with selective complaints or persistent intraocular inflammation.

4. *Posterior dislocation of IOL*, which may occur postoperatively, requires removal by a retina surgeon via a pars plana approach.

5. *Retinal detachment* and other posterior segment complications which are comparatively more common after traumatic cataract surgery need timely detection and management.

BIBLIOGRAPHY

1. Dinakaran S, Kayarkar VV. Traumatic retinal break from a viscoelastic cannula during cataract surgery. *Arch Ophthalmol.* 2004 Jun. 122(6):936.

2. Jaffe NS, Jaffe MS, Jaffe GF. Lens displacement. *Cataract Surgery and Its Complications.* 1997; 200–11.

3. Kanski JJ. *Clinical Ophthalmology: A Systematic Approach.* 1989; 257–8.

4. Kumar A, Kumar V, Dapling RB. Traumatic cataract and intralenticular foreign body. *Clin Experiment Ophthalmol.* 2005 Dec. 33(6):660–1.

5. Kumar S, Panda A, Badhu BP, Das H. Safety of primary intraocular lens insertion in unilateral childhood traumatic cataract. *JNMA J Nepal Med Assoc.* 2008 Oct-Dec. 47(172):179–85.

6. Phillips PM, Shamie N, Chen ES, Terry MA. Transscleral sulcus fixation of a small-diameter iris-diaphragm intraocular lens in combined penetrating keratoplasty and cataract extraction for correction of traumatic cataract, aniridia, and corneal scarring. *J Cataract Refract Surg.* 2008 Dec. 34(12):2170–3.

7. Rofagha S, Day S, Winn BJ, Ou JI, Bhisitkul RB, Chiu CS. Spontaneous resolution of a traumatic cataract caused by an intralenticular foreign body. *J Cataract Refract Surg.* 2008 Jun. 34(6):1033–5. Chuang LH, Lai CC. Secondary intraocular lens implantation of traumatic cataract in open-globe injury. *Can J Ophthalmol.* 2005 Aug. 40(4):454–9.

8. Sarikkola AU, Sen HN, Uusitalo RJ, Laatikainen L. Traumatic cataract and other adverse events with the implantable contact lens. *J Cataract Refract Surg.* 2005 Mar. 31(3):511–24.

5.4 TRAUMATIC SUBLUXATION AND DISLOCATION OF LENS

Pathomechanism
Clinical profile and management
- Subluxation of lens

- Dislocation of lens
- Phacoemulsification in subluxation

PATHOMECHANISM

Displacement of the lens from its normal position (in patellar fossa) results from partial or complete rupture or looseness of the lens zonules. Traumatic displacement of lens is most common of lens displacement constituting more than half of the cases.

Concussion injury to the eyeball is not infrequently associated with minimal subluxation to posterior dislocation of the lens. When blunt (non-penetrating) injury is sustained by the eye by an object moving parallel, to the visual axis, the cornea and anterior sclera is displaced backwards. This leads to a compensatory equatorial expansion (*see* Fig. 4.2). Aqueous and vitreous are relatively incompressible and transmit the force so that the ocular tissues undergo sudden expansion and possibly tearing. Zonular disruption during sudden increase in the equatorial meridian causes incomplete and symmetric lens support with resulting subluxation or dislocation.

Forces involved in causing traumatic displacement of the lens thus include:
- Backward thrust and rebounding of the lens,
- Pressure wave of the aqueous that forces root of the iris backward,
- Forcible recoil of the vitreous body, and
- Complimentary sudden enlargement of the corneoscleral ring.

Types of traumatic displacement of the lens
Depending upon the degree of zonular tear and the impact of the force, lens may be:
- *Retained in the patellar fossa*, even in the presence of zonular tear, due to its attachment to anterior vitreous phase.
- *Subluxation*, either lateral (superior, inferior, inward or outward) or axial (anteroposterior) may occur when some zonules are intact.
- *Dislocation or complete traumatic luxation of the lens* may occur at any of the following sites:

  – Anterior chamber
  – Vitreous cavity
  – Subretinal space
  – Subconjunctival space

Associations of traumatic displacement of the lens
Associations of traumatic displacement of the lens include often traumatic lesion of concussion injury to the eyeball namely commotio retinae, choroidal tear and retinal detachment.

Frenkel syndrome
Ocular contusion syndrome, characterized by subluxation of the lens associated with mydriasis and a tear of iris regulating from blunt trauma to eyeball was first described by a French ophthalmologist Henri Frenkel in 1931, and, therefore, also known as Frenkel syndrome.

CLINICAL PROFILE AND MANAGEMENT OF LENS DISPLACEMENT

Topographically, displacements of the lens may be classified as subluxation and luxation or dislocation.

SUBLUXATION OF LENS

It is partial displacement in which lens is moved sideways (up, down, medially or laterally), but remains behind the pupil. It results from partial rupture or unequal stretching of the zonules (Figs 5.4.1 and 5.4.2A).

Clinical features

Clinical features include:
- *Defective vision* occurs due to marked astigmatism or lenticular myopia.
- *Uniocular diplopia* may result from partial aphakia.
- *Anterior chamber* becomes deep and irregular.
- *Iridodonesis* (tremulous iris) is usually present.
- Dark edge of the subluxated lens is seen on distant direct ophthalmoscopy.

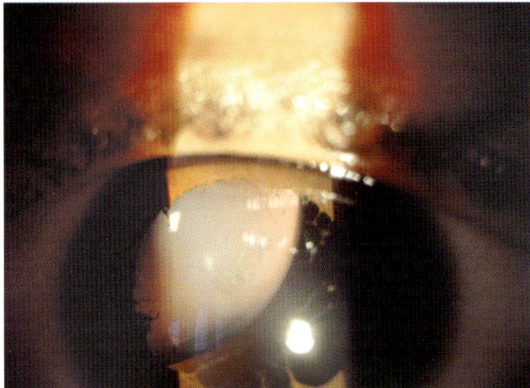

Fig. 5.4.1 *Traumatic subluxation of lens*

Complications

Complications of subluxated lens include:
- Cataractous changes,
- Uveitis,
- Complete dislocation into anterior chamber or pupil which may cause papillary block and angle closure secondary glaucoma, and
- Complete dislocation into the vitreous.

Management

A. Non-surgical management

1. *Spectacle or contact lens correction* for phakic or aphakic area (whichever gives better visual results) is helpful in many cases. Reading aid is often necessary because the subluxated lens lacks sufficient accommodation.

2. *Miotics/mydriatics* may be tried to give better visual results as per individual case.

3. *Laser pupiloplasty* has been tried with controversial results.

B. Surgical management

Indications are:
- *Decreased visual acuity*, uncorrectable by spectacles or contact lens due to either irregular astigmatism, large lenticular astigmatism, or peripheral aberration or cataractous changes.
- *Progressive posterior subluxation*, and
- *Dislocation of lens into the anterior chamber*

Surgical options for subluxated lens, each having its own indication, include:
- Lensectomy with anterior vitrectomy

- Phacoemulsification with CTR, with PCIOL
- Intracapsular lens extraction with scleral fixation PCIOL
- Intracapsular lens extraction with ACIOL.

DISLOCATION OR LUXATION OF THE LENS

In it, all the zonules are severed from the lens. A dislocated lens may be:
- Incarcerated into the pupil, or
- Present in the anterior chamber (Fig. 5.4.2B), or
- Present in the vitreous (Fig. 5.4.2C) (where it may be floating — lens nutans; or fixed to retina — lens fixata (Fig. 5.4.3)),

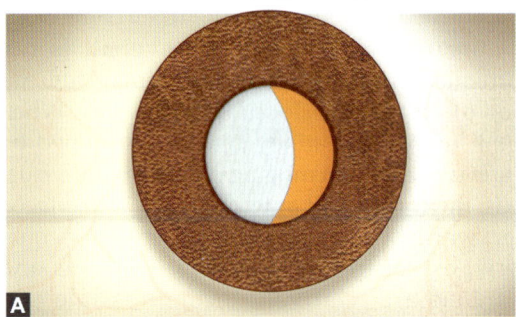

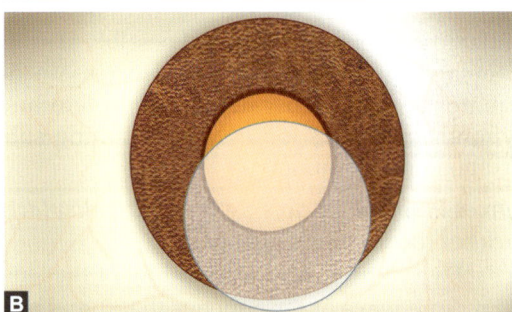

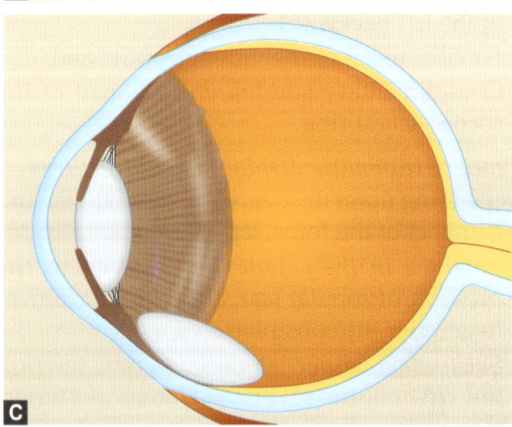

Fig. 5.4.2 *Diagrammatic depiction of displacements of lens: (A) Subluxation; (B) Anterior dislocation; and (C) Posterior dislocation*

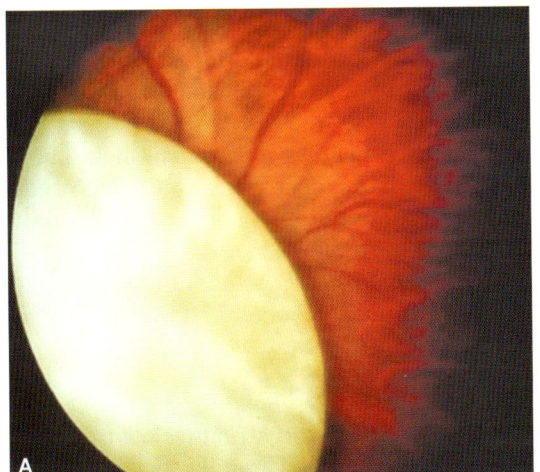

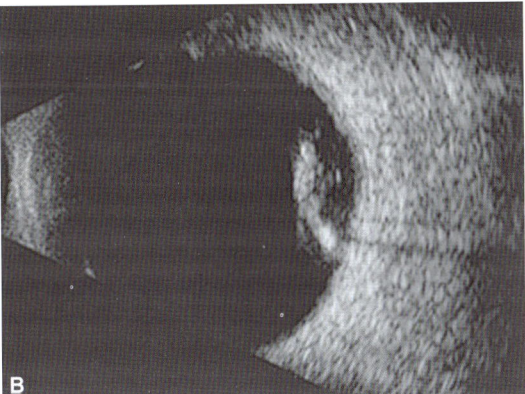

Fig. 5.4.3 *Fundus photograph (A and B) scan ultrasound, (B) showing posterior dislocation of crystalline lens*

- Present in the subretinal space, present in subscleral space or subconjunctival space (Fig. 5.4.4) or
- Extrude out of the globe, partially or completely.

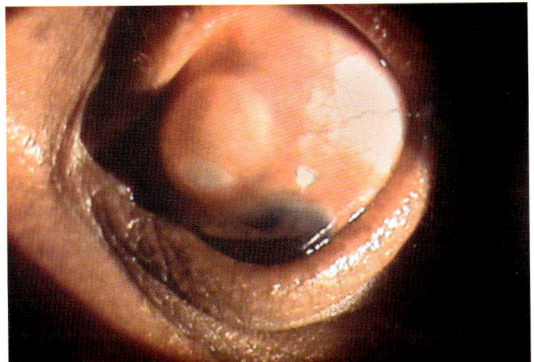

Fig. 5.4.4 *Traumatic dislocation of crystalline lens in subconjunctival space*

Clinical features

Clinical features of posterior dislocation include:

- Deep anterior chamber,
- Aphakia in pupillary area, and
- Iridodonesis
- Ophthalmoscopic examination reveals lens in the vitreous cavity.

Clinical features of anterior dislocation are:

- Deep anterior chamber, and
- Presence of lens in the anterior chamber. Clear lens looks like an oil drop in the aqueous.

Complications

Complications associated with dislocated lens are uveitis and secondary glaucoma.

Management

A. *Lens dislocated in the anterior chamber and that incarcerated in the pupil* constitutes an emergency and should be removed as early as possible.

Surgical options include intracapsular lens extraction with either anterior chamber IOL or scleral fixated posterior chamber IOL implantation.

B. *Lens dislocated posteriorly in the vitreous.*

A dislocated lens from the vitreous cavity can be removed after total vitrectomy and use of perfluorocarbon liquids (PFCL) followed by any of the following methods:

- With the help of an insulated vitreous cryoprobe, or
- By aspiration facility of vitrectomy probe (only soft cataract), or
- With phacofragmentation.

Visual rehabilitation can be achieved by any of the following methods:

- Sclera-fixated posterior chamber IOL, or
- Use of anterior chamber IOL, or
- Use of contact lens.

PHACOEMULSIFICATION IN SUBLUXATED LENS/ZONULAR DIALYSIS

A. PREOPERATIVE CONSIDERATIONS

A thorough preoperative evaluation should be carried out to:

- *Determine the associated conditions,* such as iridodialysis, sphincter tears, angle recession, cyclodialysis.
- *Zonular defect* should be characterized pre-operatively in terms of degrees/clock hours of loss.
- *Vitreous loss* is present or absent in the anterior chamber.
- *Phacodonesis* is present or absent.

B. ANAESTHETIC CONSIDERATIONS

- *General anaesthesia* in children and peribulbar anaesthesia in adults should be preferred over topical and intracameral anaesthesias.
- *Avoid stress on zonules* in the form of extensive digital massage, Pinky or Honan balloon.

C. PER-OPERATIVE CONSIDERATIONS

I. Incision

- *Incision site.* Avoid incision in the zone of subluxation to prevent enlargement of subluxation. Preferable site of incision should be in the zone opposite the subluxation to minimize traction on the zonules. However, if not possible, it may be perfomed 90° to the subluxation.
- *Scleral window* should be precut in the zone of zonular disinsertion, when the need of trans-scleral suture is anticipated to suture the IOL or capsular ring to the sulcus.

II. Capsulorhexis

- *Highly retentive viscoelastic material* should be used adequately over the area of zonular dialysis so as to tamponade the vitreous and maintain deep non-collapsing anterior chamber.
- *Vitrectomy,* if needed before capsulorhexis, should be performed with two-port system, as co-axial vitrectomy system hydrates the vitreous at the level of zonular dehiscence.
- *Initiation of capsulorhexis* should be done in the area remote from dialysis where the capsule offers sufficient resistance. Initial perforation

and creation of flap is most difficult. Effective perforation of the anterior capsule may be achieved by a sharp 15° knife or a diamond blade.

- *Advancement of capsulorhexis flap* should be in a tangential manner using 26 G bent needle or forceps. Centripetal traction can unzip the remaining zonules.
- *Size of the capsulorhexis* should be relatively large (6 mm) to counteract the tendency for further capsular contraction.

III. Hydrodissection

Gentle but thorough cortical cleavage hydrodissection should be performed carefully so as to free the nucleus maximally and lessen the stress on the zonules during phacoemulsification

IV. Phacoemulsification

Surgical recommendations based on the extent of subluxation

Before commencing nucleus management with phacoemulsification, reassess the zonular dialysis and take following measures:

- *Mild (<3 o'clock hours) zonular dialysis.* In such cases, conventional phacoemulsification can be carried out considering the below men-tioned principles.
- *Moderate (3–5 o'clock hours) zonular dialysis.* Capsular tension ring (CTR) is implanted before commencing the phacoemulsification.
- *Severe (up to 7 o'clock hours) zonular dialysis.* Modified CTR (MCTR) or Cionni's CTR is fixed to the sclera with 10–0 prolene before commencing nuclear management.

Capsular tension rings (CTRs)

Types of CTRs

Capsular tension ring (CTR) also known as 'equator ring' or 'endocapsular ring (ECR)' is made of PMMA. Though originally introduced to inhibit the proliferation of equatorial epithelial cells by *Hara et al*, the *capsular tension rings (CTRs)* are mainly used for zonular dialysis and subluxated lenses. The CTRs work on the principle of traction-expansion and stabilization. These maintain the circular contour of the bag despite zonular dehiscence. Various CTRs available presently are (Fig. 5.4.5):

- Morcher CTRs,
- Cionni CTRs,
- Henderson capsular tension ring (HCTR), and
- Ahmed capsular tension segment (CTS).

I. *Morcher capsular tension ring* (CTR). Morcher CTRs (Fig. 5.4.5A) are currently most commonly used. These are available in three types based on their diameters. Their indications are depicted in Table 5.4.1.

II. *Cionni's capsular tension ring* (Figs 5.4.5B, C and D), also called as modified capsular tension ring (MCTR), is specially designed for sclera fixation.

III. *Henderson capsular tension ring (HCTR)* is a specially designed open C-shaped loop made of a single piece of PMMA. Its unique design features eight equally spaced indentations spanning the circumference of the ring creating a sinusoidal shape (Fig. 5.4.5E). The main advantage of the ring is that the new indenta tions allow for easier nuclear and cortical matter removal while still maintaining the desired stretch of the capsular bag.

IV. *Ahmed capsular tension segment (CTS).* It is a modified design of Cionni's CTR. It is a partial ring of clear PMMA covering approxi- mately one quadrant with a hole for temporary

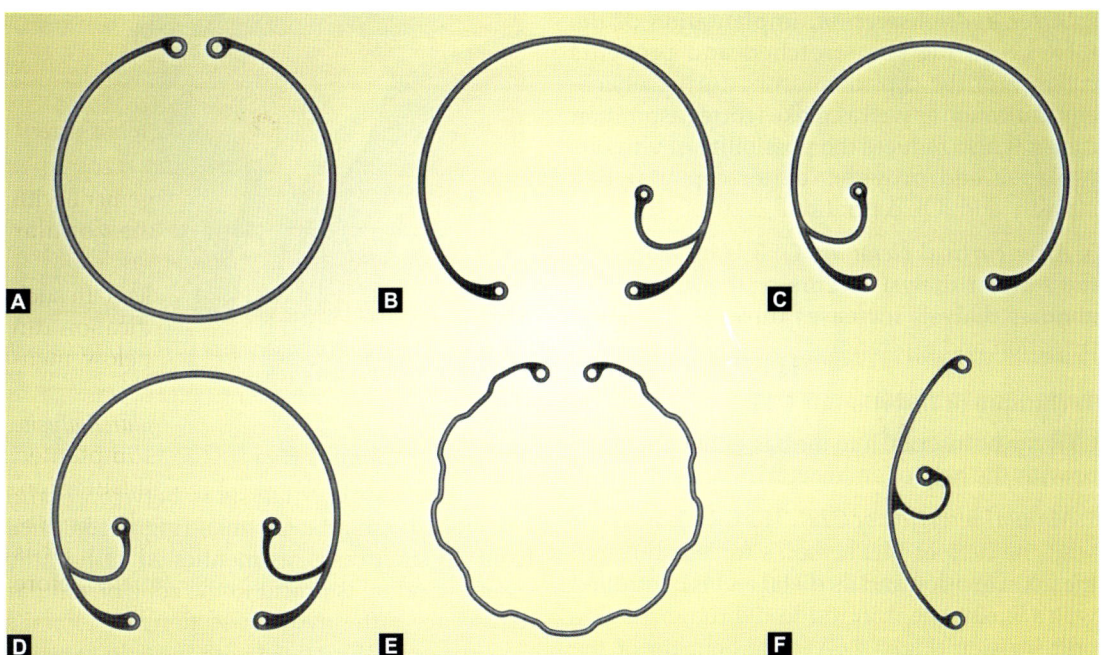

Fig. 5.4.5 *Various capsular tension rings available: (A) Morcher CTR; (B, C and D) Cionni's CTR; (E) Henderson CTR; (F) Ahmed CTS*

Table 5.4.1 *Three types of Morcher CTR and their indications*

S.no.	Type	Diameter in mm		Type of eye	Indications of use based on axial length	Corneal diameter (white to white)
		Compressed	Expanded			
1.	14	10	12.3	• Paediatric eyes • Microspherophakia	<24 mm	<11 mm
2.	14 C	11	13	• Normal eyes	24–25 mm	11–12.5 mm
3.	14 A	12	14.5	• High myopia	>25 mm	>12.5 mm

or permanent fixation (Fig. 5.4.5F), one or more CTS may be used as necessary to support the area of the capsule with weak or deficient zonules. The CTS can be used even when anterior or posterior capsular tears are present.

Time of insertion of CTR

The CTR can be inserted at variable times as below:

1. *Before hydrodissection,* the CTR implantation allows clear visualization of the anterior capsule and the proper placement of the ring. The disadvantage is that it precludes adequate cortical clean up as cortex may remain trapped between the capsule and the CTR.

2. *After hydrodissection,* implantation of the CTR keeps the bag stretched and prevents collapse of the capsular fornix during phaco-emulsification as well as makes cortex aspiration easier. It also reduces the possibility of vitreous prolapse and provides better capsular bag stability and IOL centration.

3. *After cortical clean up,* CTR is implanted, if the zonular dialysis occurs or the initial mild zonular dialysis increases during automated irrigation and aspiration.

Technique of insertion of CTR

CTR can be inserted into the bag either manually or with the help of an injector.

1. *Manual insertion of CTR.* The CTR is inserted with the help of McPherson's forceps through the main incision and its distal end is controlled with a Sinskey hook introduced through the side port incision (Fig. 5.4.6A). The bent tip of the Sinskey hook is passed in the eyelet (orifice) at the distal end of the CTR. The proximal end of the CTR is released only when it is well below the rhexis margin because if it is lost in the sulcus or the anterior chamber angle, it becomes difficult to retrieve it. The final position of the CTR should be such that the convex part of ring should abut the area of deficient zonules.

2. *Insertion of CTR with the help of injector.* The CTR can also be inserted with the help of gender capsular tension ring injector (Fig. 5.4.6B).

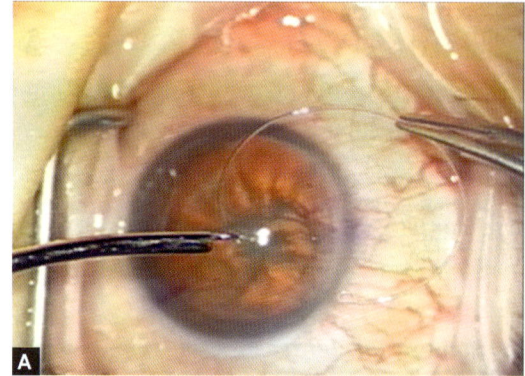

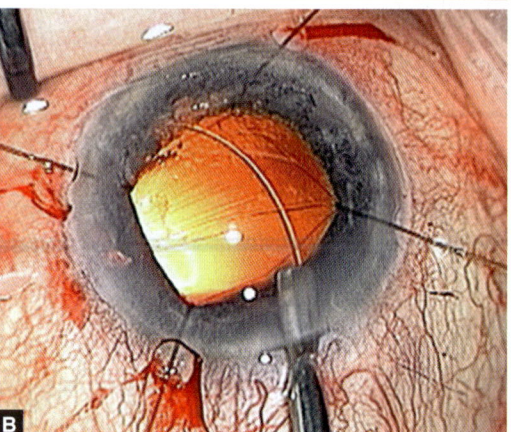

Fig. 5.4.6 *Techniques of insertion of CTR: (A) Manual with the help of McPherson's forcep; (B) with the help of an injector*

Fixation of Cionni's ring

When the zonular dialysis is between 5 and 7 o' clock hours, the Cionni's ring needs to be fixed. In such cases, as mentioned earlier, the scleral window is precut in the zone of zonular dehiscence. After hydrodissection, the Cionni's ring is inserted and fixed with the help of trans-scleral 9–0 prolene suture passed through the eyes of the ring and then through the precut scleral window. The eyelets of the Cionni's ring are at a higher plane protruding about 0.25 mm forward from the main CTR body hence lie over the anterior capsule.

Contraindications of CTR and MCTR

- Anterior capsular tear
- Posterior capsular tear
- Incomplete capsulorhexis
- Severely subluxated lens (>7 o'clock hours).

In such cases, it is often prudent to plan ICCE, followed by anterior vitrectomy and implantation of ACIOL or a scleral-fixated PCIOL (preferably).

V. Nucleus management, cortical aspiration and IOL implantation

Nuclear phacoemulsification can be performed in the bag after implantation of the CTR or outside the bag depending upon the surgeon's choice. With the latter, it is necessary to have carried out an extensive capsulorhexis, which enables nuclear prolapse either by hydro-dissection or viscoexpression.

Special points to be considered are:

- *Slow motion phaco* is recommended, i.e. vacuum, flow rate and bottle height should be kept at low to minimize the turbulence. Phaco power should be appropriate for grade of cataract.
- *For soft nuclei*, phacoaspiration or 'chip and flip' technique is recommended.
- *For moderate to hard nuclei*, phaco-chop technique is performed by many surgeons.
  Some surgeons recommend V-Kelman technique of nucleus cracking as it limits the need for rotating the nucleus and thus may prove useful.
- *Two-port anterior chamber vitrectomy* is recommended, if vitreous is detected in the AC at any stage.

Cortical aspiration. Some recommendations are:

- *Viscodissection* of cortical matter reduces stress on the zonules.
- Manual cortical aspiration is more controllable.

- *Bimanual technique* is considered better than the co-axial technique of automated aspiration.
- *Tangential traction movements* are advised when performing automated aspiration. The radial movements increase risk of traction on the ring and capsular bag.

IOL implantation. Considerations are:

- *Large diameter lens (>6 mm)* is advised to minimize the symptoms, if lens decentration occurs in the future.
- *CTR ring*, if not used earlier, may be implanted before the IOL is implanted.
- *Orientation of the haptics* parallel to the dialysis, while implanting in the bag, provides optimal zonular support. Most surgeons prefer in the bag implantation.
- *Dialling movement* should be kept to minimum.
- *Implantation on the sulcus*, where zonular support still exists along with the capturing of the optic in the capsulorhexis is recommended by some surgeons.

BIBLIOGRAPHY

1. Bilateral dislocation of the lens. SN Mitter. Br J Ophthalmol. 40(4):253; 1956 April.
2. Duker, Jay S.; Myron Yanoff MD; Yanoff, Myron; Jay S. Duker MD. *Ophthalmology*; 2009. St. Louis, Mo: Mosby/Elsevier. ISBN 0-323-04332-1.
3. Eifrig CW, Eifrig DE. "Ectopia Lentis". eMedicine. com. November 24, 2004.
4. Peter Nicholas Robinson; Maurice Godfrey (2004). *Marfan syndrome: a primer for clinicians and scientists*. Springer. pp. 5–. ISBN 978-0-306-48238-0. Retrieved 12 April 2010.

5.5 TRAUMATIC GLAUCOMA

Glaucoma in mechanical injuries
- Mechanism of traumatic glaucoma
- Profile and management

Glaucoma in non-mechanical injuries
- Glaucoma in chemical injuries
- Glaucoma in electrical injuries
- Glaucoma in radiational injuries

GLAUCOMA IN MECHANICAL INJURIES

After blunt trauma to the globe, we can divide pressure fluctuation into *EARLY* (few days to few weeks) and *LATE* (few weeks and later). Infact in many cases, intraocular pressure (IOP) may be reduced immediately following trauma because of two reasons: Firstly due to to trauma to the ciliary body the amount of aqueous secretion is reduced and secondly due to a total tear of the trabecular meshwork into Schlemm's canal the aqueous outflow is greatly exaggerated or due to a cyclodialysis developing the aqueous has been drained out via uveoscleral outflow.

Alternatively, in the short-term, the pressure may rise up for several weeks. This is due to increased resistance to the outflow of aqueous due to trabeculitis (swelling of the meshwork), due to circulating cytokines and prostaglandins.

MECHANISMS OF TRAUMATIC GLAUCOMA

Mechanisms producing traumatic glaucoma are as below:

I. *Open angle traumatic glaucoma*

1. *Acute open angle glaucomas* following trauma can occur due to:
   - Hyphema,
     - Red blood cell glaucoma, or
     - Haemorrhage glaucoma
   - Inflammatory glaucoma
   - Lens particle glaucoma
2. *Chronic open angle glaucoma* following trauma include:
   - Ghost cell glaucoma
   - Angle recession glaucoma.

II. *Angle closure traumatic glaucoma*

1. *Acute angle closure traumatic glaucoma* may occur due to:
   - Peripheral anterior synechiae,
   - Lens subluxation,
   - Lens intumescence, and
   - Uveal effusion.
2. *Chronic angle closure glaucoma* may occur due to:
   - Peripheral anterior synechiae,
   - Posterior synechiae,
   - Epithelial ingrowth , and
   - Fibrovascular downgrowth.

Note. All mechanism that can elevate IOP after closed globe trauma (blunt trauma) can also lead to increased IOP in eyes with open globe trauma (rupture or penetrating or perforating injuries). The mechanism of raised IOP pertinent to open globe trauma includes fibrous ingrowth, epithelial downgrowth and intraocular foreign bodies (IOFB).

PROFILE AND MANAGEMENT

Traumatic glaucomas can occur as following clinical types:

Early onset traumatic glaucoma

Early onset traumatic glaucoma with hyphema
- Red blood cell glaucoma
- Haemolytic glaucoma

Early onset traumatic glaucoma without hyphema
- Inflammatory glaucoma
- Lens particle glaucoma

Late onset traumatic glaucoma
- Angle recession glaucoma.
- Ghost cell glaucoma
- Haemosiderotic glaucoma
- Glaucoma with fibrous ingrowth
- Glaucoma with epithelial ingrowth

EARLY ONSET TRAUMATIC GLAUCOMA WITH HYPHEMA

RED BLOOD CELL GLAUCOMA

Mechanism of glaucoma

Obstruction of trabecular meshwork in hyphema results in secondary open angle glaucoma. Although fresh red cells are known to pass through the conventional aqueous outflow system with relative ease, it appears to be overwhelming number of cells, combined with plasma, fibrin and debris, that may lead to a transient obstruction of aqueous outflow. This is why glaucoma associated with fresh blood in the anterior chamber has also been referred to as 'red cell glaucoma' by some workers. Glaucoma is more frequent with total hyphema.

Pupil block glaucoma may also occur, though rarely in hyphema. Formation of clot (eight ball hyphema) may be associated with pupil block.

Other factors may also contribute to glaucoma in hyphema. Release of melanin into the anterior chamber with trauma may prolong the course of hyphema and affect the rate of rebleeding. Other factors associated with traumatic glaucoma may also contribute to the glaucoma associated with traumatic hyphema.

Clinical features

IOP is also reported to be raised in about 50% cases with total hyphema, in 25% cases with hyphema filling more than half of AC and in about 13% of cases with hyphema filling less than half of the AC. Although IOP may be raised after the initial bleed, but is more common in cases of recurrent haemorrhages. Acutely elevated IOP may pose as a threat for vision as a result of corneal staining or optic nerve damage.

Blood staining of the cornea may develop, if raised IOP associated with hyphema is not lowered within a few days. Cornea becomes reddish brown (Fig. 5.5.1) or greenish in colour and in later stages simulates dislocation of the clear lens in the anterior chamber. Once corneal staining occurs, it clears very slowly from the periphery towards the centre, and the whole process may take even more than 2 years.

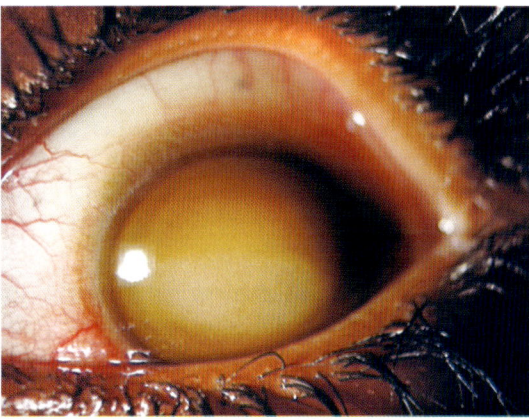

Fig. 5.5.1 *Full chamber hyphema with corneal staining*

Optic nerve damage may occur with acute rise of IOP associated with hyphema. Optic atrophy at only slightly elevated IOP has been reported in patients with hyphema associated with sickle cell haemoglobinopathies. Suboptimal blood flow to the optic nerve on the basis of sickling has been proposed as a mechanism for this sensitivity.

Management

1. *Conservative management of hyphema and medical control of IOP* include:
   • *Rest* and limiting patients ambulation
   • *Topical steroids and cycloplegics* to control inflammation
   • *Aqueous suppressants,* topical and systemic to control IOP.

2. *Measures to accelerate hyphema clearance*
   • *Hyperosmotic agents*, e.g. i.v. mannitol may accelerate resorption of clotted hyphema.
   • *Tissue plasminogen activator* (clot specific fibrinolytic agent), when given intracamerally has been reported to accelerate the clearance of experimental hyphema in rabbits, although it may increase the risk of rebleed.

3. *Prevention of rebleeding*
   • *Antifibrinolytic agents* (tranexamic acid and aminocaproic acid) have been reported to decrease the incidence of rebleed by delaying the natural lysis of the clot.
   • *Lowering of systemic blood pressure and elevation of head end of bed* are also reported to decrease rebleed and accelerate clearance of hyphema.

- *Avoidance* of aspirin and NSAIDs for the first week after hyphema or till hyphema clears is useful.

4. **Surgical removal of hyphema.** When conservative measures fail to prevent vision loss from damage to optic nerve and corneal staining, surgical measures are required to remove hyphema and control the IOP.

Proposed guideline for surgical removal of hyphema is that an IOP threatening the optic nerve, like 60 mm Hg for 2 days or 50 mm Hg for 5 days or 35 mm Hg for 7 days, requires intervention.

Timing for surgical intervention. It is advisable (if possible), to delay the evacuation of hyphema until the 4th day, because at this time, the clot is somewhat retracted and less adherent to the surrounding structures.

Surgical techniques used in the literature include: Anterior chamber washout, clot expression, delivery of the clot with a cryoprobe, automated hyphaemectomy and ultrasonic emulsification and aspiration.

- *Paracentesis and manual irrigation-aspiration* using two-way Simcoe's cannula is a simple and safe procedure.
- *Viscodissection of the clot* from the iris and expression of the anterior chamber may be used for a clot.
- *Removal of the clot with vitrectomy instruments* is also considered a safe and effective procedure.

5. **Adjunctive surgical procedure along with hyphema removal** has included:

- *Peripheral iridotomy* in the setting of pupillary block resulting from the clot.
- *Trabeculectomy* has also been used for control of IOP.
- *Cyclodiathermy* to control recurrent bleeding has also been described.

HAEMOLYTIC GLAUCOMA

Haemolytic glaucoma, described first of all by Fenton and Zimmerman (1963), is a type of glaucoma associated with intraocular haemorrhage.

Pathogenesis

It is an acute secondary open angle glaucoma due to the obstruct ion (clogging) of the trabecular meshwork caused by macrophages laden with lysed RBC debris.

Pathology

Microscopic study of the enucleated eyes with haemolytic glaucoma revealed the trabecular meshwork to be occluded by RBCs, debris and macrophages laden with blood pigments. The endothelial cells of trabecular meshwork were degenerated and had phagocytosed the blood.

Clinical features

- *IOP* is acutely raised causing pain, nausea and even vomiting.
- *Cornea* may show oedema.
- *Anterior chamber* is normal in depth and on slit-lamp examination shows numerous reddish cells in the aqueous humour.
- *Angle of anterior chamber* on gonioscopy is open, with reddish-brown pigment covering the trabecular meshwork.

Diagnosis

Clinical diagnosis is made from the history suggestive of intraocular haemorrhage associated with the above signs.

Confirmation of diagnosis is made by anterior chamber paracentesis, which reveals pigment-containing macrophages laden with rather than khaki-coloured ghost cells.

Management

1. **Medical therapy** is the form of topical and systemic aqueous suppressants, may be needed for sometime to control IOP, otherwise, the condition is self-limiting and does not need prolonged therapy.

2. **Surgical therapy** is rarely needed:
i. *Anterior chamber* washout may be required in occasional cases, where IOP is not controlled by medical therapy
ii. *Filtration surgery* may be considered in non-responsive cases.
iii. *Cyclodestructive procedures* may be required in painful blind eyes.

EARLY ONSET TRAUMATIC GLAUCOMA WITHOUT HYPHEMA

INFLAMMATORY GLAUCOMA

Caused by acute uveal and trabecular inflammation induced by trauma due to circulating cytokine and prostaglandins.

Characterized by acute rise in IOP associated with presence of inflammatory cells in the anterior chamber, which transiently obscure the intertrabecular spaces.

Treatment includes a short course of topical steroids, timolol maleate and oral acetazolamide.

LENS PARTICLE GLAUCOMA

Pathogenesis. It is a type of secondary open angle glaucoma, in which trabecular meshwork is blocked by the lens particles floating in the aqueous humour. It occurs due to lens particles or following traumatic rupture of the lens. However, the associated inflammation, whether in response to the trauma or retained lens material, may also contribute to glaucoma in this condition.

Clinical features. Symptoms of acute rise in IOP associated with lens particles in the anterior chamber (Fig. 5.5.2).

Management includes:
• *Medical therapy* to lower IOP.
• *Irrigation-aspiration* of the lens particles from the anterior chamber may be required.
• *Cycloplegics and topical steroids* to control inflammation.

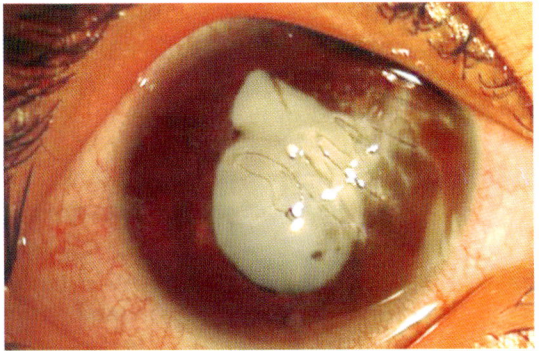

Fig. 5.5.2 *Lens particle glaucoma secondary to post-traumatic rupture of anterior lens capsule*

PHACOANTIGENIC GLAUCOMA

Pathogenesis. As in the case of lens particle glaucoma, there is usually a preceding disruption of lens capsule by injury, leading to release of lens proteins. Distinguishing feature is a latent period during which sensitization to the lens proteins occurs. IOP is then raised due to inflammatory reaction of the uveal tissue excited by the lens matter. Basically, it is also a type of secondary open angle glaucoma where trabecular meshwork is clogged by both inflammatory cells and the lens particles.

Clinical features. Phacoantigenic glaucoma (previously known as phacoanaphylaxis) is a rare entity. In this condition, there occurs:
• *Fulminating acute/inflammatory* reaction due to antigen (lens protein)–antibody reaction.
• Typical finding is a granulomatous inflammation in the involved eye after it gets trauma.
• *KPs* are present on the corneal endothelium and the anterior lens surface. In addition, a low grade vitritis, synechial formation and residual lens material in the anterior chamber may be found.

Management consists of:
• *Medical therapy* to lower IOP.
• *Treatment of iridocyclitis* with steroids and cycloplegics.
• *Irrigation-aspiration* of the lens matter from anterior chamber (if required) should always be done after proper control of inflammation.

PHACOMORPHIC GLAUCOMA

Phacomorphic glaucoma is an acute secondary angle-closure glaucoma caused by intumescent lens, i.e. swollen cataractous lens due to rapid maturation of cataract following traumatic rupture of capsule.

Pathogenesis. The swollen lens pushes the iris forward and oblitrates the angle resulting in secondary acute angle closure glaucoma. Further, the increased iridolenticular contact also causes potential pupillary block and iris bombe formation.

Clinical presentation. Phacomorphic glaucoma presents as an acute congestive glaucoma with features almost similar to acute primary angle-

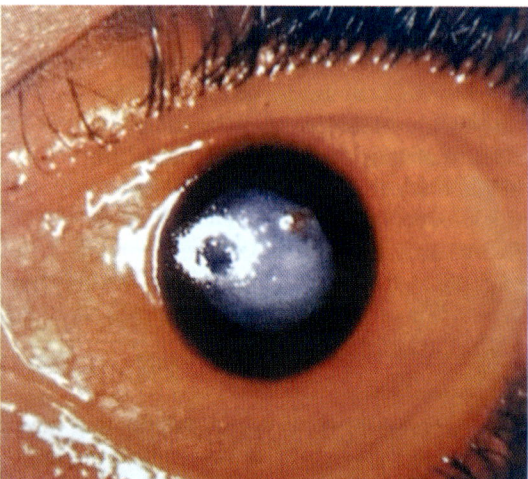

Fig. 5.5.3 *Phacomorphic glaucoma due to intumiscent cataractous lens triggered by trauma*

closure except that the lens is always cataractous and swollen (Fig. 5.5.3).

Treatment should be immediate and consists of:

- *Medical treatment* to control IOP by i.v. mannitol, systemic acetazolamide and topical beta blockers and steroids.
- Laser iridotomy may be effective in breaking the angle closure attack.
- Cataract extraction with implantation of PCIOL (which is the main treatment of phacomorphic glaucoma) should be performed once the eye becomes quiet.

GLAUCOMA DUE TO SUBLUXATED LENS

Subluxation (partial zonular dehiscence) of the lens may cause lens-induced angle closure glaucoma (Fig. 5.5.4).

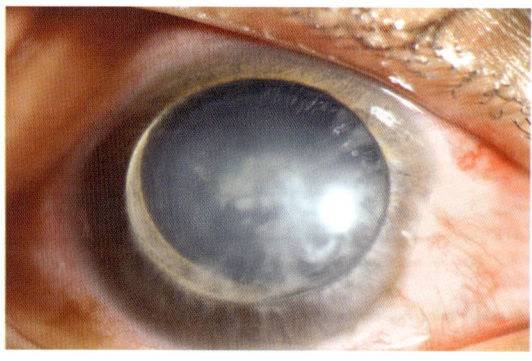

Fig. 5.5.4 *Subluxated cataractous lens causing glaucoma*

Mechanism of glaucoma

- *Pupil block* may be caused by a lens dislocated into the pupil or anterior chamber or subluxated or tilted forward against the iris without entering the anterior chamber. Pupillary block may also be caused by the vitreous herniation.
- *Peripheral anterior* synechiae may develop from a long-standing pupillary block and produce chronic IOP elevation.

Management

- *Antiglaucoma medical treatment* with hyperosmotic agents, carbonic anhydrase inhibitors and β-blockers may be helpful in breaking the attack.
- *Cycloplegics* may relieve the attack by dilating the pupil, when the lens has subluxated into the pupil.
- *Laser PI* helps by providing bypass to aqueous in the presence of pupillary block.
- *Surgical removal* of the lens may be required when the lens is in anterior chamber or lens extraction is needed to relieve the glaucoma or improve vision. Patient must be informed about the surgical risks with guarded prognosis.

LATE ONSET TRAUMATIC GLAUCOMAS

TRAUMATIC ANGLE RECESSION GLAUCOMA

Angle recession glaucoma is also known as posttraumatic angle recession glaucoma or contusion angle recession glaucoma or contusion angle deformity.

Angle recession refers to rupture in the ciliary body face between scleral spur and iris root (Fig. 5.5.5).

Treacher Collins described the micropathology of angle recession glaucoma as a "split into the ciliary muscles in its entire circumference so that angle of the chamber was prolonged out". In 1945, D'Ombrain postulated that angle recession led to increased intraocular tension.

Angle recession may be associated with dislocation or subluxation of the lens, traumatic cataract, iridodialysis, cyclodialysis, hyphema and retinal detachment, extraocular muscle avulsion, orbital trauma and globe rupture in extreme cases. Unilateral open angle glaucoma usually occurs after years (may be 10 years) of blunt trauma. Angle recession is not the cause of glaucoma but just indicator of old trauma. Glaucoma occurs due to slowly induced fibrosis of trabecular meshwork.

Lifetime risk of developing glaucoma in patients with angle recession is as below:

• Angle recession <180%: 4%
• Angle recession >180%: 22%
• Fellow eye has a 50% greater risk of developing glaucoma.

Clinical profile

Incidence. Incidence is reported inconsistently. The presence of angle recession does not necessarily mean the onset of raised IOP and nerve head pathology. Studies have indicated that 6–20% of all individuals with angle recession went on to develop late onset glaucoma. A 3:1 to 4:1 male preponderance was noted by some studies.

Slit-lamp findings. Anterior chamber of the injured eye appears deeper than the other eye. Other features of blunt trauma, such as phaco-donesis, iridodialysis and hyphema, might be seen.

Gonioscopic findings. Gonioscopically, angle recession is characterized by widening of the ciliary body and prominence of the ciliary spur. Sometimes trabecular meshwork tears are seen along with iridodialysis and cyclodialysis.

After the injury scar tissue may fill the angle recession cleft confounding the diagnosis at later follow-ups. So, as soon as blunt trauma is noted and the cornea is clear enough and the patient cooperative enough, a gonioscopy should be carried out.

Angle recession may be:

• *Shallow.* Characterized by increased visibility of the ciliary body and the scleral spur.
• *Moderate.* Tear extends between the longitu-dinal and circular fibres of the ciliary bodies.
• *Deep. Gonioscopically,* angle recession is chara-cterized by an irregular widening of the ciliary body band (Fig. 5.5.5).

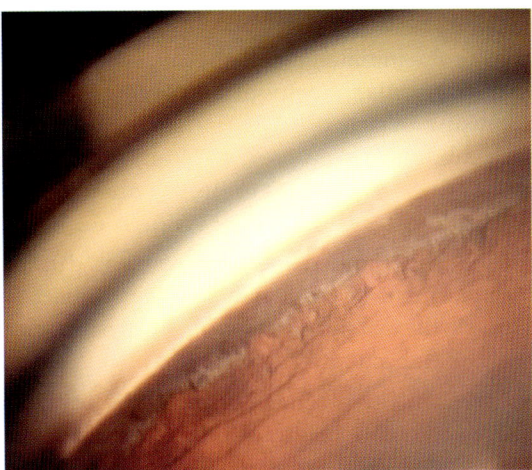

Fig. 5.5.5 *Traumatic angle recession (gonioscopic view)*

Ultrasound biomicroscopy produces high-resolution images of the anterior segment, providing cross-sectional views of the angle in vivo similar to those of a histologic section (Fig. 5.5.6). This non-invasive procedure is readily performed in a clinical setting in an intact globe. High-resolution images of angle recession, iridodialysis and cyclodialysis have been described.

Anterior segment OCT is another way to diag-nose, which can study the angle.

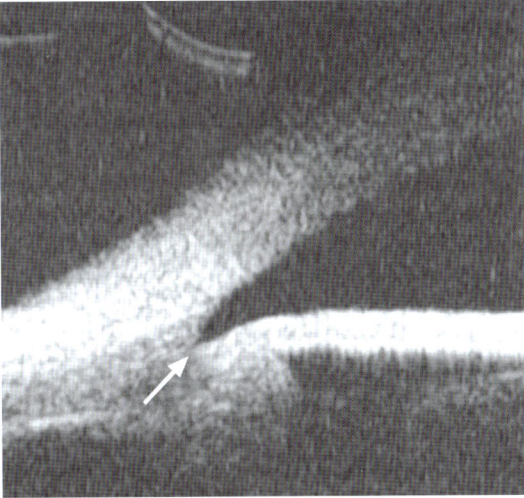

Fig. 5.5.6 *Ultrasound biomicroscopy (UMB) depicting angle recession*

Pathology

- After the initial injury to the ciliary body and or trabecular meshwork, scarring occurs, causing obstruction. Also a Descemet's like membrane is seen growing from the cornea over the angle similar to the membrane seen in iridocorneal endothelial syndrome.

- Chandler claimed that glaucoma is due to impairment of the action of ciliary muscles, due to the tear in its body, which open the pore of the trabecular meshwork.

- Cases with involvement of lesser area of angle showed no rise of intraocular pressure during the follow-up period. This agrees with the findings of Alter who observed glaucoma to be associated more commonly in cases having 240° or more of angle involvement. It is usually agreed that more than 180° of angle involvement is required for pressure elevation in most cases.

- It is interesting to note that the other eye in unilateral angle recession glaucoma is more likely to have elevated IOP as well as be steroid responders.

- It is safe to conclude that eyes with a tendency to develop higher IOP have a greater tendency to develop glaucoma after blunt trauma.

Management

Medical treatment. In angle recession glaucoma, beta blockers—like timolol, alpha agonists—like brimonidine, prostaglandin analogues—like latanoprost and carbonic anhydrase inhibitors—like dorzolamide, all can help lower intraocular pressure.

However, pilocarpine and other miotic are contraindicated as they decrease uveoscleral outflow. The meshwork in scarred uveoscleral outflow is the predominant pathway for aqueous egress.

Surgical treatment is as below:

- *Filtering surgery* is less effective in angle recession glaucoma eyes than in eyes with chronic simple glaucoma. Mitomycin-C application increases the success rate in some studies to beyond 50% for 5 years.

- *Valve implants,* such as the Molteno and Ahmed, have proved to be successful with certain studies showing 57% survival rate at 5 years.

- *Other modalities,* like trabeculoplasty, non-penetrating surgeries or trabeculopuncture, are found ineffective.

Continual follow-up with effective medical and surgical management is the key to long-term glaucoma management in these cases.

GHOST CELL GLAUCOMA

Ghost cell glaucoma, initially described by Campbell et al (1976), is a type of secondary open angle glaucoma in which the trabecular meshwork is blocked by ghost cells (described below) and is associated with vitreous haemorrhage.

Mechanism of glaucoma

One to three weeks after traumatic vitreous haemorrhage, the RBCs degenerate, loose their pliability and become *khaki-coloured* cells called the *ghost cells.* Histopathologically, ghost cells have thin walls and appear hollow except for clumps of denatured haemoglobin called 'Heinz bodies' (Fig. 5.5.7). Once developed, the ghost cells remain in the vitreous cavity for months. Whenever there occurs disruption of the anterior hyaloid face (situations as mentioned below), the ghost cells pass from the vitreous into the anterior chamber unlike fresh RBCs, the ghost cells are not able to pass through the trabecular meshwork causing its blockage, leading to rise in IOP.

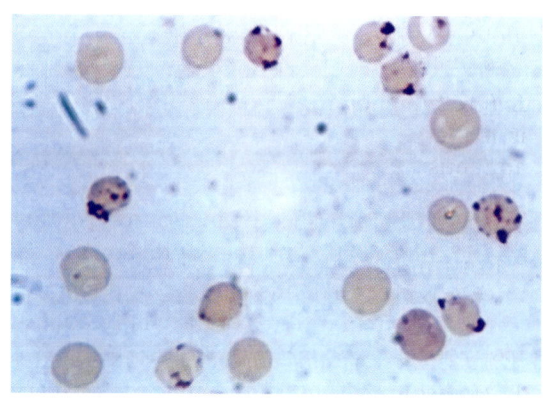

Fig. 5.5.7 *Heinz bodies in ghost cell glaucoma*

Specific situations for disruption of anterior hyaloid face include:
- Trauma with presumed disruption of anterior hyaloid face.
- Pre-existing pseudophakia or aphakia (before vitreous haemorrhage).
- Cataract surgery performed after vitreous haemorrhage.
- Vitrectomy operation.

Clinical features

1. *IOP,* depending upon the number of ghost cells in the anterior chamber, may vary from normal to marked elevation associated with pain and corneal oedema.

2. *Cornea* may show oedema and/or characteristic khaki-coloured cells on the endothelium.

3. *Anterior chamber,* on slit-lamp examination, may reveal:
- *Ghost cells* in the aqueous humour
- *Pseudohypopyon* may occur due to settling down of ghost cells when present in abundance. Pseudohypopyon may occasionally be associated with a layer of fresh RBCs (known as *'Candy-stripe sign'*)

4. *Angle of anterior chamber,* on gonioscopy, is open and may appear normal or may show a layer of deposited khaki-coloured cells.

Differential diagnosis

Differential diagnosis needs to be made from phacolytic glaucoma, haemosiderotic glaucoma, and inflammatory glaucoma.

Clinically, diagnosis of ghost cell glaucoma is made from the typical history and signs on examination as described above.

Laboratory confirmation of ghost cell glaucoma is made on examination of ghost cells in the aqueous aspirate. This examination may be performed with:
- Phase contrast microscopy, or
- Routine light microscopy of a paraffin embedded specimen stained with H and E.

Management

1. *Medical therapy,* similar to POAG, may be effective in more than half of the cases.

2. *Surgical therapy* may be required when medical therapy fails:
i. *Anterior chamber wash,* using two-way irrigation-aspiration cannula, is the surgery of choice and is most effective. It may be repeated when required.
ii. *Pars plana vitrectomy* may be required in unresponsive patients to ensure complete removal of blood components trapped in the vitreous body.
iii. *Trabeculectomy* is sparingly required.

HAEMOSIDEROTIC GLAUCOMA

Haemosiderotic glaucoma is a rare secondary open angle glaucoma associated with *intraocular haemorrhage.*

Pathogenesis. It is a rare variety of secondary glaucoma occurring due to sclerotic changes in trabecular meshwork caused by the iron from the phagocytosed haemoglobin by the endothelial cells of trabeculum. Thus, we can say that haemosiderosis is similar to siderosis bulbi, except that the source of iron in haemosiderosis is degenerating RBCs rather than a retained intraocular foreign body.

Clinical features of this rare secondary open angle glaucoma are similar to POAG, except that it is associated with a history of intraocular haemorrhage.

Management includes:
1. *Medical therapy* with aqueous suppressants to control the IOP.
2. *Trabeculectomy* may be required in non-responsive cases.

HAEMOLYTIC GLAUCOMA

It is an acute secondary open angle glaucoma due to the obstruct ion (clogging) of the trabecular meshwork caused by macrophages laden with lysed RBC debris.

GLAUCOMA ASSOCIATED WITH EPITHELIAL INGROWTH AND FIBROUS DOWNGROWTH

Epithelial downgrowth or fibrous ingrowth or both together may occur following any anterior segment incisional surgery (e.g. cataract surgery, glaucoma surgery, penetrating keratoplasty, etc.) or penetrating trauma. Of course, their incidence has decreased markedly in recent years owing to improved microincisional surgery and suturing techniques.

Epithelial ingrowth

Pathogenesis

Conjunctival and corneal epithelial cells may ingrow into the anterior chamber following either surgical or traumatic wound under the following conditions:

- *Penetration of epithelium* into the anterior chamber usually occurs through a fistula which may be associated with incarceration of iris, lens material or vitreous strands in the wound *implantation of epithelial cells* into the anterior chamber from surgical instruments or sutures.

Clinical features

Epithelial ingrowth into the anterior chamber may proliferate in three forms: pearl tumour, epithelial cyst and epithelial downgrowth:

- *Pearl tumours* usually occur after penetrating trauma associated with implantation of a cilium along with epithelial elements. The epithelial walls of the pearl tumour are keratinized and so give a pearly appearance. The pearl tumours may remain stationary for a long time or may enlarge till the anterior chamber and cause secondary angle closure glaucoma.

- *Epithelial cysts,* also known as epithelial inclusion cysts, are formed when the surface epithelial cells are implanted in the anterior chamber following surgical or accidental trauma. It is believed that iris tissue provides nutritional support for the epithelial cells to grow as a cyst in months or even years. These cysts appear as translucent, non-vascular anterior chamber cysts. The cyst wall shows varying degrees of pigmentation. The cysts may remain stationary or may enlarge to fill the pupil and anterior chamber.

- *Epithelial ingrowth* (Fig. 5.5.8) presents as greyish sheet with rolled edges, growing from the wound margin along the posterior surface of the cornea, trabecular meshwork, iris surface and ciliary body. This sheet is formed when the surface epithelium gets opportunity

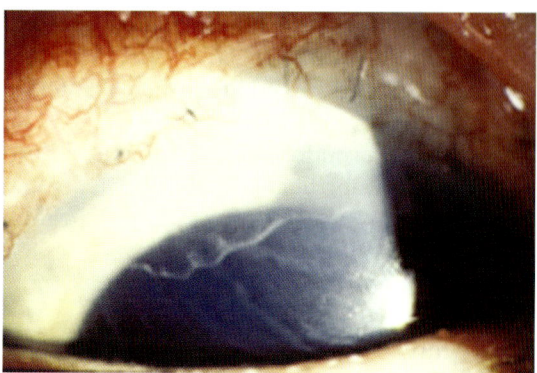

Fig. 5.5.8 *Post-traumatic epithelial ingrowth causing raised intraocular pressure*

to grow into the anterior chamber through the wound which is not properly closed, e.g. when iris tissue or vitreous strands are incarcerated. It is usually associated with persistent inflammation that does not respond to steroid therapy. It was common occurrence after cataract surgery when the wound size used to be large and non-valvular closed with 3 to 7 sutures. The suspected epithelialization can be confirmed by applying a shot of argon laser photocoagulation to the iris which turns white.

Specular microscopy and confocal microscopy allow direct visualization of epithelial cells.

Mechanism of glaucoma. Epithelial downgrowth may cause glaucoma by following mechanisms:

- *Secondary open angle glaucoma*, due to epithelial membrane covering the trabecular meshwork.
- *Secondary angle closure glaucoma,* following contraction of the membrane with PAS formation.
- *Pupillary block glaucoma* may occur when the epithelial membrane advances across the pupil to the anterior vitreous face.

Management

Treatment of epithelial downgrowth is often frustrating. An early diagnosis is essential to avoid later enucleation. It is advisable to determine the extent of epithelialization by applying argon laser shots before taking up any of the following surgical measures to treat the epithelial downgrowth:

- *Surgical excision* of the membrane through a limbal incision along with fistulectomy (when present).
- *Cryotherapy* of the involved posterior corneal surface using a double freeze-thaw technique.
- *Swabing with absolute alcohol* of the involved corneal surface.
- *Scrapping the membrane* off the corneal surface.
- *Pars plana vitrectomy approach* to remove the iris membrane off the ciliary body combined with unipolar diathermy and end photo-coagulation. Alternatively, after removal of membrane and involved iris, intraocular air may be inserted and cryotherapy applied in the transcorneal and transcleral fashion.

Postoperative treatment to control inflammation and IOP should include topical:
- *Steroid* eyedrops,
- *Cycloplegic* eyedrops, and
- *Aqueous* supplements.

Treatment of pearl tumours and epithelial cysts
- *Pearl tumours* rarely need treatment, as they remain stationary for a long period.
- *En bloc surgical excision of* an anterior chamber cyst and involved iris is indicated when enlargement threatens other intraocular structures. Post-traumatic epithelial cysts usually require surgical excision for progressive enlargement.

Surgical treatment of glaucoma is often required and is mostly difficult:
- *Filtration surgery* with intraoperative use of mitomycin C or postoperative 5-fluorouracil may be tried.
- *Glaucoma drainage device* may be the treatment of choice in many cases with glaucoma secondary to epithelial downgrowth.
- *Enucleation* was required in the past, in many eyes with painful blind eye due to intractable glaucoma associated with epithelial downgrowth. However, with improved diagnosis and early treatment, the need for enucleation is decreasing.

Fibrous downgrowth

Fibrous downgrowth, also known as stromal ingrowth or stromal outgrowth, occurs under similar circumstances as epithelial downgrowth and may occur alone or in association with epithelial downgrowth. Unlike epithelial downgrowth, the fibrous ingrowth is slow to progress and may be self-limited. Because of this relatively indolent nature of fibrous ingrowth, vis-à-vis epithelial downgrowth, comparatively a smaller number of eyes require enucleation.

Pathogenesis

Two forms of this condition have been described: fibrous ingrowth and retrocorneal membrane.

1. *Pathogenesis of fibrous ingrowth.* Like epithelial downgrowth, the fibrous ingrowth also occurs when there is inadequate wound closure after intraocular surgery or penetrating trauma. It follows a break in the corneal endothelium and Descemet's membrane, which allows fibroblasts to enter the anterior chamber from subepithelial connective tissue or from corneal or limbal stroma. The ingrowth of connective tissue is inhibited when the inner wound margins are bridged by the endothelium by the second postoperative break. Thus, one can say that damged corneal endothelium is also a risk factor for stromal ingrowth even after well-opposed wound.

2. *Pathogenesis of retrocorneal membrane.* Inflammatory and traumatic insults to the cornea are reported to result in the formation of retrocorneal membrane. Descemet's membrane is typically intact and the metaplastic corneal endothelium and blood mononuclear cells are believed to contribute the fibrous tissue.

Clinical features

Fibrous ingrowth presents as a thick greyish white, translucent vascular, retrocorneal membrane. The edges of this membrane have tongue-like projections rather than scalloped edges of epithelial membrane. Overall the appearance of fibrous membrane resembles a woven cloth.

Glaucoma. Initially, secondary open angle glaucoma develops from associated inflammation and haemorrhage. But the frequent complication is secondary angle closure glaucoma which occurs when the fibrous ingrowth involves the angle and, on contraction leads to formation of PAS and the destruction of trabecular meshwork.

Posterior segment involvement may occur due to tractional forces produced by the fibrous membrane and induce retinal tears or detachments and cystoid macular oedema.

Management

Fibrous ingrowth has no specific treatment per se. Therefore, attention needs to be given to the complicating sequelae without efforts to eradicate the membrane.

Glaucoma should be managed medically or surgically as necessary.

Release of vitreous traction by vitrectomy or Nd:YAG laser lysis may be required to prevent further posterior segment complications.

Penetrating keratoplasty may be required for visual rehabilitation.

GLAUCOMA IN NON-MECHANICAL INJURIES

GLAUCOMA IN CHEMICAL INJURIES

Glaucoma is more common after alkali burns but also seen after severe acid burns.

Mechanism of glaucoma

1. *Early rise of IOP* is caused by:
   - Shrinkage of collagen tissue cornea and sclera, and
   - Increase in uveal blood flow.
2. *Intermediate rise of IOP* is caused by intraocular inflammatory changes. Hypopyon may also develop and contribute to rise of IOP.
3. *Late rise of IOP* is caused by intraocular damage and formation of PAS or other intraocular scarring. Delayed pressure rise in also caused by prostaglandin release.

Management

I. Medical therapy

1. *Antiglaucoma agents,* especially topical and systemic aqueous suppressants, are quite useful. Miotics and prostaglandin should usually be avoided.

2. *Antiprostaglandins.* The presence of prostaglandins during the delayed pressure rise suggests that the early use of drugs, such as indomethacin and imidazoles, which inhibit prostaglandin synthesis, may be beneficial.

II. Surgical therapy

1. *Filtration surgery* may be required, but may be differential due to scarring of conjunctiva and episcleral tissue.
2. *Glaucoma drainage device procedure,* such as Ahmed or Molteno valve, should be considered when external scarring is present.
3. *Cyclodestructive procedures* may be considered as a last resort.

GLAUCOMA IN ELECTRICAL INJURIES

Transient rise of IOP is reported after electrical injury, cardioversion, and electroshock therapy.

Mechanisms of glaucoma in electric shock includes;
- *Venous dilatation*
- *Contraction of the extraocular muscle*, and
- *Pigment dispersion*

Treatment. Usually no treatment is required as the rise in IOP is transient. If required, topical and systemic aqueous suppressants may be given. Miotics and prostaglandin are usually avoided.

GLAUCOMA IN RADIATIONAL INJURIES

Rise in IOP has been reported after radiation injury to the eyeball following radiation therapy to the structures near the eye.

Mechanism of rise in IOP following radiation injury to the eyeball includes:
- *Neovascularization of the angle*
- *Structural damage to trabecular meshwork* causing secondary open angle glaucoma associated with diffuse conjunctival telangiectasia.
- *Ghost cell glaucoma* following radiation retinopathy and intraocular haemorrhage.

Management includes:
- *Medical therapy* with topical and systemic aqueous suppressants may be useful.
- *Surgical therapy needed* includes:
  - *Filtration surgery*, chances of success are less.
  - *Cyclodestructive procedures* are often required to control IOP.

BIBLIOGRAPHY

1. Bai HQ, Yao L, Wang DB, Jin R, Wang YX. Causes and treatments of traumatic secondary glaucoma. Eur J Ophthalmol. 2009;19(2):201–206.

2. Campbell D, Shields MB, Liebmann JM. Ghost cell glaucoma. In: Ritch R, Shields B, Krupin T, eds. The Glaucomas. Vol 2. 1989:1239–1247.

3. Campbell DG, Simmons RJ, Grant WM: Ghost cells as a cause of glaucoma. Am J Ophthalmol 1976:81–441.

4. Ellant JP, Obstbaum SA. Lens-induced glaucoma. Doc Ophthalmol. 1992;81(3):317–338.

5. Gadia R, Sihota R, Dada T, Gupta V. Current profile of secondary glaucomas. Indian J Ophthalmol. Jul-Aug 2008;56(4):285–289.

6. Manners T, Salmon JF, Barron A, Willies C, Murray AD. Trabeculectomy with mitomycin C in the treatment of post-traumatic angle recession glaucoma. Br J Ophthalmol. 2001;85(2):159–63.

7. Moisseiev E, Kinori M, Glovinsky Y, Loewenstein A, Moisseiev J, Barak A. Retained lens fragments: nucleus fragments are associated with worse prognosis than cortex or epinucleus fragments. Eur J Ophthalmol. Nov-Dec 2011;21(6):741–747.

8. Rosenbaum JT, Samples JR, Seymour B, Langlois L, David L. Chemotactic activity of lens proteins and the pathogenesis of phacolytic glaucoma. Arch Ophthalmol. Nov 1987;105(11):1582–1584.

9. Schaal S, Barr CC. Management of retained lens fragments after cataract surgery with and without pars plana vitrectomy. J Cataract Refract Surg. May 2009;35(5):863–867.

10. Shields MB. Glaucomas associated with intra-ocular hemorrhage and glaucomas associated with ocular trauma. In: Textbook of Glaucoma. 1992:381–399.

11. Shingleton BJ, Hersh PS. Traumatic hyphema. In: Eye Trauma. 1991:104–116.

12. Walton W, Von Hagen S, Grigorian R, Zarbin M. Management of traumatic hyphema. Surv Ophthalmol. 2002;47(4):297–334.

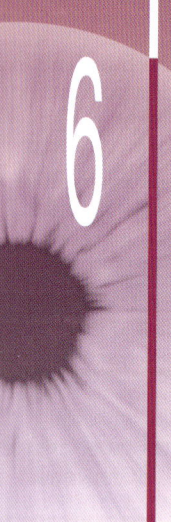

POSTERIOR SEGMENT TRAUMA

6

6.1 TRAUMATIC LESIONS OF RETINA AND VITREOUS

INTRODUCTION AND PATHOPHYSIOLOGY

INTRODUCTION

Both blunt as well as penetrating traumas can lead to retinal tears, detachment and vitreous haemorrhage. As per one estimate in US, the rate of retinal involvement in various eye injuries is 30% and that of vitreoretinal involvement is about 40%. Traumatic retinal detachments are also not uncommon; these constitute about 10–12% of all rhegmatogenous detachments which are mostly observed in males that too in the relatively younger age group. Traumatic retinal tears are precursors of RD which are usually observed near the vitreous base in countrecoup injury and at the site of impact in coup (direct) injury. It is, therefore, all the more important to diagnose and treat these breaks by periodic indirect ophthalmoscopy so that subsequent RDs can be prevented.

PATHOPHYSIOLOGY

Before actually describing the tears as a result of blunt trauma, it is important to discuss the mechanism of their formation as shown in Fig. 6.1.1. Blunt trauma to the eye (e.g. cricket ball injury) comes with a velocity that compresses the eyeball, decreasing its axial length and expanding its equatorial diameter known as *compression phase*. This is followed rapidly by decompression when eyeball tends to come back to normal axial length and equatorial diameter known as *decompression phase*. However, it overshoots in the process of decompression when axial length increases and equatorial diameter decreases known as

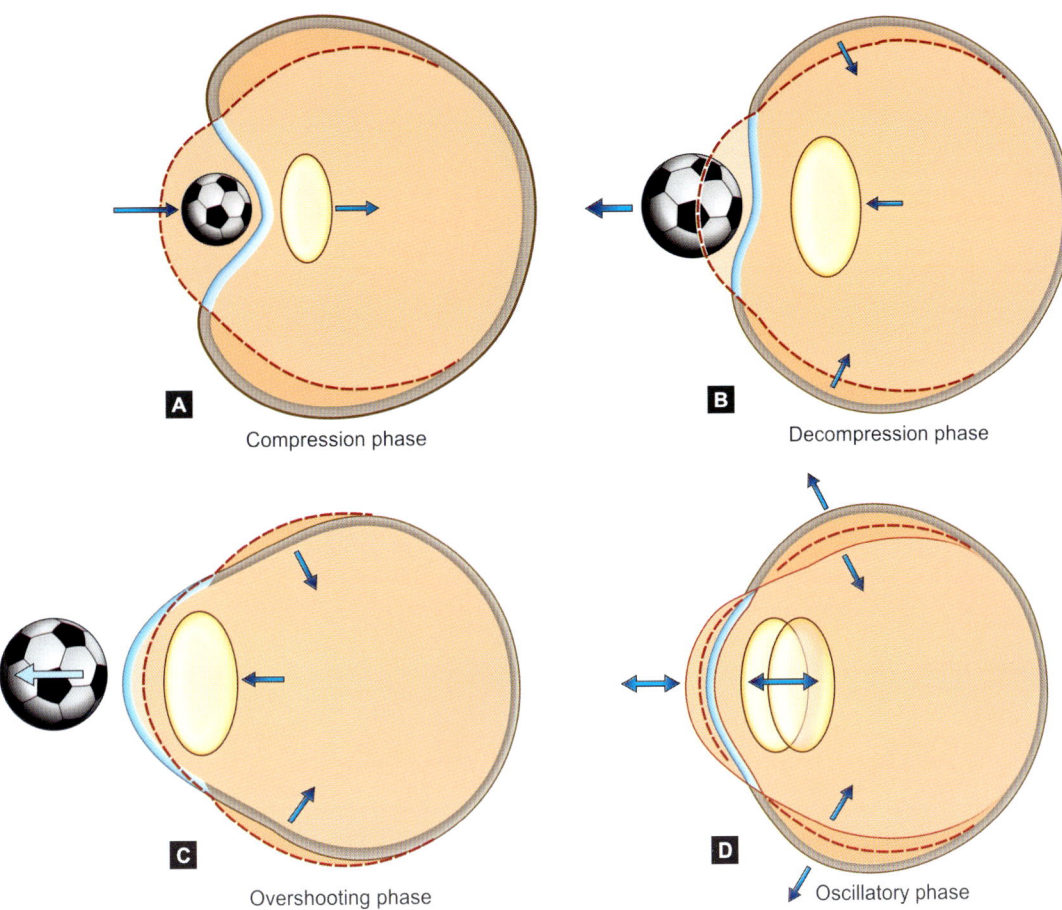

A Compression phase

B Decompression phase

C Overshooting phase

D Oscillatory phase

Fig. 6.1.1 *Various phases of deformation of the eyeball when struck by a blunt object*

overshooting phase. Finally, there is *oscillatory phase* wherein there are small cyclical increases and decreases in the axial length and equatorial diameter of the eyeball which gradually dampens until the eye becomes stationary.

From the above description, it is obvious that the sudden deformation of the global, as is seen in blunt missile striking the cornea at a high speed, induces tractional force on the vitreous base and peripheral retina leading to tears at anterior and posterior borders of vitreous base. Such tractional forces may also work at abnormal vitreoretinal adhesions as in lattice degeneration and chorioretinal scars and may result in retinal tears.

The eyeball is least protected inferotemporally and it rolls upwards due to Bell's phenomenon, a protective reflex, whenever a noxious stimulus approaches the eye. Therefore, majority of blunt objects strike the eye inferotemporally thereby producing retinal breaks at the site of direct impact (coup mechanism) and directly opposite superonasally by countrecoup mechanism. This explains why retinal dialysis and tears are quite frequent in these two quadrants.

TRAUMATIC RETINAL LESIONS

TRAUMATIC RETINAL TEARS

A variety of retinal breaks and vitreous lesions can occur in closed globe injury as a result of blunt trauma. It is important to diagnose and treat them before they progress to rhegmato-genous retinal detachment. Hence indirect ophthalmoscopy is must in each and every case of closed globe injury provided the media permits otherwise such cases should be subjected to B-scan ultrasonography. It is pertinent to mention here that the subjects of trauma are predominantly males that too of younger age group. In addition, myopic eyes are more likely to develop retinal tears as compared to emmetropic eyes after trauma.

Types of retinal tears

Irregular tears

When a blunt object strikes the eye posterior to the ora serrata, the direct coup effect on the retina may cause full-thickness retinal necrosis and fragmentation with subsequent retinal detachment. The underlying RPE is usually damaged as well. These are usually seen in inferotemporal quadrant and are irregular in configuration mostly associated with peri-retinal haemorrhage (Fig. 6.1.2).

Peripheral retinal tears

The horseshoe tears are of common occurrence. The location and configuration of these tears tend to mimic those which are seen after posterior vitreous detachment (PVD) in non-traumatic rhegmatogenous retinal detachment, implying thereby that these are secondary to vitreous traction following trauma-induced posterior vitreous detachment (Fig. 6.1.3).

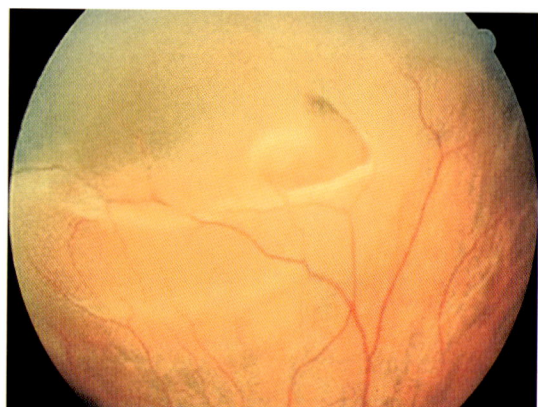

Fig. 6.1.3 *Fundus photograph showing horseshoe tear with retinal detachment following PVD*

Giant retinal tears

Giant retinal tear (GRT) is defined as peripheral break extending through 90° or more of the retinal circumference in which the vitreous gel is attached essentially to the anterior flap thereby allowing independent mobility of the posterior edge of tear. GRTs are idiopathic in 70%, traumatic in 20% and in 10% at the posterior edge of chorioretinal degeneration. GRT needs to be differentiated from dialysis. Dialysis is a disinsertion of retina from ora seratta which could be of variable extent. Vitreous is attached to the posterior margin of the dialysis and posterior vitreous detachment is absent thus preventing it from inversion. In giant retinal tears, vitreous remains strongly attached to the anterior margin of the tear; the posterior margin without any vitreous attachment is free to move and inverts towards disc due to gravity (Fig. 6.1.4).

Retinal dialysis

Retinal dialysis are most common infero-temporally followed by superonasally, the former is by direct injury and the later is because of countrecoup injury. When located supero-nasally, they are nearly always caused by trauma. All dialyses, even inferotemporal ones, are traumatic. These are most frequent traumatic retinal breaks. However, many are familial, bilateral, or found in patients with no historical evidence of injury. In these cases, there is

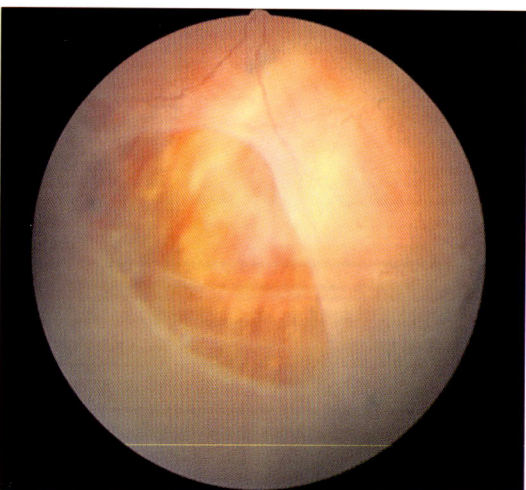

Fig. 6.1.2 *Irregular retinal breaks in the inferotemporal quadrant following blunt trauma*

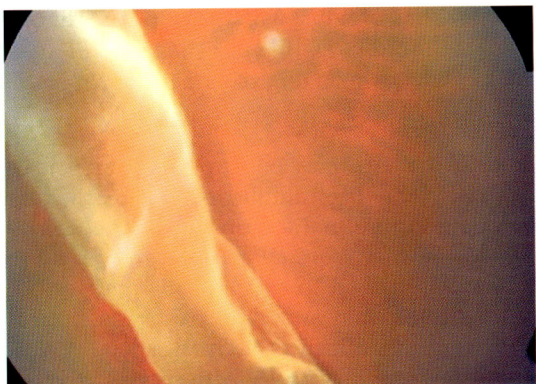

Fig. 6.1.4 *Giant retinal tear with inverted flap following blunt trauma*

probably a developmental abnormality of the inferotemporal peripheral retina and vitreous base. All retinal dialyses do not lead to RRD. Retinal dialyses progress to RRD after few weeks to few months. The slow progression is due to formed vitreous in the young and the attachment of the vitreous to the posterior edge of dialysis providing stability and making detachment less likely, this is in contrast to GRT where RD is almost instantaneous (Fig. 6.1.5).

Stretch tears

Occasionally, rapid horizontal expansion of the eye can produce a stretch tear of the retina. These curvilinear breaks are usually concentric to the optic nerve. They can cause retinal detachment, but they are mostly self-sealing.

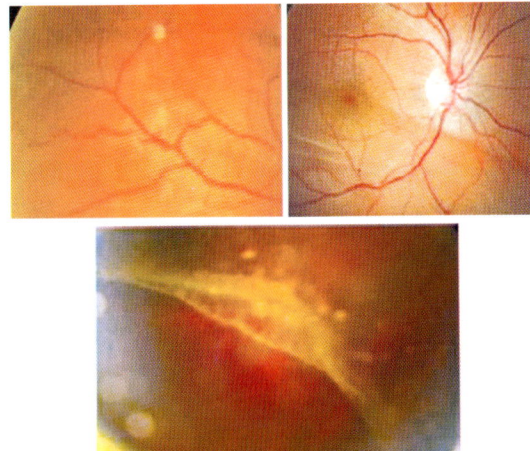

Fig. 6.1.5 *Traumatic RD with inferotemporal retinal dialysis*

Traumatic macular holes

(See page 99)

Management of traumatic retinal tears

Periodic examination of the posterior segment by indirect ophthalmoscopy has already been emphasized. It is of great importance particularly in cases of retinal dialysis since these may not be evident on initial examination and indirect ophthalmoscopy with scleral depression is usually avoided and is resented by the patient sometime in the early stage of trauma because of pain. At the subsequent visit, never forget to exhaustively screen inferotemporal and superonasal quadrants by depressor indirect ophthalmoscopy, however, thorough screening of entire ora serrata is necessary.

In the absence of retinal detachment most retinal breaks are treated either by cryoretinopexy or laser retinopexy. The latter is preferred as it is an outdoor procedure and leads to minimal periocular reaction. Some of the retinal dialysis may also be self-sealing due to vigorous chorioretinal inflammation and scarring, however, meticulous periodic examination is must.

In the presence of retinal detachment, these are treated as any other case of rhegmatogenous RD.

TRAUMATIC RHEGMATOGENOUS RETINAL DETACHMENT

Trauma accounts for up to 12% of rhegmatogenous retinal detachments and thus is the leading cause of retinal detachment in children and adolescents. Men and boys are most likely to be engaged in fights or contact sports and they form at least three-fourths of the patients with traumatic retinal detachment. Traumatic RD occurs secondary to the occurrence of the above said traumatic breaks and trauma-induced liquefaction of vitreous and posterior vitreous detachment. Although the breaks occur at the time of injury but the detachment may not follow simultaneously as the patients are young and the vitreous is in gel-form. Except for giant retinal tears, in the rest of the breaks, there is a latent period between the occurrence of break and progression to RD. This latent period is smaller in peripheral and irregular necrotic breaks as compared to retinal dialysis. In the latter, the RD may not develop since the dialysis is supported by formed vitreous at its base and its edge remains attached to the vitreous.

Clinical types of traumatic RD

Thus depending upon the type, location and status of the vitreous, three types of RDs may be seen as under.

Retinal detachment with horseshoe retinal tear

Horseshoe-shaped peripheral retinal breaks progress to RD more quickly and are bullous in nature. These usually have same sign and symptoms of flashes, floaters, field defects and failing vision. The line of management is the same as non-traumatic RDs.

Retinal detachment with giant retinal tears

Giant retinal tears (GRT) is invariably and almost instantaneously associated with RD. GRT has well-defined anterior and posterior edges and the vitreous is not attached to the posterior edge, being unsupported curls on itself and gets inverted. It should be operated as early as possible otherwise it is going to be complicated by severe proliferative vitreoretinopathy (PVR) as denuded RPE is in direct contact with vitreous cavity (Fig. 6.1.6). GRT is treated by 240 encircling band fixation 14 mm behind limbus followed by pars plana vitrectomy, releasing of

inverted flap of retina with the help of perfluoro-carbon liquid (PFCL), cryo-/laser-retinopexy and PFCL – silicon oil exchange.

Retinal detachment with retinal dialysis

Retinal dialysis may or may not be associated with RD. It has been amply discussed earlier that in case chorioretinal scarring heals the dialysis, the RD may not occur as the edge of dialysis remains attached to the vitreous and formed vitreous base may support the dialysis, thereby retina remains attached. Such cases require close monitoring and prophylactic cryo- or laser-retinopexy. However, the dialysis might remain open and retinal detachment follows.

Characteristically, detachments following retinal dialysis progress slowly since gel vitreous in young patients liquefies gradually. There is always a latent period of few weeks to few months sometime, few years following trauma that RD develops. These are shallow and chronic RDs and patient usually becomes aware of it once the macula is involved particularly in inferotemporal retinal dialyses (Fig. 6.1.7). Role of exhaustive screening by indirect ophthalmo-scopy is of paramount importance so that early diagnosis and prompt treatment is considered in such cases. One may observe on examination demarcation lines, RPE atrophy, subretinal precipitates and intraretinal macrocysts. Proliferative vitreoretinopathy is uncommon so the prognosis of reattachment is usually excellent following scleral buckling and sub-retinal fluid drainage.

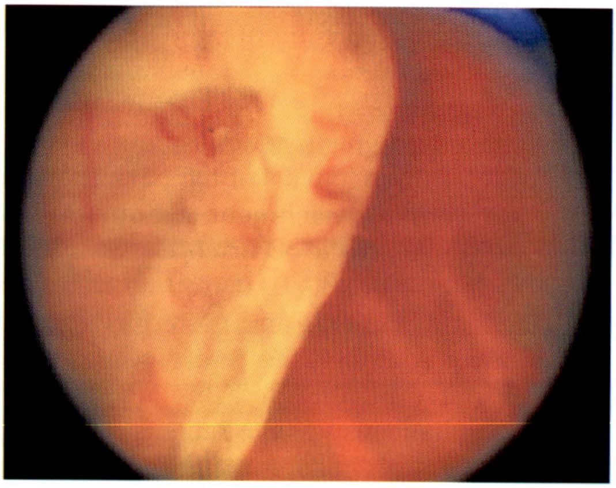

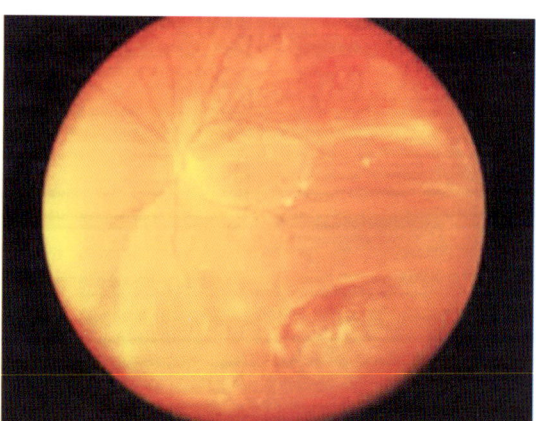

Fig. 6.1.6 *Giant retinal tear with proliferative vitreoretino-pathy*

Fig. 6.1.7 *Traumatic inferoretinal dialysis with retinal detachment involving macula*

TRAUMATIC LESIONS OF VITREOUS

POSTERIOR VITREOUS DETACHMENT (PVD)

Closed globe injury can cause PVD either immediately or after 2–3 weeks depending upon the severity of injury. In case of very severe injury, the cascade of events of concussion injury leading to sequential changes in the antero-posterior and circumferential diameters of the eye are responsible for detachment of posterior hyaloid membrane from the optic nerve head and fovea centralis. One can see a ring of tissue in the separated vitreous by 90 D slit-lamp examination which represents the attachment of vitreous to the optic nerve head and is called as Weiss ring (Fig. 6.1.8). It is diagnostic sign of PVD. An OCT picture vividly depicts PVD (Fig. 6.1.9). In less severe injuries, the blunt trauma leads to synchysis (fluid) followed by syneresis (collapse of framework of vitreous) of the vitreous body resulting in PVD. During the process of posterior vitreous separation, tears may form at the site of abnormal vitreoretinal adhesions which may progress to RD.

AVULSION OF VITREOUS BASE

This is pathognomonic of blunt trauma, the avulsed vitreous base looks like a ribbon floating in the vitreous cavity (bucket handle sign) (Fig. 6.1.10). Unfortunately, the vitreous base does not separate cleanly from the retina and pars plana epithelium. The retina can be torn along the posterior margin of the vitreous base, or the nonpigmented pars plana epithelium can be torn along the anterior margin of the vitreous base, or both can be torn simultaneously. Similarly, if the vitreous is strongly adherent to either lattice degeneration or a vitreoretinal scar posterior to the vitreous base, a posterior flap tear may occur. These tears can cause retinal detachment. However, vitreous base avulsion without any break does not need any treatment only close monitoring is required by periodic indirect ophthalmoscopy.

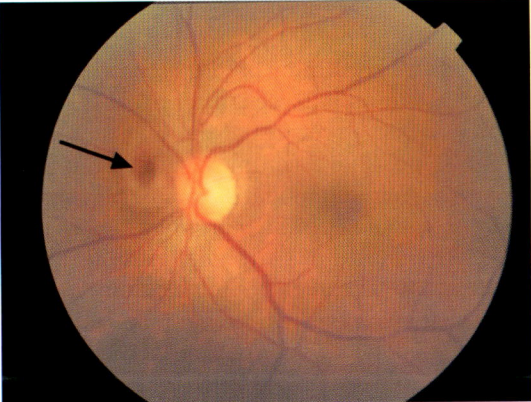

Fig. 6.1.8 *Fundus photograph showing PVD with Weiss' ring*

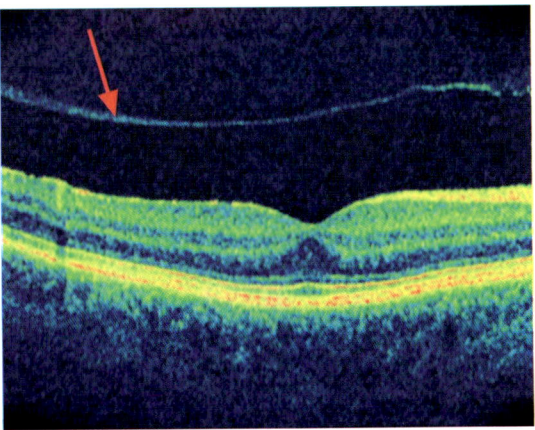

Fig. 6.1.9 *OCT picture showing PVD*

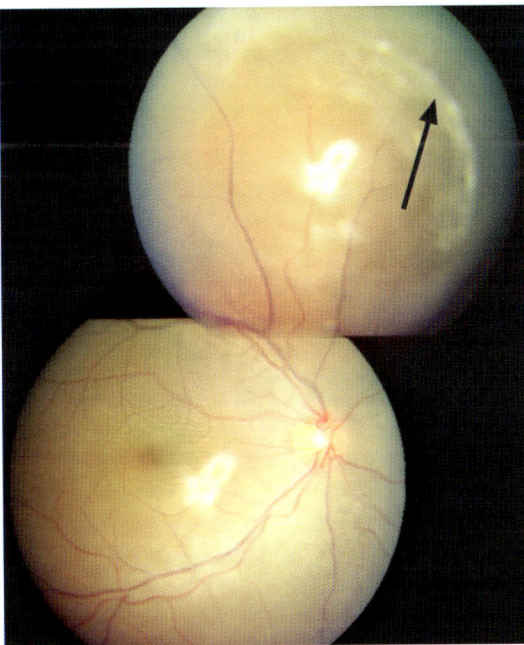

Fig. 6.1.10 *Avulsion of vitreous base with bucket handle sign (arrow)*

VITREOUS HAEMORRHAGE

It may be associated with closed globe or open globe injury. Following closed globe injury the retina is torn, blood vessels that bridge tears may bleed into the vitreous. Vitreous haemorrhage can also result from acute PVD, avulsion of superficial retinal vessels and possible mechanism is rupture of the ciliary body (Fig. 6.1.11). Ultrasound examination is indicated, if the posterior segment is obscured by haemorrhage to rule out retinal tear or detachment, choroidal detachment, posterior vitreous detachment, or occult globe rupture. Bed rest with head elevation is recommended, as it encourages the blood to settle and improves the view of the fundus. Early intervention by pars plana vitrectomy is desired in case of associated retinal detachment and ghost cell glaucoma. In addition, the blood in the vitreous cavity promotes PVR which further warrants early intervention.

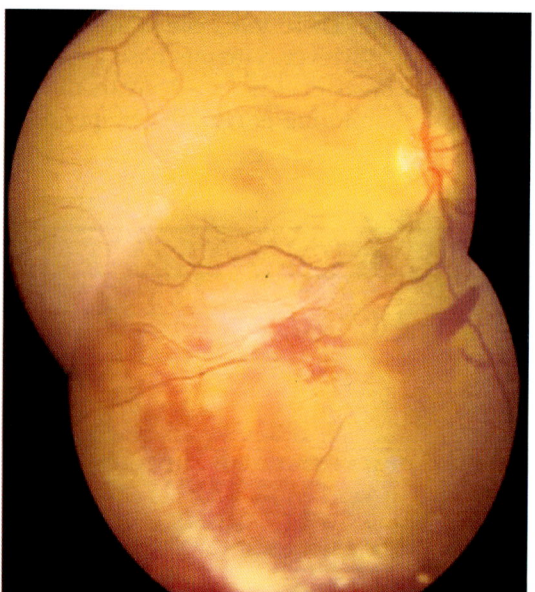

Fig. 6.1.11 *Fundus photograph showing resolving vitreous haemorrhage who on follow-up showed inferior retinal detachment*

Vitreous haemorrhage associated with open globe injury

It is an ominous sign since it has much poorer prognosis than those associated with closed globe injury. It incites devastating sequence of events which ultimately lead to tractional/rhegmatogenous retinal detachment. Following open globe injury involving posterior segment, cellular proliferation starts at the site of penetration within first few days which subsequently leads to the formation of cyclitic, epiretinal and subretinal membranes. The proliferation begins to occur along the vitreous incarceration as well, in the mean time posterior vitreous starts separating from ILM. Ultimately contraction of these proliferating membranes particularly in the presence of blood leads to tractional RD or rhegmatogenous RD or combined RD.

Management

Management involves the primary repair followed by PPV. The timing of PPV is controversial. Majority favours 1–2 weeks after primary repair whereas other advocates at the time of repair. As far as possible a complete vitrectomy with posterior hyaloid removal should be performed in order to avoid epiretinal proliferation. In case complete removal of peripheral vitreous is not possible, 240 silicon encircling element may be applied. Outcome is favourable only if there is no associated retinal, optic nerve or corneal injury.

BIBLIOGRAPHY

1. Cooling RJ. Traumatic retinal detachment – mechanisms and management. Trans Ophthalmol Soc UK 1986; 105:575–579.
2. Hollander DA, Irvine AR, Poothullil AM, Bhisitkul RB. Distinguishing features of non-traumatic and traumatic retinal dialysis. Retina 2004; 24:669–675.
3. Shunmugam M, Ang GS, Lois N. Giant retinal tears. Surv Ophthalmol 2014; 59:192–216.

6.2 TRAUMATIC MACULOPATHY

Introduction
Traumatic macular lesions
• Commotio retinae

• Choroidal rupture
• Traumatic macular hole
• Retinitis sclopetaria

INTRODUCTION

Despite increasing awareness by variety of educational programmes through various media and issuing of warning signals, the incidence of ocular injuries is not decreasing on the contrary it is increasing. The posterior segment manifestations of severe ocular trauma are the foremost cause of permanent visual morbidity. In fact the involvement of retina is second only to the cornea as the most frequently involved tissue of the eye in the ocular injuries. The scenario is more disappointing when it is known that most eye injuries are preventable provided the persons at work wear eye protection.

Blunt trauma can damage the eye at the site of direct impact called as coup injury and at the site opposite to the direct impact by a countrecoup mechanism. The retina is particularly vulnerable to countrecoup injury.

Closed globe injuries resulting from blunt trauma can affect the macula and result in a variety of maculopathies. Blunt trauma leads to anteroposterior compression of eyeball and since the volume of the eyeball is fixed, this results into its equatorial expansion thereby severely stretching posterior segment structures and causing:
• Commotio retinae,
• Choroidal ruptures,
• Macular holes, and
• Retinitis sclopetaria.

TRAUMATIC MACULAR LESIONS

COMMOTIO RETINAE

Commotio retinae is a countrecoup contusive injury to the retina following blunt trauma to anterior segment of eye. It may or may not be accompanied by choroidal rupture. It was first described by Berlin in 1873. It can occur centrally or peripherally, and when it involves the macula, it is called *Berlin's oedema*.

Pathogenesis

Berlin's oedema is not a true oedema. Swelling and disorganization of the outer retinal layers cause the opaqueness. There are various contradictory studies for intracellular and extracellular oedemas. The studies have shown disruption of photoreceptor outer segment and retinal pigment epithelium (RPE) which is outer blood retinal barrier. *FFA* may show masking of the choroidal fluorescence in early stage and window defect in late stage of the disease.

Clinical features

Immediately after trauma, the retina appears normal on examination although the patient may complain of decreased vision. The affected area becomes white and opaque usually hours after the trauma. It consists of a geographic pattern of grey white cloudy opacification of the outer retina. The oedema may be confined to posterior pole, peripapillary region or peripheral retina. If the posterior pole is involved, it may present as pseudo cherry red spot (Fig. 6.2.1).

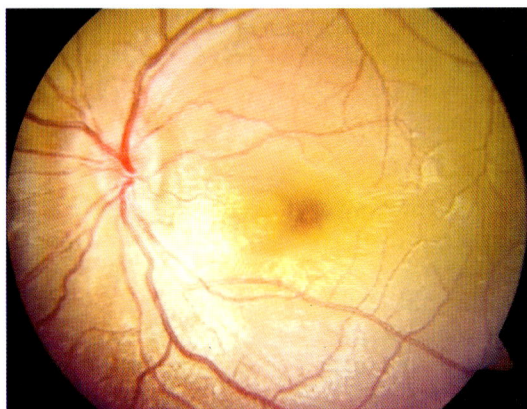

Fig. 6.2.1 *Fundus picture showing Berlin's oedema characterized by white opacification at level of deep sensory retina, mild disc oedema and internal limiting membrane folds (pseudo cherry red spot)*

- *Visual acuity* in commotio retinae varies from 20/20 to 20/400 and does not always correlate with the degree of retinal opacification.
- *Late manifestations of blunt injury to the RPE* vary from minor atrophic changes to massive hyperplasia and migration resulting in bone corpuscular and granular pigmentation that resembles retinitis pigmentosa.
- *Cystoid macular oedema* is seen in rare cases which can progress to a macular hole.

Management and prognosis

Management. Berlin's oedema is usually self-limiting and resolves without sequelae and there is no known intervention that alters its course and prognosis.

Prognosis is usually good except in cases with associated subfoveolar choroidal rupture and/or subfoveolar haemorrhage. *Poor outcome* is seen in severe retinal pigment epithelial damage involving hyperplasia or migration of RPE and serous retinal detachment.

CHOROIDAL RUPTURE

Pathogenesis

Approximately, 5–10% of patients with blunt trauma develop a choroidal rupture. Choroidal rupture can be secondary to indirect or direct trauma.

After blunt trauma, the ocular globe undergoes mechanical compression and then sudden hyperextension. The sclera has tensile strength to resist this insult; the retina is also protected because of its elasticity. The Bruch membrane neither has elasticity nor tensile strength; therefore, it breaks.

Clinical features

Cases secondary to direct trauma tend to be located more anteriorly and at the site of impact and parallel to the ora, whereas those secondary to indirect trauma occur posteriorly. Most eyes have a single rupture, but up to 25% of eyes have multiple ruptures. These ruptures have a crescent shape and are concentric to the optic disc (Figs 6.2.2 and 6.2.3). Indirect choroidal ruptures are almost four times more common than direct ruptures. Mostly ruptures occur temporal to the disc, and 66% involve the macula.

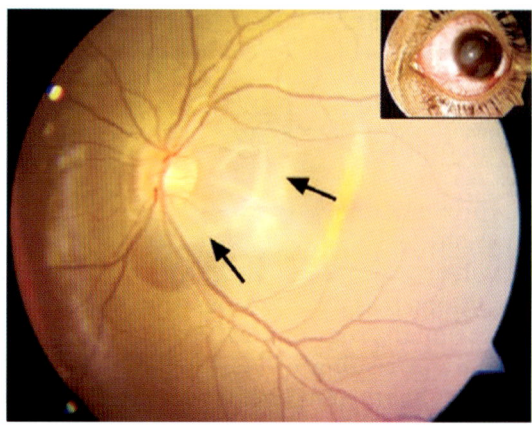

Fig. 6.2.2 *Fundus photograph of two crescent-shaped choroidal ruptures concentric to disc and subretinal bleed (arrows). Inset shows anterior segment picture of the same patient showing iridodialysis*

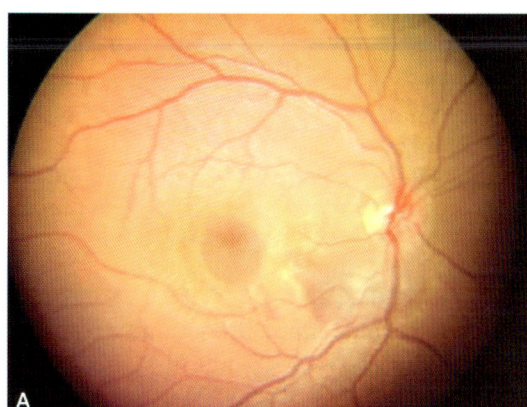

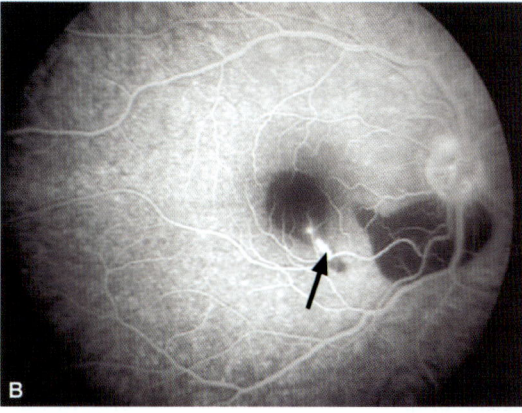

Fig. 6.2.3 *Coloured picture (A) and FFA (B) showing choroidal rupture, resolving subretinal bleed and FFA showing hyperfluorescence due to choroidal neovascular membrane (black arrow)*

During the acute phase, the small capillaries in the choriocapillaris are damaged, leading to subretinal or sub-RPE haemorrhage, which in conjunction with retinal oedema may obscure the choroidal rupture. The deep choroidal vessels are usually spared. As the blood clears, a white, curvilinear, crescent-shaped streak concentric to the optic nerve is seen. Fibroblast activity is seen by 4–14 days.

During the healing phase, choroidal neovascularization (CNV) is a universal phenomenon. In most cases, it involutes spontaneously but in 15–30% of patients, CNV may arise again and lead to a haemorrhagic or serous macular detachment with concomitant visual loss.

Risk factors for CNV include older age, the length of the rupture, and the distance of the rupture from the centre of the fovea.

- *Ocular examination* must be thorough to rule out orbital fractures or globe ruptures.
- *CT scan and MRI* of the eye and orbit should be considered under appropriate circumstances.
- *Fluorescein angiography* and *indocyanine green* ICG may be a useful adjunct to detect CNV.

Management

If fovea is not involved, prognosis is good. If CNV is extrafoveal, it may be treated successfully with laser photocoagulation and anti-VEGF therapy for subfoveal CNVM.

TRAUMATIC MACULAR HOLES

It is a common manifestation of contusive injury and account for about 10% of all macular holes. Fovea being devoid of inner layers is extremely thin and without any blood supply and has attachment with the vitreous. It is thus predisposed to full thickness hole formation following contusion. It has also been reported in association with accidental laser injury, electric shock and lightening strike.

Pathogenesis

Pathogenesis is not well established, possibly the acute compression–decompression force exerted on the globe cause local posterior vitreous detachment, leading to dehiscence in the fovea or to avulsion of a small operculum. It may occur within hours of accident.

With laser injury, the macular hole is caused by coagulation necrosis following the intense laser burn, and the hole can develop in the days or weeks following the injury.

Clinical features

Traumatic macular hole ranges in size from 300 to 750 µ and may be oval or round in shape. In contrast to age-related idiopathic macular hole, posterior vitreous detachment is typically absent since the subjects involved tend to be young. These are often associated with other signs of injury, like adjacent RPE disturbance and epiretinal proliferation (Fig. 6.2.4).

Surgical management

Surgical management of traumatic macular holes is similar to that of idiopathic macular holes, and includes — vitrectomy, ILM peeling, and fluid–gas exchange followed by prone posture. Selection of cases and timing of surgery are important, and outcome often depends on associated trauma-related ocular pathologies. Spontaneous closure of the hole can occur but is not common, and surgery should not be deferred for too long, as long-standing holes are associated with a poor prognosis.

RETINITIS SCLOPETARIA

Pathogenesis

Retinitis sclopetaria a distinct closed globe injury typically caused by transmitted shock waves

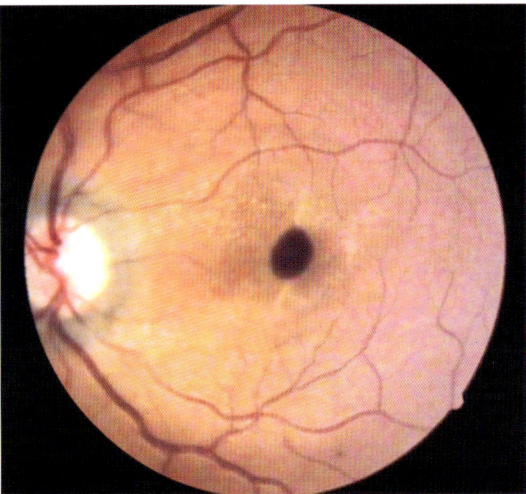

Fig. 6.2.4 *Fundus photograph showing traumatic macular hole*

generated by passage of a high-velocity missile through the orbit without directly striking the eye. This causes rupture of the choroid or retina and leads to irregular ragged holes. The holes are result of mechanical disruption and fragmentation of retina.

Clinical features

Initially, a subretinal or vitreous haemorrhage may be seen. Profoundly decreased vision is seen in optic nerve damage. In severe cases, massive amounts of fibrous tissue proliferate into the eye as seen in Fig. 6.2.5. A claw-like break is often seen in Bruch's membrane and in the choriocapillaris. It is tempting to intervene due to frightening size and posterior location of the breaks but retinal detachment rarely occurs due to inflammation at the edges of necrotic retina which causes firm chorioretinal adhesions, but late detachment from a break at a distal site can occur. In addition, patients tend to be relatively young and have formed vitreous, thus lowering the risk of RD.

Management

The attending ophthalmologist should be aware of this condition so that unwarranted surgical intervention is avoided.

Visual prognosis depends on macular involvement, if there is macular scaring it is poor but, return of 6/6 vision has also been reported.

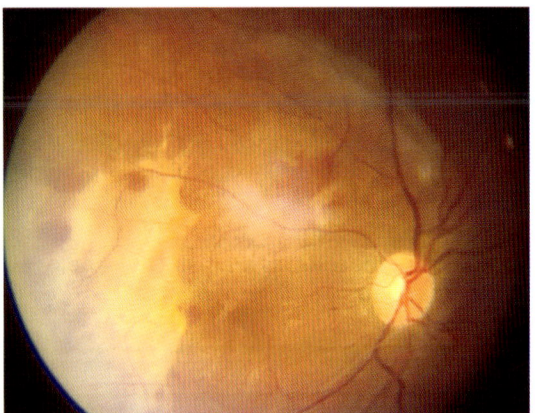

Fig. 6.2.5 *Fundus photograph showing retinal holes in the posterior retina with subretinal fibrosis suggestive of retinitis sclopetaria in a young patient*

BIBLIOGRAPHY

1. Blanch RJ, Good PA, Shah P, Bishop JR, Logan A, Scott RA. Visual outcomes after blunt ocular trauma. Ophthalmology 2013; 120:1588–1591.

2. Fraiser EI, Hang SJ, Mc Donald HR. Clinical presentation of chorio-retinitis scloptreia. Retina cases brief reports 2014; 8(4):257–259.

3. Miller JB, Yonekawa Y, Elliot D, Vavvas DG. A review of traumatic macular hole: Diagnosis and Treatment. Int Ophthalmol Clin 2013; 53: 59–67.

4. Raman SV, Desai UR, Anderson S, Samuel MA. Visual prognosis in patients with traumatic choroidal rupture. Can J Ophtalmol 2004; 39:260–266.

6.3 RETINAL MANIFESTATIONS OF TRAUMA ELSEWHERE

Introduction
Retinal syndromes with trauma elsewhere
- Purtscher's retinopathy
- Valsalva's retinopathy

- Shaken baby syndrome
- Terson's syndrome
- Fat embolism syndrome

INTRODUCTION

There are certain conditions which have their manifestations in the eyes but are caused by mechanical impact elsewhere in the body. These may be because of embolization or sudden increase of the intravascular pressure. There are many of these, however, the ones which are commonly seen in the day-to-day practice discussed in this chapter include:

- Purtscher's retinopathy
- Valsalva's retinopathy
- Shaken baby syndrome
- Terson's syndrome
- Fat embolism syndrome

RETINAL SYNDROMES WITH TRAUMA ELSEWHERE

PURTSCHER'S RETINOPATHY

Purtscher's retinopathy has been associated with traumatic injury, primarily blunt thoracic trauma and head trauma, and numerous nontraumatic diseases. Purtscher's retinopathy is haemorrhagic and vaso-occlusive vasculopathy syndrome of severe vision loss with multiple patches of superficial retinal whitening and retinal haemorrhages.

Pathogenesis

The most accepted mechanism is leucoembolization that causes arteriolar occlusion and infarction of the microvascular bed. Leucocyte aggregation, which is induced by complement 5a, is believed to be the most likely mechanism of embolization. Traumatic chest compression and increased intracranial tension after blunt head trauma are common causes. Besides trauma, it is also seen in cases of acute pancreatitis, long bone fractures, postpartum period, pre-eclampsia shock, disseminated intravascular coagulopathy, fat embolization and

vasculitic diseases. The degree is not necessarily indicative of the risk of developing retinopathy.

Clinical features

The patients may present with unilateral or bilateral vision loss (possibly severe) generally within 2 days. Decreased vision occurs in the affected eyes, generally in the range of 20/200 to counting fingers. Vision often improves over several months to a range of 20/30 to 20/200, depending on the severity of the retinal damage. The retinal findings in Purtscher's retinopathy are cotton-wool spots, areas of retinal whitening around the optic nerve, and intraretinal haemorrhages. Less common reported findings include serous detachment of the macula, preretinal haemorrhages, dilated vessels, and optic disc oedema. Confluence of cotton-wool spots in the central macula may simulate the cherry-red spot that is seen in central retinal artery occlusion. Macular cotton-wool spots and intraretinal haemorrhages in patients with this history of trauma are diagnostic of the condition. Typically, there is sparing of the retinal whitening immediately adjacent to the larger retinal vessels (Fig. 6.3.1).

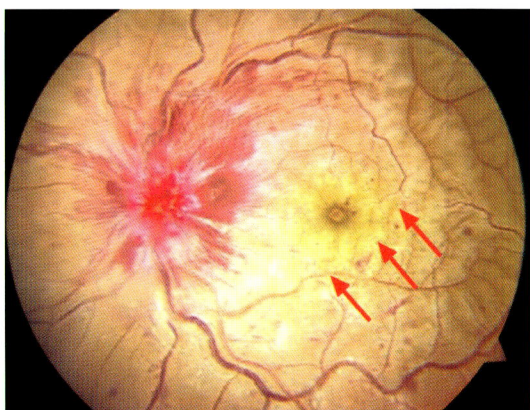

Fig. 6.3.1 *Fundus picture showing superficial retinal haemorrhages and retinal whitening suggestive of Purtscher's retinopathy*

Differential diagnosis

Differential diagnoses of Purtscher's retinopathy include central retinal artery occlusion, giant cell arteritis, hypertension, ocular manifestations of HIV, syphilis, Sjögren's syndrome and Terson's syndrome. If the patient has a history of head trauma or thoracic trauma, obtain appropriate X-ray films or imaging studies—skull or rib fractures may be present. These injuries may require more extensive investigations. Fundus fluorescein angiography studies (early in the disease) demonstrate capillary leakage and staining of the retinal arterioles, venules and capillaries. In severe disease, nonperfusion of the small arterioles that surround the central macula, perivenous staining, venous dilation are often noted.

Treatment

No proven treatment exists for Purtscher's retinopathy that occurs after traumatic injury however, provide surgical care as required for trauma. When it is because of cause other than trauma then the treatment is the control the underlying disease.

VALSALVA'S RETINOPATHY

The retinopathy caused by increased intra-thoracic pressure at Valsalva's manoeuvre which is forceful exhalation against a closed glottis, like straining at stools, coughing, heavy weight-lifting. The veins above the heart have no valves. A rapid rise in the intrathoracic pressure induces a rapid rise in the intravenous pressure leading to the rupture of various vessels in and around the eye.

It is characterized by a well-circumscribed red blood under internal limiting membrane, which is usually boat-shaped, in or near macular region. The colour of blood may alter with time (Fig. 6.3.2). The individuals with tortuosity of 2nd or 3rd order arterioles are predisposed to it

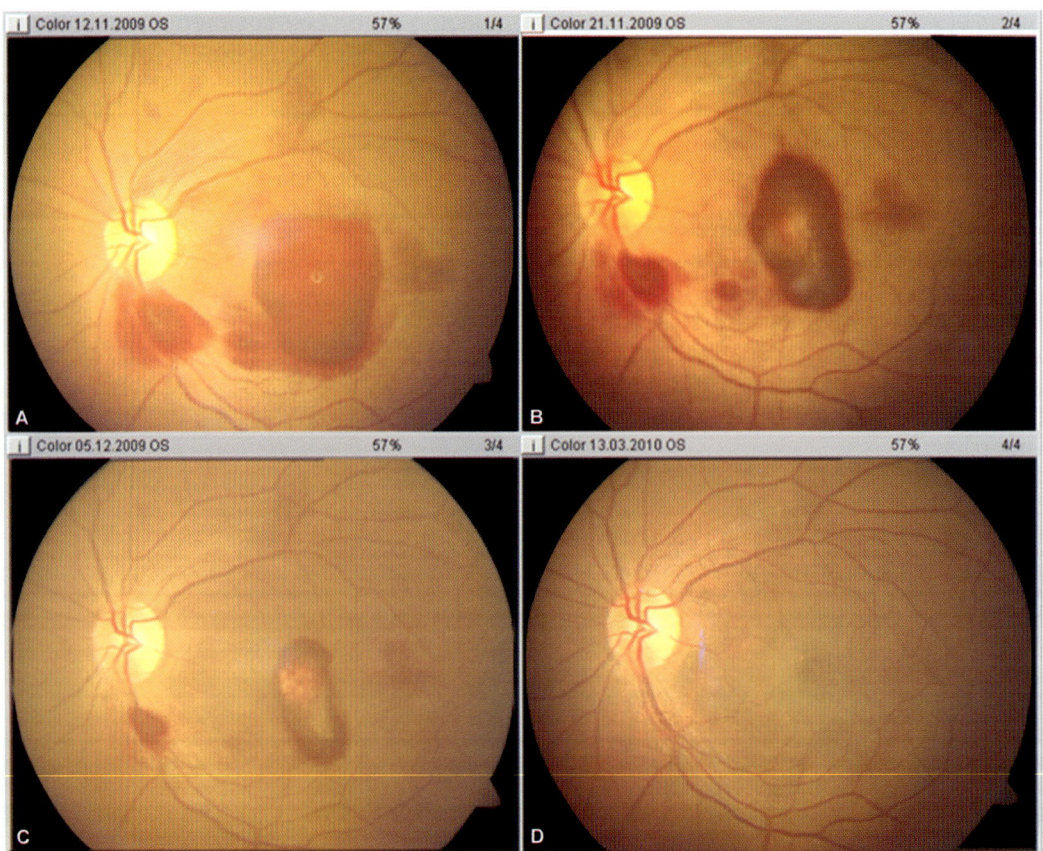

Fig. 6.3.2 *Sequential fundus photographs (A to D) showing resolution of Valsalva's retinopathy over a follow-up of 4 months*

which is inherited as autosomal dominant trait. It clears on its own and only reassurance is required. It is initially red, but eventually with the loss of haemoglobin, it may appear yellow. If it does not clear, a pars plana vitrectomy may be planned. Laser hyaloidotomy may be considered, however, it may lead to epiretinal membrane formation. Nevertheless, it leads to instantaneous trickling of blood inferiorly into the vitreous cavity thereby restoring the vision.

SHAKEN BABY SYNDROME

Child abuse is a major public health issue. It is well recognized that shaken baby may not show the classic stigmata of child abuse, such as fractures, bruises and other visible injuries which may pose difficulty in the actual recognition of child abuse victims. Thus the ophthalmologist has an important role in diagnosing child abuse in the absence of visible marks of injury. Shaken baby syndrome is largely restricted to children <3 years of age with majority in the first year of life.

Pathogenesis

The most accepted mechanism is sudden indirect acceleration–deceleration traction stresses combined with forceful striking of the head against a soft surface, the latter may not leave behind visible marks of injury.

Clinical features

Retinal haemorrhages are found in 65 to 95% of patients. These may vary from focal haemorrhages in one layer to massive haemorrhages in all the layers of retina with extension into the vitreous. The massive haemorrhages are almost invariably associated with brain haemorrhage and with retinal detachment. Traumatic retinoschisis is particularly diagnostic lesion caused by traction applied to retina by the vitreous gel as the child is submitted to repetitive acceleration–deceleration forces. The retina splits creating a blood filled cystic cavity, not reported in otherwise healthy children except shaken baby syndrome victims. In addition, depending upon the quantum of injury, the child may have hyphaema, angle recession and cataract in the anterior segment and signs of periorbital injury.

Diagnosis

If the classical physical findings as mentioned above are present, then the diagnosis is easy. However, the presence of only retinal haemorrhages makes the diagnosis difficult. The other causes of non-accidental trauma, such as coagulopathy and actual accidental injury, should be explored. It should always be kept in mind that shaken baby syndrome by and large is a diagnosis of exclusion. The diagnosis needs to be considered and vigorously explored, if the facts and circumstantial evidence do not explain the nature or extent of injury.

Treatment

Most of the ocular lesions are self-limiting, only close monitoring and observation is required.

TERSON'S SYNDROME

Terson in 1900 described intraocular haemorrhage in association with any form of intracranial haemorrhage; this is known as Terson's syndrome. The most common cause of Terson's syndrome is acute subarachnoid haemorrhage resulting from a ruptured intracranial aneurysm. Mostly it is unilateral but bilateral involvement is common.

Pathogenesis

Intracranial haemorrhage leads to acute rise of intracranial pressure which is transmitted via vaginal sheaths of optic nerve to the central retinal vein. This in turn causes rise of intraocular venous pressure, distention and rupture of capillaries resulting in retinal and vitreal haemorrhage.

Clinical features

In acute stage, one may see multiple preretinal, intraretinal and subretinal haemorrhages. Vitreous haemorrhage is seen in about 3 to 8% patients following subarachnoid haemorrhage. The preretinal haemorrhage is characteristically boat-shaped (D-shaped) between the internal limiting membrane and posterior hyaloid surface. It is also known as subhyaloid haemorrhage.

Management

The vitreous haemorrhage is treated on lines as followed in other instances. It is logical to wait for 2 months which not only facilitates PVD but will have minimal deleterious effect on the retina. If the vitreous haemorrhage does not resolve within that period, patient is subjected to pars plana vitrectomy.

Subhyaloid haemorrhage at the posterior pole mostly covers macula thereby diminishing the vision markedly. The vision can be restored almost instantaneously by subjecting the patient to hyaloidotomy with YAG laser at the lowest dependent part of the haemorrhage. The haemorrhage gravitates inferiorly into the vitreous which resolves spontaneously leaving behind clear macula. Subretinal and intraretinal haemorrhages resolve in due course of time.

FAT EMBOLISM SYNDROME (FES)

It was described in 1861 as part of clinical findings in certain patients suffering from fractures of long bones, particularly thigh bones. It is clinically observed in about 50% patients of long bone fractures and may have adverse outcome in about 20% of severe cases. FES is associated with respiratory failure, hypoxia, petechial rash, pyrexia and altered mental state.

Signs and symptoms begin 12–72 hrs after the trauma.

The ocular findings are similar to Purtscher's retinopathy which has been reported after chest compression injury. The fundus findings include cotton-wool spots and retinal haemorrhages and retinal whitening. The visual prognosis for patients of FES is generally good because of macular sparing, however, permanent visual scotomata has been reported.

BIBLIOGRAPHY

1. Clerk AM, Sunavala JD, Katrak SM, Kothari SS. Fat embolism syndrome after polytrauma. J Assoc Physicians India 2005; 53:193.

2. De Maeyer K, Van Ginderdeuren R, Postelmans L, Stalmans P, Van Calster J. Sub-inner limiting membrane haemorrhage: causes and treatment with vitrectomy. Br J Ophthalmol 2007; 91: 869–872.

3. Garcia-Arumi J, Corcostegui B, Tallada N, Salvador F. Epiretinal membranes in tersons syndrome—A clinic-pathologic study. Retina 1994; 14:351–355.

4. Squier W. The shaken baby syndrome: Pathology and mechanism. Acta Neuropthal 2011; 122: 519–542.

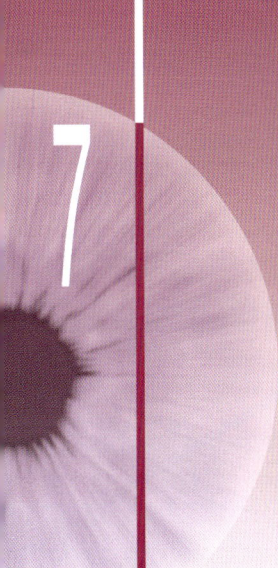

7

INTRAOCULAR FOREIGN BODIES

GENERAL CONSIDERATIONS

Open globe injuries with a retained intraocular foreign body (IOFB) may cause severe vision loss, either due to the trauma or due to secondary events related to IOFB. The modern safe and refined technique of pars plana vitrectomy and microsurgical techniques have led to favourable visual outcome. The combination of a standard 3-port pars plana vitrectomy with a wide-field viewing system, xenon illumination, and IOFB forceps, rare earth endomagnets allows the surgeon to efficiently and safely remove an IOFB, thus reducing the rate of complications. Furthermore, the addition of newer generation broad-spectrum systemic antibiotics has led to reduced rate of post-traumatic endophthalmitis.

CLASSIFICATION

Ocular foreign bodies may be classified as intra-ocular and extraocular foreign bodies. Intra-ocular foreign bodies have been conventionally termed as retained intraocular foreign bodies (RIOFB). These are further divided into anterior

and posterior segment RIOFB. The extraocular foreign bodies may get lodged in the orbit, lids and on the surface of conjunctiva and cornea. These have been dealt in the respective chapters. In this chapters, anterior and posterior segment RIOFB will be discussed.

Ocular foreign bodies
Extraocular foreign bodies
- Conjunctival
- Corneal
- Lids
- Orbital

Intraocular foreign bodies
- Anterior segment RIOFB
- Posterior segment RIOFB

DEMOGRAPHIC FEATURES

The incidence of RIOFB ranges from 20 to 40% among open globe injuries. It occurs primarily in younger age group since about two-thirds cases are observed in the age group of 21 to 40 yrs. There is male predominance as 90–100% patients belong to the male sex. Most common activities at the time of inflicting of foreign body are chisel and hammer injury, industrial work, roadside accidents, weapon-related and blast injuries. Most common retained intraocular foreign bodies are iron and steel. The other less common foreign bodies are particles of glass, stone, lead pellets, copper percussion caps, aluminium, plastic and wood.

MODES AND PROFILE OF OCULAR LESIONS

MODES OF DAMAGE

A penetrating/perforating injury with retained intraocular foreign body may damage the ocular structures by the following modes:

- Mechanical effects.
- Introduction of infection.
- Reaction of foreign bodies.
- Sympathetic ophthalmitis (*see* Chapter 8)

PROFILE OF OCULAR LESIONS WITH RIOFB

A. MECHANICAL EFFECTS

Mechanical effects depend upon the size, velocity and type of the foreign body. Foreign bodies greater than 2 mm in size cause extensive damage. The lesions caused also depend upon the route of entry and the site up to which a foreign body has travelled and in general these include:

- Corneal or/and scleral perforation,
- Hyphema
- Iris hole
- Rupture of the lens and traumatic cataract
- Vitreous haemorrhage and/or degeneration;
- Choroidal rupture, haemorrhage and in- flammation
- Retinal hole, haemorrhages, oedema and detachment.

Location of IOFB

Having entered the eye through the cornea or sclera, a foreign body may be retained in any of the following sites (Fig. 7.1):

1. *Anterior chamber*. In the anterior chamber, the IOFB usually sinks at the bottom. A tiny foreign body may be concealed in the angle of anterior chamber, and visualized only on gonioscopy. A piece of glass in anterior chamber

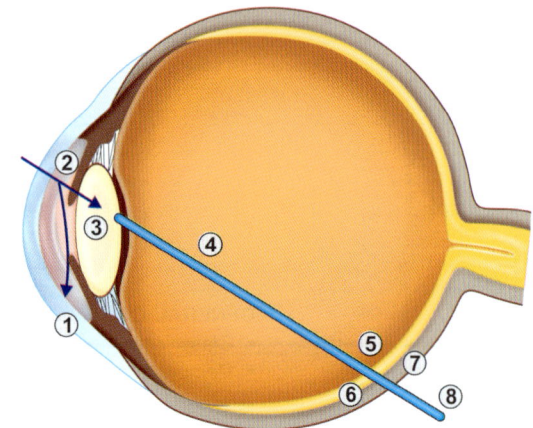

Fig. 7.1 *Common sites for retention of an intraocular foreign body: (1) anterior chamber, (2) iris, (3) lens, (4) vitreous, (5) retina, (6) choroid, (7) sclera, (8) orbital cavity*

is exceptionally difficult to detect because its refractive index differs so little from that of surrounding media, however, it can be diagnosed by ultrasonic biomicroscope.

2. *Iris*. Here the foreign body is usually entangled in the stroma and can be seen only by slit-lamp.

3. *Posterior chamber*. Rarely a foreign body may sink behind the iris after entering through pupil or after making a hole in the iris. The hole in the iris is diagnostic of a retained intraocular foreign body and in the presence of a normal lens one may see the red glow through the iris hole on retroillumination.

4. *Lens*. Foreign body may be present on the anterior surface or inside the lens. Either an opaque track may be seen in the lens or the lens may become completely cataractous.

5. *Vitreous cavity*. A foreign body may reach here through various routes, which are depicted in Fig. 7.2. If it comes to rest in the vitreous, it may remain suspended for some time in the gel vitreous and later as the vitreous becomes fluid, it sinks to the bottom. If the media is clear, the foreign body in the vitreous can be seen by indirect ophthalmoscopy. The tract through the vitreous is often seen as grey line in the initial stages.

6. *Retina, choroid and sclera*. A foreign body may obtain access to these structures through corneal route or directly from scleral perforation and after coursing through the vitreous it may

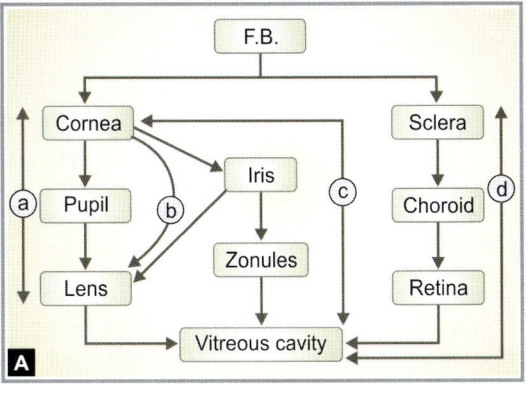

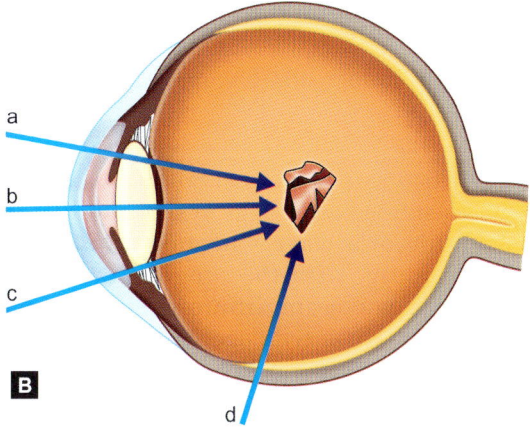

Fig. 7.2 *Logarthmic (A) and diagrammatic (B) depiction of routes of access of a foreign body in the vitreous, through: (a) cornea, pupil, lens; (b) cornea, iris, lens; (c) cornea, iris, zonules; (d) sclera, choroid, retina*

lodge on the retina where it may ricochet once or twice and then rest on the retina. While sitting on the retina it is seen as a black substance with metallic sheen. It is usually surrounded by yellowish white exudates and red blood clot and in the mean time gets encapsulated by fibrous tissue, in case timely removal is not carried out. Subsequently, retina in the neighbourhood becomes heavily pigmented. Ultimately, the vitreous becomes fluid and bands of fibrous tissue may form along the traversing path of the foreign body in the vitreous. These bands may contract and cause tractional retinal detachment. In addition because of concussion, pigmentary disturbance at the macula may deteriorate central vision.

7. Orbital cavity. A foreign body piercing the eyeball may occasionally cause double perforation and come to rest in the orbital tissue.

B. INTRODUCTION OF INFECTION

Intraocular infection is the real danger to the eyeball. Fortunately, small flying metallic foreign bodies are usually sterile due to the heat generated on their commission. However, pieces of the wood and stones carry a great chance of infection. Unfortunately, once intraocular infection is established it usually ends in endophthalmitis or even panophthalmitis. The details of post-traumatic endophthalmitis have been discussed in Chapter 9.

C. REACTIONS OF THE FOREIGN BODY

I. Inorganic foreign body

Depending upon its chemical nature, following 4 types of reaction are noted in the ocular tissues:

1. *No reaction* is produced by the inert substances which include glass, plastic, porcelain, gold, silver and platinum.
2. *Local irritative reaction* leading to encapsulation of the foreign body occurs with lead and aluminium particles.
3. *Suppurative reaction* is excited by pure copper, zinc, nickel and mercury particles.
4. *Specific reactions* are produced by iron (siderosis bulbi) and copper alloys (chalcosis).

Siderosis bulbi

Iron is the most commonly retained metallic intraocular foreign body. The severity of toxicity of iron foreign body depends on the content of iron, i.e. pure iron is more toxic than the alloy of iron. In case, iron foreign body is not removed and continues to be in eye, it leads to degenerative changes in various tissues of the eye and the condition is called as siderosis bulbi. By and large, it occurs within 2 months to 2 years of stay of the iron foreign body in the eye. However, earliest changes have been reported after 9 days of trauma.

Mechanism

The iron particle undergoes electrolytic dissociation by the current of rest and its ions are disseminated throughout the eye. These ions combine with the intracellular proteins, thus damaging especially the epithelial cells causing atrophy. The intraocular tissues are not uniformly affected. It involves the epithelium of lens and iris, retinal pigment epithelium (RPE) and Müller cells of retina and cells of trabecular meshwork. The tissue damage in siderosis is mainly because of cytoplasmic deposition of iron ion leading to alteration of cell membrane permeability, breakdown of lysosomes and liberation of enzymes and cell degeneration.

Clinical features

1. *Lens*: It is involved first of all where oval-shaped rusty deposits are seen in the anterior epithelium arranged radially around a ring corresponding to the edges of dilated pupil. This appearance is pathognomonic and called as siderotic cataract, and eventually the whole lens becomes cataractous (Fig. 7.3).

2. *Iris*: The colour of the iris changes and is different from the other eye and the condition is called as heterochromia iridis. It is first stained greenish and then turns reddish brown which is more evident in light pigmented irides. The iron ions get deposited in the sphincter of pupil causing mid-dilatation first and absence of reaction later on. These changes recover partially only in the initial stages after the removal of foreign body.

3. *Retina*: Retinal changes resemble the changes seen in pigmentary retinal dystrophy which starts in the periphery and then extend posteriorly with attenuation of vessels. Gradually night blindness and concentric visual field loss

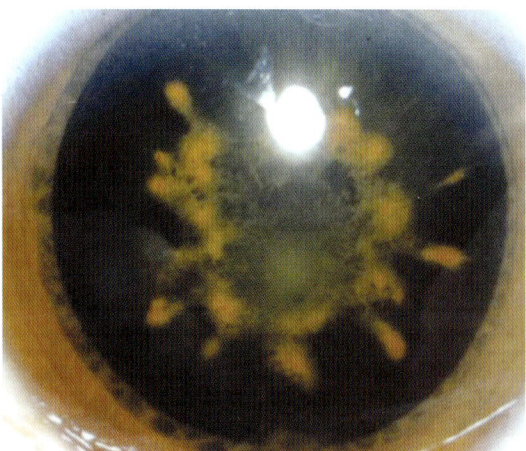

Fig. 7.3 *Siderotic cataract in case of a retained intraocular iron foreign body*

follows. Finally pigmentary changes also involve the macula.

4. *Glaucoma*: Secondary open angle glaucoma occurs as a late complication, unless foreign body gets encapsulated or removed in time. The mechanism is unknown but probably is related to the infiltration of iron in the trabecular meshwork.

Note. If untreated, the patient loses vision because of cataract, glaucomatous optic atrophy and retinal degeneration. The changes are by and large irreversible unless the foreign body is removed in the early stages.

Electrophysiology and histopathology

Electroretinogram. The condition can be monitored by ERG which is more sensitive test for evaluating retinal function than assessing visual acuity. In early stage, it shows increased amplitude of a wave with normal b-wave. Subsequently, with the progression of the disease, b-wave amplitude decreases and ultimately in advanced stage, it becomes flat. As per one estimate, up to 50% b-wave reduction, the changes of siderosis appears to be reversible. Hence, timely removal of the RIOFB can only salvage siderosis bulbi.

Histopathology. The iron deposits in the various ocular tissues can be revealed by Prussian blue reaction. There is always intense blue colouration around the foreign body. The pathognomonic blue stain is found particularly in the corneal corpuscles, in the trabecular meshwork, anterior layers of iris, subcapsularly in the anterior surface of lens, on the inner surface of ciliary body and in the retina where the entire retinal vascular system is clearly marked out.

Chalcosis

Retained copper intraocular foreign body is less common than iron. It occurs mostly in copper industry (zambia), copper wire injuries, shell explosions (made of brass).

As for iron, the reaction of copper shown by ocular tissue, varies with the content of copper. If the copper is pure, severe acute inflammatory reaction associated with hypopyon occurs which may lead to phthisis bulbi, if left untreated. In case, there are brass and bronze which are alloys of copper, the reaction is less severe rather chronic and this is called as chalcosis.

Mechanism

Copper ions from alloy are dissociated electrolytically and deposited on the limiting membranes — Descemet's membrane of cornea, lens capsule and internal limiting membrane of retina. This is in contrast to iron that copper ions do not enter into a chemical combination with intracellular proteins of the cells and hence in chalcosis, degenerative changes are not seen. This may explain why the vision remains indefinitely good despite apparent changes of chalcosis.

Clinical features

1. *Cornea:* There is deposition of tiny granules of copper near Descemet's membrane in the deep stroma near the limbus usually involving the entire circumference of cornea in a ring shaped manner called as Kayser–Fleischer ring. It is greenish-blue in colour.

2. *Lens:* In the lens, the deposition occurs under the lens capsule giving the appearance of sunflower cataract which is golden-green in colour and pathognomonic of chalcosis. It is arranged like petal of sunflower and does not usually impair vision (Fig. 7.4).

Anterior chamber and vitreous may show brightly refractile microscopic particles.

3. *Iris:* It may become greenish in colour and poorly responds to mydriatics.

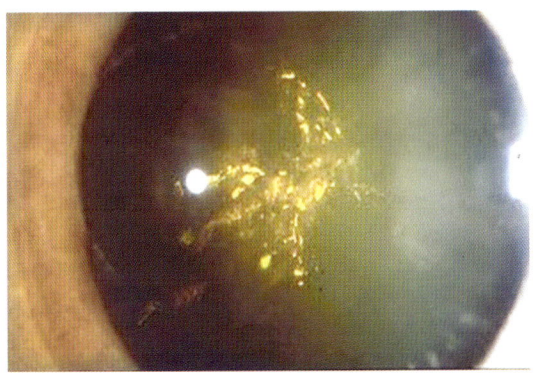

Fig. 7.4 *Sunflower cataract in chalcosis bulbi*

4. *Retina:* Occasionally, on the retina at the posterior pole, metallic sheen of lustrous golden plaques are seen.

Note. The established picture of chalcosis is that of exquisitely beautiful brilliant golden eye with above mentioned features. Most of the features are reversible after the removal of foreign body. ERG may be carried out for monitoring the visual function which mostly remains good.

Non-reactive or encapsulated and fixed intraocular foreign bodies

Occasionally, there might be some delayed presentation of retained intraocular foreign body where the foreign body although metallic but with well-formed encapsulation, or totally inert foreign bodies, like large graphite foreign bodies (pencil leads), rubber pellets which are fixed in the vitreous or a few foreign bodies which have pierced in the optic nerve head and carry a huge risk of torrential haemorrhage with attempted removal, these kind of foreign bodies can be safely left alone and the patient can be monitored with clinical examination and electrophysiological tests, like electroretinogram (ERG) and VER (visually evoked potentials). Intervention can be planned, if there is a risk of retinal detachment/endophthalmitis.

D. SYMPATHETIC OPHTHALMITIS

See Chapter 8.

MANAGEMENT OF RETAINED INTRA-OCULAR FOREIGN BODIES (RIOFB)

DIAGNOSIS AND LOCALIZATION OF IOFB

Diagnosis

It is of extreme importance to ascertain about the retention of the foreign body in the eye after an open globe injury. One should inquire a detailed history, examination and subject the patient to certain diagnostic tests to arrive at the diagnosis of RIOFB. Even if the facilities of CT scan and ultrasonography are not existing, ophthalmologist must order a simple plain X-ray orbits (AP view) to rule out foreign body in the presence of history suggestive of RIOFB. This is despite the fact that the vision is 6/6 and eye is apparently without any signs of inflammation as quite often patient is unaware that something has entered in the eye. This will safeguard against any medicolegal claim under Consumer Protection Act. Following stepwise approach should be taken in order to come to a correct diagnosis.

History

A careful history regarding the actual activity being performed by the patient at the time of afflicting with the injury must be recorded. It may provide a clue about the type and nature of IOFB.

Ocular examination

1. *Slit-lamp examination.* A thorough ocular examination with slit-lamp including gonioscopy should be carried out.

Signs which may give some indication about IOFB are: subconjunctival haemorrhage, uveal show under the conjunctiva, corneal scar, holes in the iris, and opaque track through the lens.

2. *Fundus examination.* With clear media, sometimes IOFB may be seen on indirect ophthalmoscopy in the vitreous or on the retina (Fig. 7.5).

3. *Gonioscopy.* IOFB lodged in the angle of anterior chamber may be visualized by gonioscopy. If it is suspected in the posterior chamber in the presence of a hole in the iris, it may be detected by ultrasound biomicroscopy and anterior segment OCT.

Plain X-ray orbit

Anteroposterior and lateral views are still being recommended for the location of IOFB, as most foreign bodies are radio-opaque. However, many workers feel there is no use of plain film radiography (PFR), as CT images are required for suspected IOFB, even PFR is negative.

Localization of IOFB

Once IOFB is suspected clinically and later confirmed, on fundus examination and/or X-rays, its exact localization is mandatory to plan the proper removal. Following techniques may be used:

1. Radiographic localization

Before the advent of ultrasonography and CT scan, different specialized radiographic techniques were used to localize IOFBs; which are now obsolete. However, a simple limbal ring method which is still used is described below.

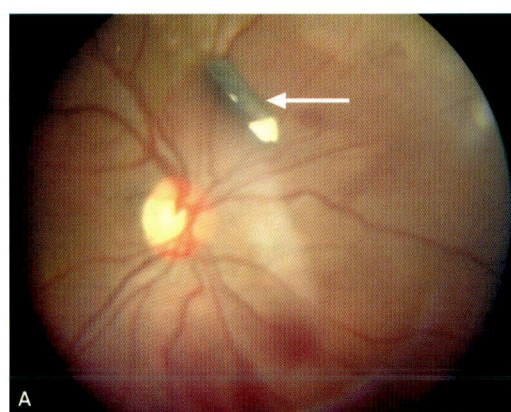

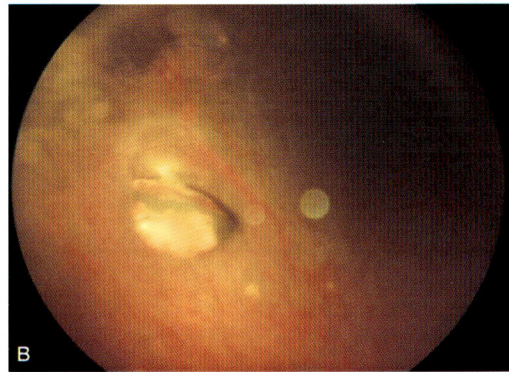

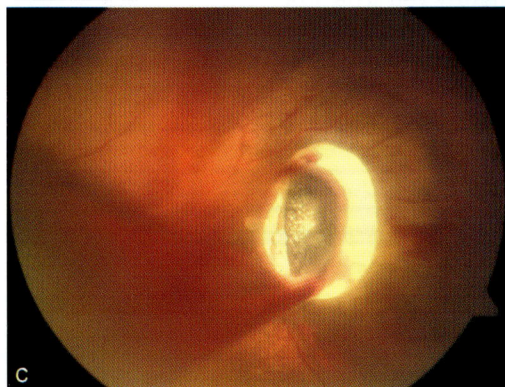

Fig. 7.5 *Fundus photograph showing retained iron foreign body (A) In the vitreous cavity with vitreous haemorrhage inferiorly; (B) Foreign body an retinal surface with surrounding siderotic changes; (C) Foreign body covered by fibrous capsule with associated vitreous haemorrhage*

Limbal ring method. It is most simple but nowadays, sparingly employed technique. A metallic ring of the corneal diameter is stitched at the limbus and X-rays are taken (Fig. 7.6). One exposure is taken in the anteroposterior view which tells about the quadrant in which the foreign body is lying. In the lateral view, three exposures are made one each while the patient is looking straight, upwards and downwards, respectively. The position of the foreign body is then estimated from its relationship with the metallic ring in different positions by drawing a schematic eye keeping in account the magnification factor of the metallic ring (Fig. 7.7).

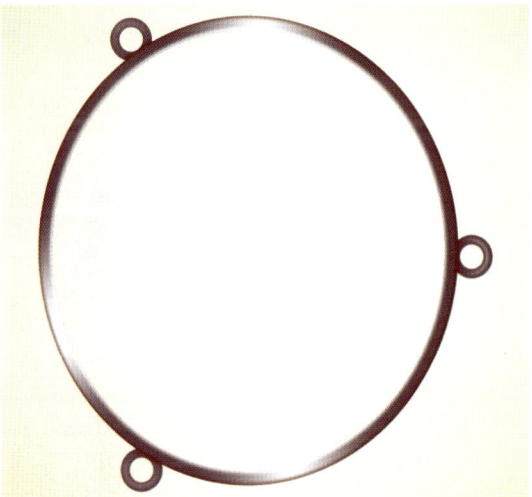

Fig. 7.6 *Limbal ring used for localization of an intraocular foreign body*

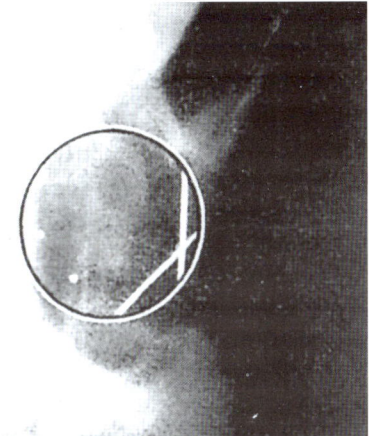

Fig. 7.7 *Limbal ring method of radiographic localization of IOFB: Lateral view with eyeball in straight position; superimposed over lateral view with eyeball in down gaze*

2. Ultrasonographic localization

It is being used increasingly these days. It can tell the position of even non-radio-opaque foreign bodies. It is the best indirect method to find out the associated tissue injuries, such as choroidal and vitreous haemorrhages and retinal detachment and to monitor the eye during the follow up after primary repair. It is avoided after open globe injury. It tends to overestimate the size of the RIOFB and should not be used for measuring purpose. False negative results are possible, if the IOFB is small, wooden or of vegetative matter and false positive results may be found in the presence of air bubble. Ultrasound biomicroscopy is superior to CT, MRI and contact B scan ultrasonography in localizing small non-metallic IOFBs in the anterior segment (Fig. 7.8). Occasionally multiple intraocular foreign bodies can be present and the sonologist should keep this in mind.

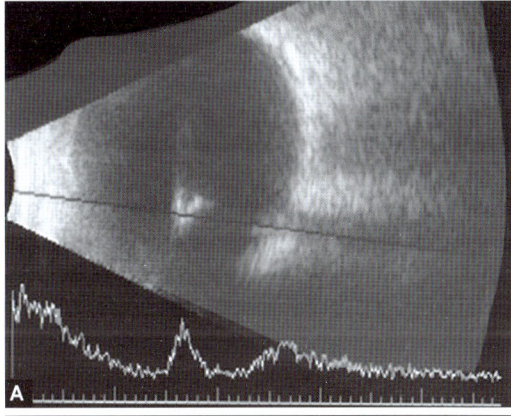

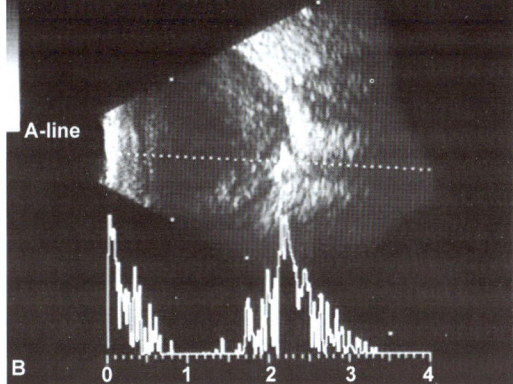

Fig. 7.8 *(A) USG showing a hyperechoic RIOFB in the vitreous cavity with post-acoustic shadowing; (B) Ultrasound showing vitreous echoes with intraocular foreign body on the retinal surface with after shadowing*

3. CT scan

With axial and coronal cuts, CT scan is presently the best method of IOFB localization. It provides cross-sectional images with a sensitivity and specificity that are superior to plain radiography and ultrasonography. CT cannot distinguish various types of metals and it can miss plastic IOFBs. In case too wide cuts are taken or the patient moves the eye during the procedure even the metallic IOFBs are missed. Helical (spiral) CT provides image superior to conventional CT. The former has a shorter examination time, has the ability to reconstruct coronal/sagittal images without further scanning and reduces motion artifacts and radiation. It can detect IOFB as small as 0.625 mm. In case of doubt whether IOFB is intraocular or extraocular or in the eyewall, spiral CT may help (Fig. 7.9).

4. MRI

It is a powerful tool for cross-sectional and soft tissue analysis. However, it is *avoided in metallic IOFBs* since the movement of foreign body during the procedure may damage the eye structures. The available literature is confusing regarding its safety in iron IOFBs. Some reports say the movement of foreign body is rare, the other say it is common.

TREATMENT

After ascertaining the presence and location of the foreign body, it should always be removed except in the following rare circumstances:
• It is inert and sterile

• The process of removal is invariably going to affect vision drastically

Technique of removal of foreign body will depend upon the location of the foreign body, whether it is retained in the anterior segment or posterior segment.

Removal of foreign body from anterior segment

Usually, it is carried out under local anaesthesia as a second stage procedure after the primary repair. However, foreign bodies in anterior chamber and in the iris may be removed at the time of primary repair itself.

In general, magnetic foreign bodies are easier to be removed than non-magnetic foreign bodies in the anterior segment.

1. *Foreign body in the mid-corneal stroma* can be removed under operating microscope with the help of 26 No. hypodermic needle mounted on 2cc syringe. Foreign body deep in the stroma needs to be supported posteriorly with the iris repositor introduced in the anterior chamber which will safeguard against the falling of foreign body in the angle of anterior chamber during its manipulation.

2. *Foreign body in the anterior chamber* can be removed with the help of a magnet in case it is magnetic (Fig. 7.10). The incision is made on

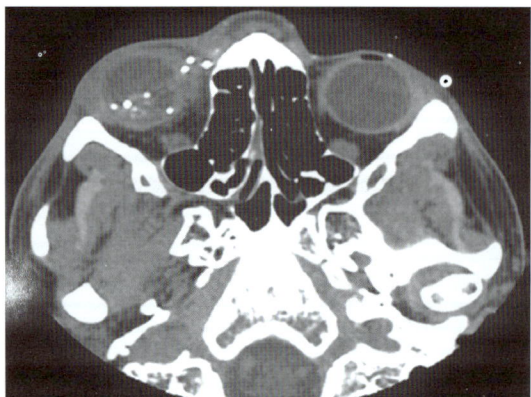

Fig. 7.9 *Axial CT scan of the orbit showing multiple foreign bodies*

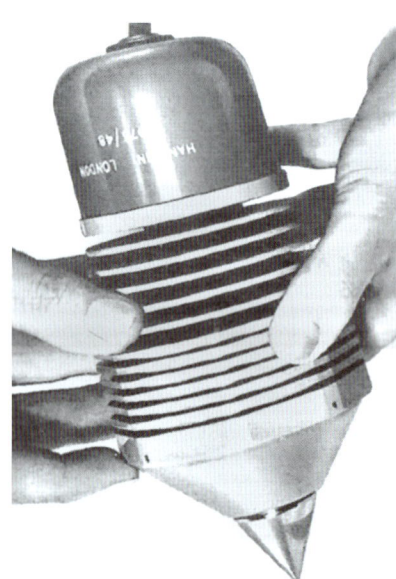

Fig. 7.10 *Hand-held magnet*

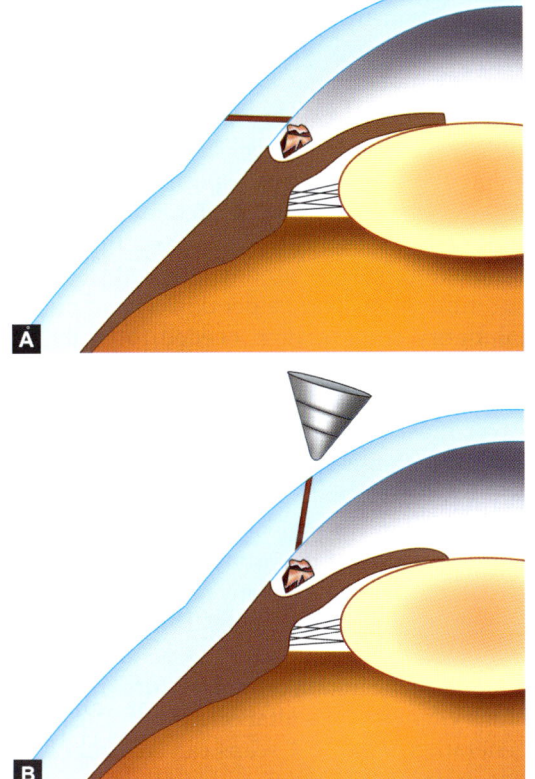

Fig. 7.11 *Removal of a magnetic intraocular foreign, body from the anterior chamber: (A) the wrong incision; (B) correct incision*

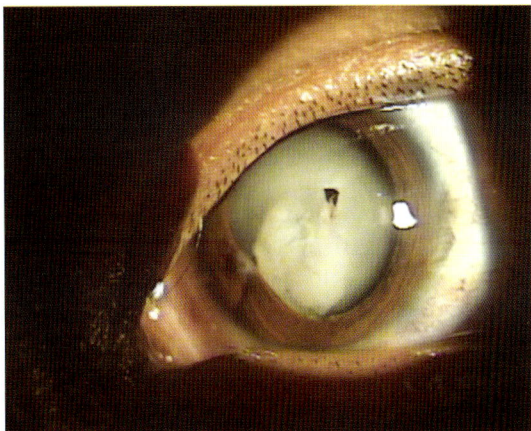

Fig. 7.12 *Lenticular foreign body with traumatic cataract*

cornea in the quadrant of foreign body 3 mm inside the limbus which is directed toward foreign body (Fig. 7.11). Non-magnetic foreign bodies are picked up with the help of toothless forceps after filling the anterior chamber with viscoelastic substance.

3. *Foreign body entangled in the iris tissue* whether magnetic or non-magnetic is removed by performing sector iridectomy of the part of the iris containing the foreign body through a suitably placed keratome incision. In case it is lying on the iris, it can be picked up with a toothless forceps.

4. *Foreign body in the lens:* Intralenticular foreign bodies usually lead to traumatic cataract warranting cataract extraction (Fig. 7.12). Magnet extraction of magnetic foreign bodies is usually difficult in intralenticular foreign bodies. Therefore, all foreign bodies in the lens are treated as non-magnetic foreign bodies and extracapsular cataract extraction may be by phacoemulsification should be planned along with IOL implantation. The foreign body is usually evacuated along with lens matter or may be removed with the help of forceps after filling the AC with viscoelastic substance. The surgeon should be careful in the presence of posterior capsular rent observed during surgery lest foreign body drop should occur in the vitreous cavity.

Removal of foreign body from posterior segment

Historical perspective of RIOFB removal

Historically, intraocular foreign bodies (magnetic) were removed through the pars plana using an external magnet, after a thorough and meticulous localization with a limbal ring as a reference plane and radiograms taken in anteroposterior, and lateral views in various gazes. However, external magnetic extraction of metallic IOFB was associated with a high incidence of intraocular damage. With the development of the pars plana vitrectomy (PPV) and the addition of vitrectomy instrumentation and IOFB forceps, both magnetic and non-magnetic IOFBs could be removed from the vitreous cavity with minimum collateral damage.

Intraocular foreign body removal was originally localized using scout films of the orbit. This technique has long been replaced by improvements in ultrasonography and computed tomography (CT) technology. The advances in CT have enabled better preoperative planning by using improved resolution to determine the exact location and size of an IOFB.

Williams et al published the first large series of visual outcomes using PPV microsurgical techniques, with 60% retaining better than 20/40 best-corrected visual acuity. Chow and colleagues found no difference in visual acuity when comparing an external magnet versus an internal PPV approach for IOFB removal. Over the last 10 years, numerous authors have published their experiences with IOFB removal using a PPV approach. Current IOFB removal techniques incorporate the most recent advances in PPV microsurgical instrumentation and technology.

Methodical stepwise approach for open globe injury with possible IOFB

Open globe injury with a possible IOFB should start with an extensive methodical stepwise approach.

Preoperative planning, testing and management

First step is the IOFB preoperative planning and testing. An open globe injury with a suspected retained IOFB needs a systemic evaluation to rule out any life-threatening emergency, if necessary (not needed in a chisel hammer type of injury but mandatory in blast victims). After ruling out any concomitant injury that may require more emergent attention, an extensive history should be obtained in the patient who is conscious and able to communicate. The surgeon should document the etiology of the injury; the type of material that may have entered the eye, such as metallic (magnetic/nonmagnetic), nonorganic (stone), organic (plant/wood), or autologous (bone, cilia); time of injury; last meal; and allergy to penicillin.

Complete ophthalmic examination should include an initial visual acuity, pupillary examination to rule out an afferent pupillary defect, a slit-lamp examination to rule out endophthalmitis, and a dilated fundus examination by indirect ophthalmoscope to possibly visualize the IOFB and rule out a retinal detachment. Intraocular pressure and B-scan ultrasonography may be deferred until the primary globe repair is completed to evaluate the retina and the choroid.

Prophylactic antibodies. The surgeon should immediately order broad-spectrum antibiotics. Today's top choices for IOFB endophthalmitis prophylaxis include moxifloxacin 400 mg intravenously once per day or levofloxacin 500 mg intravenously once per day. The minimum inhibitory concentration needed to inhibit the growth of 90% of organisms (MIC90) of these 2 antibiotics penetrating into the vitreous will cover most bacterial causes of post-traumatic endophthalmitis except *Pseudomonas aeruginosa* and *Bacillus cereus*.

CT scan orbit. The patient should have an urgent CT helical scan of the orbits and the brain. The surgeon should rule out any intracranial foreign bodies or roof fractures that may need neurosurgical consultation. Depending on the etiology of the injury, orbital fractures may need otolaryngology consultation as well. The newer generation helical CT scans can reformat IOFB images in axial, coronal, and sagittal views. The high-resolution CT scan generate images as thin as 0.625 mm (Fig. 7.9). The patient with a suspected open-globe injury without a foreign body on the CT scan, can then proceed to the operating room for primary globe repair.

Ultrasonography. Although CT scan is very sensitive in picking up RIOFB, ultrasonography gives valuable information regarding site of impaction of foreign body, status of posterior vitreous detachment, any associated retinal detachment, presence of concurrent vitreous haemorrhage or endophthalmitis (Fig. 7.8).

Primary repair versus two-stage operation?

Timing and type of surgery are the next major decisions in the management of an IOFB. The surgeon can either primarily close the open globe and secondarily remove the IOFB or combine both surgeries at the same time. The patient with an open globe injury with a retained IOFB must be stable for extended surgery, if both the globe repair and IOFB are planned together. An open globe repair, IOFB removal, and intravitreal antibiotics are necessary with a post-traumatic endophthalmitis. Important determining factors are:

- *Availability of trained operating room personnel* who are skilled in assisting during very complicated and lengthy primary open-globe closure and IOFB removal cases is a very important factor. Operating with unskilled personnel after hours may not be the safest setting for an IOFB removal; therefore, primary globe closure with secondary IOFB removal may be a safer option in such circumstances.

- *Corneal clarity* is also a very important consideration when determining primary globe closure with or without IOFB removal. Corneal oedema and stromal haze improve dramatically from 7 to 10 days after primary globe repair. In such a situation, two-stage surgery is preferred.

Pars plana vitrectomy

Once the surgeon decides to remove an IOFB, the operating room planning must include the necessary equipment and supplies needed for the surgical case.

Retained IOFBs in the posterior segment will require a PPV. The vitreoretinal surgeon may choose from a 20-gauge PPV or a small gauge 23/25-gauge PPV. Very small IOFBs less than 0.5 mm can be removed through the cannulas without enlarging the sclerotomy wounds. And in case of larger foreign bodies, a hybrid 23 (two ports) and a 20-gauge port at the surgeons active hand may be used.

Conventional 20-gauge versus small gauge vitrectomy

The 20-gauge PPV uses a microvitreoretinal (MVR) blade to create an incision in the sclera which can be enlarged, if needed to remove the IOFB. The 20-gauge sutured sclerotomy PPV is better suited for most IOFB injuries, than the 23/25-gauge vitrectomy.

Trocar insertion in small gauge vitrectomy may exacerbate a traumatic optic neuropathy, worsen corneal oedema, and cause wound leakage from a recent primary globe closure (all these complications are often pre-existing in cases with RIOFB).

Therefore, 20-gauge PPV is preferred over small gauge vitrectomy.

Suprachoroidal haemorrhage has been documented in 6% of IOFB cases. Visual outcome after a suprachoroidal haemorrhage are extremely poor, with high rates of no light perception visual acuity, chronic postoperative hypotony, and non-repairable retinal detachment.

It is not possible to perform small gauge PPV in suprachoroidal haemorrhage. 20-gauge PPV may be performed either with 6 mm long cannula or after drainage of suprachoroidal haemorrhage.

At the beginning of the PPV, a vitreous sample can be obtained and sent for immediate Gram stain and culture. Intraocular foreign body removal will start with a pars plana lensectomy, if associated with a traumatic cataract. The anterior capsule not damaged by the IOFB should be endevoured to keep intact for possible future intraocular lens implantation (IOL).

The most conservative approach is to leave the eye surgically aphakic and return for secondary IOL implantation 3 to 6 months after IOFB removal. The other option in case of an RIOFB with no evidence of endophthalmitis is a preparatory phacoemulsification which can be done with IOL, provided the foreign body is less than 5 mm × 5 mm × 5 mm.

IOL implantation at the time of IOFB has many pitfalls. The IOL may be subluxated postoperative by the gas tamponade used for retinal detachment repair. The IOL may develop synechiae to the iris during the immediate postoperative period, with permanent changes in the pupil. The artificial IOL implant may lead to a higher risk of delayed endophthalmitis, considering the fact that a contaminated foreign body was removed from the eye at the time of IOL implantation.

Once core vitrectomy is performed, it is important to achieve a complete posterior hyaloid separation from the posterior pole and also from the foreign body site (Fig. 7.13) so as to prevent iatrogenic breaks while performing foreign body retrieval. The methods of posterior hyaloid separation are beyond the scope of this chapter.

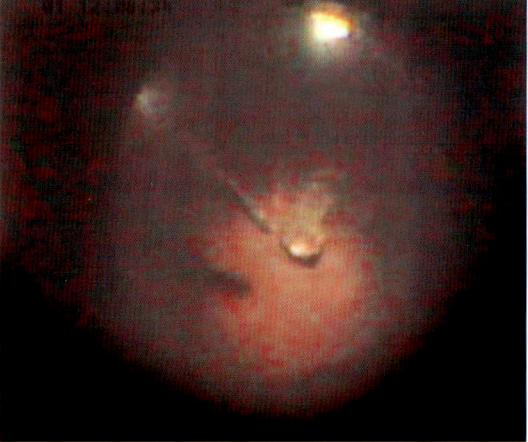

Fig. 7.13 *Vitrectomy being performed around a stone intravitreal foreign body*

Size of the IOFB is the most important factor in determining the instrumentation for IOFB removal.

- *A magnetic metallic IOFB less than 1 × 1 × 1 mm* in dimension is most easily removed using a positive action IOFB endomagnet (Grieshaber). This instrument uses the magnet to capture the small IOFB and retracts the IOFB into a sleeve before removal from the sclerotomy site. This prevents the IOFB from catching on the edge of sclerotomy and falling back into the eye.

- *Intravitreal foreign body ranging in size from 1 to 3 mm* regardless of composition is best removed with a Grieshaber Pannarale basket forceps (Fig. 7.14).

- The Grieshaber Machemer diamond-coated foreign body forceps (Fig. 7.15) are very commonly used in our set-up and they are

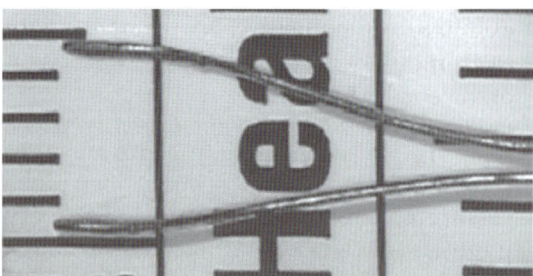

Fig. 7.15 *Diamond dusted Machemer foreign body forceps*

useful for grabbing an IOFB that is 3 to 5 mm in smallest dimension and are necessary when removing large pieces of glass off the macula. The diamond coating prevents slippage of smooth glass foreign bodies during retrieval.

Intraretinal and subretinal foreign bodies. The moment the foreign bodies, which are mostly metallic, get lodged in these locations, the fibrous tissue reaction starts and they get encapsulated in a matter of days. At this stage, the foreign bodies are often invisible and are detected by the imaging techniques only. The era of retrieval of magnetic foreign body by external earth magnetic is over. These are removed by vitreous surgery may be with the help of intraoperative magnetic/vitreous forceps after incising the capsule and mobilization of the foreign body.

Subretinal IOFBs, commmonly hidden by blood, can be removed through an adjacently prepared retinotomy or through a peripheral pre-existing retinal break. The subretinal use of viscoelastics may help in protecting the photoreceptors.

Prophylactic retinopexy around the break is considered, only if there is vitreoretinal traction due to incomplete removal of posterior hyaloid membrane. It is probably unnecessary, if there is complete removal of vitreous. Laser is preferred over cryo since the latter stimulates surface proliferation. However, the more anterior is the location of break the more retinopexy is desired.

Prophylactic scleral buckling used to be considered in the bygone era when intraretinal foreign body used to be removed through the scleral incision adjoining the foreign body by

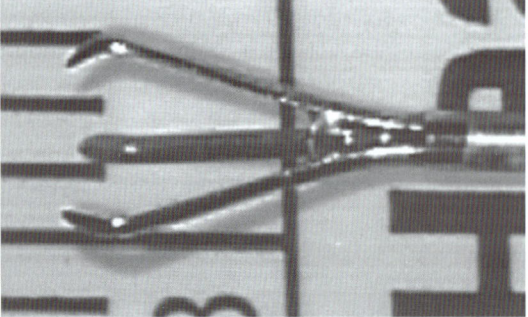

Fig. 7.14 *Pannarale basket foreign body retrieval forceps*

external earth magnetic. Now, the foreign bodies are removed by PPV with complete removal of vitreous, therefore, the consensus is not in favour of prophylactic sclera buckle, however, it may be considered in cases where peripheral vitrectomy cannot be performed satisfactorily and the threat of PVR is significant as in vitreous haemorrhage and foreign bodies more than 4 mm.

Sclerotomy incisions larger than 5 mm tend to leak fluid faster than infusion through a 20-gauge infusion line. Globe collapse prevents observation and safe removal of an IOFB. Therefore, IOFBs requiring larger than 5 mm sclerotomy should be retrieved through a sclera tunnel/limbal incision so that globe does not collapse.

Corneal clarity is the most important aspect of intraocular foreign body removal. Injured corneas become more oedematous as IOFB cases progress. Particular attention to intraocular pressure is imperative to reduce progression of corneal oedema.

Illumination of the retina during PPV has significantly improved visualization of IOFBs and retinal tear. Most of the vitrectomy systems now come with in built illumination system. In older machines a separate endoilluminator was used (Fig. 7.16). The newer generation xenon light sources enable the surgeon to see past an oedematous cornea and safely retrieve IOFBs. Xenon-illuminated laser probes enable the management of retinal tears and detachments especially when used in conjunction with perfluoro-n-octane. Chandelier light sources are also commercially available to perform bimanual removal of large IOFBs.

Preservative-free intraoperative triamcinolone is extremely useful in identifying residual cortical vitreous through an oedematous cornea.

Without signs of retinal injury, the globe can be left with balanced salt solution, and the sclerotomies closed with vicryl 7–0. Air may be used as a tamponade after laser retinopexy for retinal tears. Postoperatively a scar may be formed in some cases due to impact of foreign body (Fig. 7.17).

After IOFB removal, retinal detachments may be repaired in the standard fashion with or without an encircling band. Intraocular foreign body related retinal detachments can be repaired with sulfur hexafluoride (SF6), per-fluoropropane (C3F8), or silicone oil (1000 or 5000 centistoke) depending on the severity of the injury. The most severe IOFB-related retinal detachments and perforating injuries need silicone oil for long-term tamponade to prevent the effects of proliferative vitreoretinopathy.

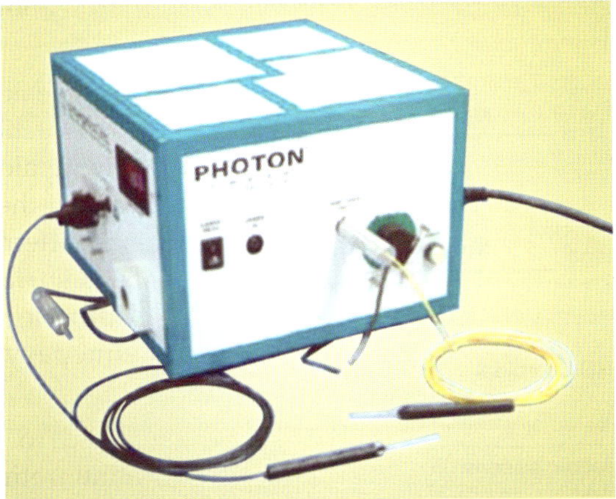

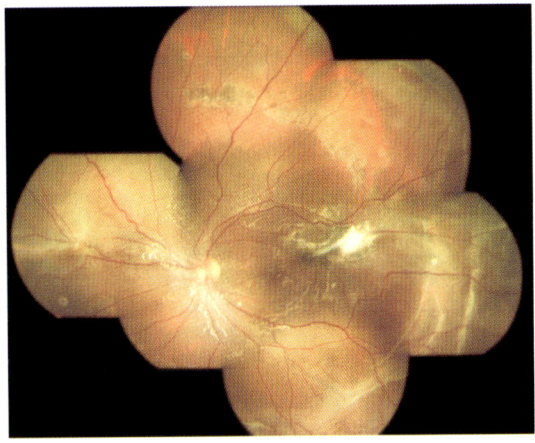

Fig. 7.16 *Illumination system (endoilluminator light probe and chandeliers)*

Fig. 7.17 *Fundus photograph montage of the left eye of a patient who underwent vitrectomy with intraocular foreign body removal. The scar at the posterior pole is due to the impact of foreign body*

Schematic outlines for management of intraocular foreign body

Fig. 7.18 summarizes the schematic outlines for intraocular foreign body management.

IMPORTANT ASPECTS RELATED TO IOFB

Visual outcomes after IOFB injury can vary depending on other concomitant globe injuries. Preoperative visual acuity is usually reduced by

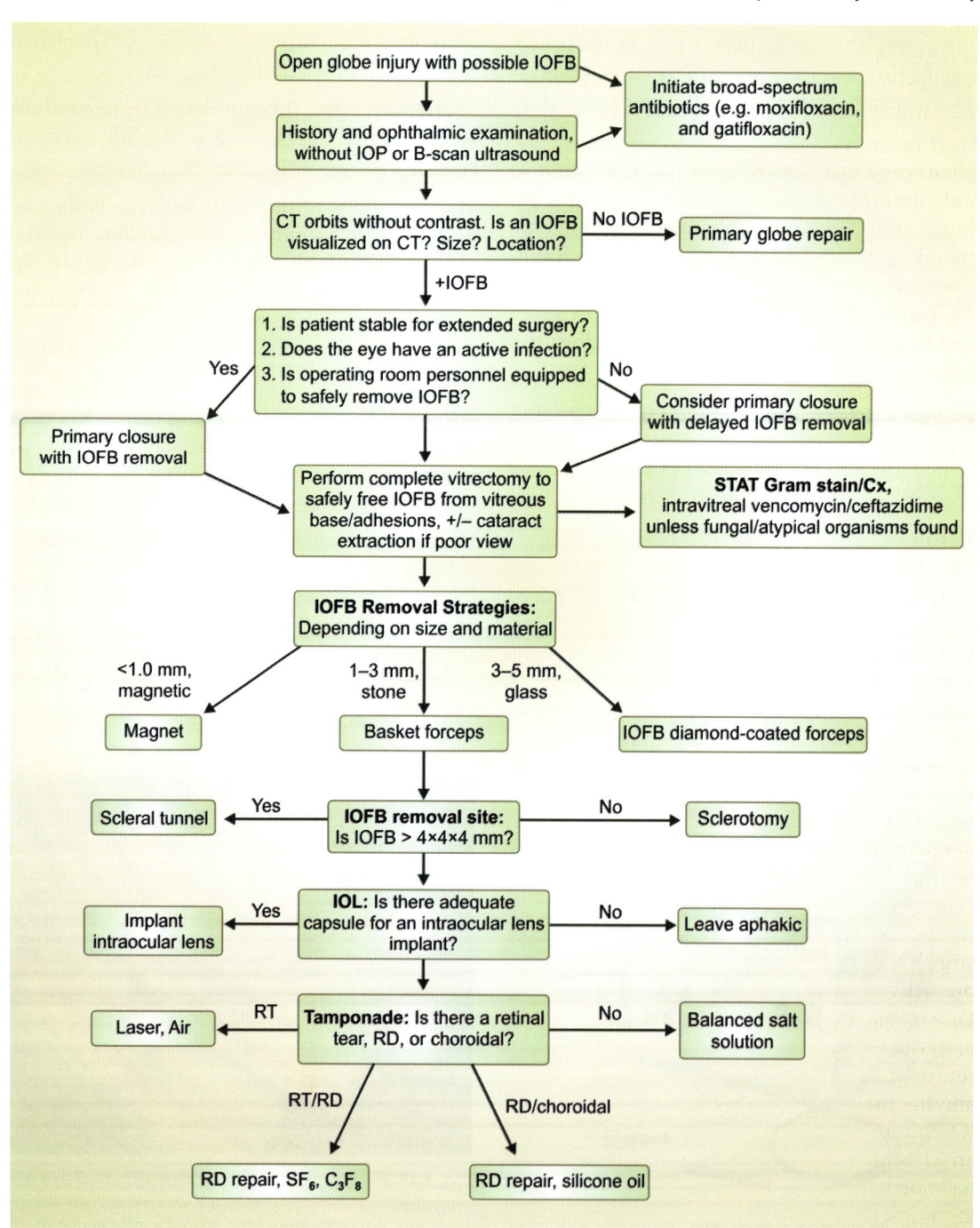

Fig. 7.18 *Schematic outline for management of IOFB*

traumatic cataract or vitreous haemorrhage. These two media opacities are removed during IOFB removal. The major contributing factors for long-term poor visual acuity are traumatic optic neuropathy, corneal scarring, residual effects of post-traumatic endophthalmitis, and suprachoroidal haemorrhage as well as proliferative vitreoretinopathy (PVR) causing irreparable chronic retinal detachment.

Most common type of IOFB injury involves a small corneal laceration with traumatic cataract and vitreous haemorrhage in more than 50% of these cases. These IOFB injuries have excellent visual recovery, with most obtaining best-corrected visual acuity 20/40.

Corneal scarring and astigmatism are significant factors for vision loss after an IOFB injury. Anterior segment reconstruction for a traumatic iridodialysis is commonly repaired using a double-armed McCannel suture to repair a sectoral iris defect. Aniridia IOL can be used to manage traumatic aniridia with symptomatic photophobia. Traumatic optic neuropathy can be followed using visual field or multifocal visual evoked potential testing.

Rate of preoperative retinal detachment associated with an IOFB has been reported at 31%. Intraocular foreign body removal associated with a retinal detachment can be extremely complicated, especially with subretinal IOFBs located away from the entry site of the IOFB. It has been found that an IOFB left in the subretinal space after PPV is a nidus for PVR formation regardless of IOFB composition and recommend removing a subretinal IOFB through the existing retinal hole or another retinotomy site. Postoperative IOFB-related retinal detachment can also contribute to poor visual outcome, with large IOFB and endophthalmitis as the strongest predictive factors.

Late rhegmatogenous retinal detachments have been documented after posterior segment IOFB removal. Proliferative vitreoretinopathy is another major risk factor for vision loss after an IOFB injury. Cardillo and colleagues reported an 11% rate of PVR after IOFB, with vitreous haemorrhage as a major risk factor. PVR can lead to chronic non-repairable total retinal detachment, with resulting phthisis bulbi requiring enuclea-

tion. Increased depth of IOFB penetration and more extensive, intraocular injuries are associated with higher rates of PVR. Intraocular foreign body injuries, which penetrate through the retina, develop PVR in up to 75% of the cases. On the contrary, an IOFB, that penetrates into the vitreous cavity or ricochets off the retina surface, only carries roughly a 5% rate of PVR formation.

Post-traumatic endophthalmitis has historically averaged 4 to 8% of all IOFB injuries, with up to 30% in rural settings. Bacteria, such as *B. cereus, Staphylococcus aureus, Streptococcus pneumoniae,* and *Pseudomonas aeruginosa* can lead to extremely poor visual results. Reported risk factors for post-traumatic endophthalmitis include delay in primary closure, delay in IOFB removal, disruption of the crystalline lens, and sustaining ocular trauma in a rural setting.

- *Clinical features associated with favourable visual acuity* outcomes in post-traumatic endophthalmitis include better presenting visual acuity, culture of a non-virulent organism, lack of a retinal detachment, absence of clinical endophthalmitis, and shorter wound length.

- *Broad-spectrum systemic antibiotics* with third- or fourth-generation fluoroquinolones have been increasingly used by ophthalmologists after open globe injuries. The levels of orally administered fluoroquinolones in the aqueous and vitreous have been shown to exceed the MIC90 of the major organisms causing post-traumatic endophthalmitis.

- *A meta-analysis of all published post-traumatic endophthalmitis* cases reported an average rate of 8.7% in open globe injuries. Recent published studies have suggested a reduction in this rate of post-traumatic endophthalmitis to 1–2% over the last 10 years.

CONCLUSION

Current IOFB removal techniques have advanced with improving retinal imaging using ultrasound and helical CT scan for localization and preoperative planning and improved PPV techniques and instrumentation combined with newer broad-spectrum antibiotics. All these put together have improved the visual outcome and mitigated complications from IOFB injuries.

BIBLIOGRAPHY

1. Al-Omran AM, Abboud EB, Abu El-Asrar AM. Microbiologic spectrum and visual outcome of post-traumatic endophthalmitis. Retina 2007; 27(2): 236–242.
2. Boldt HC, Pulido JS, Blodi CF, et al. Rural endophthalmitis. Ophthalmology 1989; 96(12): 1722–1726.
3. Chow DR, Garretson BR, Kuczynski B, et al. External versus internal approach to the removal of metallic intraocular foreign bodies. Retina. 2000; 20(4):364–369.
4. Coleman DJ, Lucas BC, Rondeau MJ, et al. Management of intraocular foreign bodies. Ophthalmology 1987; 94(12):1647–1653.
5. Colyer MH, Weber ED, Weichel ED, et al. Delayed intraocular foreign body removal without endophthalmitis during Operations Iraqi Freedom and Enduring Freedom. Ophthalmology 2007; 114(8):1439–1447.
6. de Smet MD, Mura M. Minimally invasive surgery vs endoscopic retinal detachment repair in patients with media opacities. Eye 2008; 22(5):662–665.
7. De Souza S, Howcroft MJ. Management of posterior segment intraocular foreign bodies: 14 years' experience. Can J Ophthalmol 1999; 34(1):23–29.
8. El-Asrar AM, Al-Amro SA, Khan NM, et al. Retinal detachment after posterior segment intra-ocular foreign body injuries. Int Ophthalmol 1998; 22(6):369–375.
9. El-Asrar AM, Al-Amro SA, Khan NM, et al. Visual outcome and prognostic factors after vitrectomy for posterior segment foreign bodies. Eur J Ophthalmol 2000; 10(4):304–311.
10. Ersanli D, Sonmez M, Unal M, et al. Management of retinal detachment due to closed globe injury by pars plana vitrectomy with and without scleral buckling. Retina 2006; 26(1):32–36.
11. Fison PN, Chignell AH. Diplopia after retinal detachment surgery. Br J Ophthalmol 1987; 71(7):521–525.
12. Gallemore RP, Bokosky JE. Penetrating kerato-plasty with vitreoretinal surgery using the Eckardt temporary keratoprosthesis: modified technique allowing use of larger corneal grafts. Cornea 1995; 14(1):33–38.
13. Gelender H, Vaiser A, Snyder WB, et al. Temporary keratoprosthesis for combined penetrating keratoplasty, pars plana vitrectomy, and repair of retinal detachment. Ophthalmology 1988; 95(7):897–901.
14. Greven CM, Engelbrecht NE, Slusher MM, et al. Intraocular foreign bodies: management, prognostic factors, and visual outcomes. Ophthalmology 2000; 107(3):608–612.
15. Hariprasad SM, Shah GK, Mieler WF, et al. Vitreous and aqueous penetration of orally administered moxifloxacin in humans. Arch Ophthalmol 2006; 124(2):178–182.
16. Imrie FR, Cox A, Foot B, et al. Surveillance of intra-ocular foreign bodies in the UK. Eye. May 25, 2007.
17. Irvine AR. Old and new techniques combined in the management of intraocular foreign bodies. Ann Ophthalmol 1981; 13(1):41–47.
18. Jonas JB, Budde WM. Early versus late removal of retained intraocular foreign bodies. Retina 1999; 19(3):193–197.
19. Jonas JB, Knorr HL, Budde WM. Prognostic factors inocular injuries caused by intraocular or retrobulbar foreignbodies. Ophthalmology 2000; 107(5):823–828.
20. Klistorner A, Fraser C, Garrick R, et al. Correlation between full-field and multifocal VEPs in optic neuritis. Doc Ophthalmol 2008; 116(1):19–27.
21. Kramer M, Kramer MR, Blau H, et al. Intravitreal Voriconazole for the treatment of endogenous Aspergillus endophthalmitis. Ophthalmology 2006; 113(7):1184–1186.
22. Kuhn F, Morris R. Posterior segment intraocular foreign bodies: management in the vitrectomy era. Ophthalmology 2000; 107(5):821–822.
23. Kwong JS, Munk PL, Lin DT, et al. Real-time Sonography in ocular trauma. AJR Am J Roentgenol 1992; 158(1) 179–182.
24. Lakits A, Prokesch R, Scholda C, et al. Multi-planar imaging in the preoperative assessment of metallic intraocular foreign bodies. Helical computed tomography versus conventional computed tomography. Ophthalmology 1998; 105(9):1679–1685.
25. Lieb DF, Scott IU, Flynn HW Jr, et al. Open globe injurieswith positive intraocular cultures: factors influencing final visual acuity outcomes. Ophthalmology 2003; 110(8):1560–1566.
26. Machemer R. A new concept for vitreous surgery; Surgical technique and complications. Am J Ophthalmol 1972; 74(6):1022–1033.
27. Pavlovic S. Primary intraocular lens implanta-tion duringpars plana vitrectomy and intraretinal foreign body removal. Retina 1999; 19(5): 430–436.

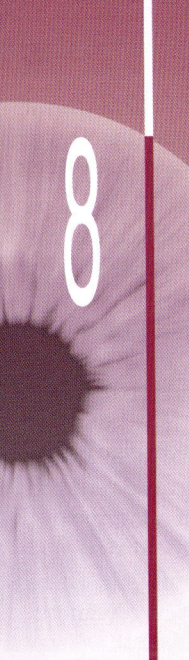

8

SYMPATHETIC OPHTHALMITIS

INTRODUCTION AND EPIDEMIOLOGY

INTRODUCTION

It is a bilateral, diffuse, chronic, non-necrotizing granulomatous inflammation of the uveal tract in one eye following injury or surgery to the contralateral eye. The injured eye is known as exciting eye and the fellow eye developing inflammation weeks to years later is called as sympathizing eye. Earliest clinical description of the disease was reported by William Mackenzie in 1840. Later on Ernst Fuchs in 1905 described the disease in detail including the uveal nodules, which had been noted earlier by Dalen, and so now known as 'Dalen-Fuchs' nodules.

EPIDEMIOLOGY

As the disease is very rare, its incidence remains speculative with estimated incidence ranging from 0.2 to 0.5% after penetrating ocular injury. Gass reported the incidence after trauma as 0.06%. The incidence after intraocular surgery is estimated to be 0.01%. In a prospective study from Ireland, estimated incidence of 0.03 in 100,000 population was calculated. Vitreoretinal surgery has been documented to be the major inciting factor for the development of sympathetic ophthalmia during recent times with trauma being the second on the list. The incidence with the vitreoretinal surgery has been estimated to be about every 1 in 800 cases undergoing posterior segment surgery. Rare causative factors include anterior segment surgeries, laser therapies, plaque brachytherapy, intravitreal injections and post-irradiation of ocular tumours. No racial predilection has been noted, however, following factors increase the propensity to develop sympathetic ophthalmia:
- Penetrating trauma with uveal incarceration,
- Surgical repair—48 hrs or more after initial injury,
- Site of penetrating injury—ciliary body,
- Size of wound larger than 5 mm, and
- Age of patient—first decade of life.

ETIOLOGY AND PATHOLOGY

ETIOLOGY

Delayed hypersensitivity to uveal–retinal pigment. The definitive etiological factors are still not established, however, experimental evidence suggests an autoimmune, *delayed hypersensitivity reaction to uveal–retinal antigen.*

Debate continues regarding the specific antigen involved. Various antigens implicated are uveal melanin, S antigen derived from retinal rod photoreceptor segments, cellular antigens of RPE and choroidal melanocytes.

Genetic predispositions have also been identified. The disease has strong association with HLA-A11, Cw, –DRB1*04, –DQB1*04, –DR4, –DQw3 and –DRw53.

PATHOLOGY

Typically, it is a granulomatous inflammation of the uveal tract characterized by diffuse lymphocytic infiltration and of epitheloid cells and giant cells the later having phagocytosed pigment. There is classic sparing of choriocapillaris in contrast to VKH. Dalen-Fuchs nodules consist of monocyte-derived cells and hyperplastic RPE cells. The predominance of T lymphocytes in the choroidal infiltrate supports the theory of a T cell-mediated delayed hypersensitivity reaction (Fig. 8.1).

CLINICO-INVESTIGATIVE PROFILE

CLINICAL FEATURES

The time period from injury to presentation can vary from 5 days to even 50 years with about 90% of patients presenting within a year.

The injured and the contralateral eye is referred to as an 'exciting eye' and a 'sympathizing eye', respectively.

Presenting symptoms include mild pain, decreased vision more so involving near vision due to paresis of accommodation, lacrimation and photophobia in sympathizing eye associated with increasing inflammation in the exciting eye. Examination reveals ciliary flush, anterior chamber cells and flare. Anterior chamber reaction ranges from mild to severe with large mutton fat keratic precipitates, inflammatory thickening of iris and broad based posterior synechiae. Although trabecular meshwork blockage can lead to raised IOP, ciliary body shutdown may also cause reduced IOP. Posterior segment lesions include vitritis, papillitis and mid-equitorial multifocal choroiditis which may become confluent. There may be peripapillary choroidal involvement. Exudative retinal detachment and macular oedema may also be present. The typical Dalen-Fuchs nodules are small hypopigmented yellowish creamy circular spots at the level of RPE which histologically appear as choroidal granulomata (Fig. 8.2). They are composed of macrophages, lymphocytes and epithelioid cells. Though typical, and found in 30% cases but are not pathognomonic of sympathetic ophthalmia since they are also seen in Vogt-Koyanagi-Harada disease, sarcoidosis and tubercular uveitis.

Complications include secondary angle closure or open angle glaucoma, complicated cataract, chronic macular oedema and choroidal neovascularization. Eventually in untreated cases atrophy of the choroid, retina and optic nerve sets in, which may eventually lead to phthisis bulbi.

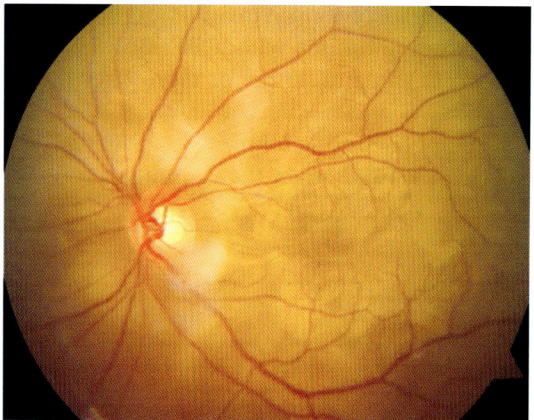

Fig. 8.1 *Fundus photograph of a patient with sympathetic ophthalmitis showing yellowish creamy circular spots at the level of RPE suggestive of typical Dalen–Fuchs nodules*

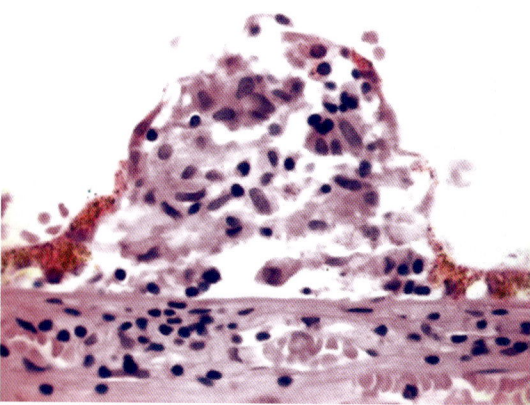

Fig. 8.2 Histopathology of Dalen-Fuchs nodule

INVESTIGATIONS

No clinical diagnostic tests can reliably confirm the diagnosis of sympathetic ophthalmia. The diagnosis is initially based on conspicuous clinical features, history of trauma and ultimately on histopathological examination which is rarely possible. However, following tests may help in narrowing down the diagnosis.

1. *FFA.* Two types of patterns are seen. Most frequently during the acute phase of the disease multifocal hyperfluorescent dots seen in early phase of angiogram which leak during late phase. In advanced cases, if pigment epithelium is severely damaged, pooling of dye under neurosensory retinal detachment is observed as in VKH (Fig. 8.3). Late staining of the disc may be seen, even if the disc does not show oedema.

The second less common pattern is characterized by lesions that block fluorescence during the early phase and hyperfluorescence during the late phases as in APMPPE. Dalen-Fuchs nodules may appear as hypo- or hyperfluorescent lesions. During the chronic stage of disease, absence of RPE is seen as 'window defects'.

2. *ICGA.* It also shows two patterns. Active lesions show hypocyanescence in the inter-mediate phase of the angiogram which fades in later phases. In atrophic areas, hypocyanescence remains till the late phases. It has been used to document and monitor response to therapy.

3. *OCT.* It is useful for monitoring the retinal detachment and retinal oedema.

4. *USG.* B-scan demonstrates the extent of choroidal thickening (Fig. 8.4).

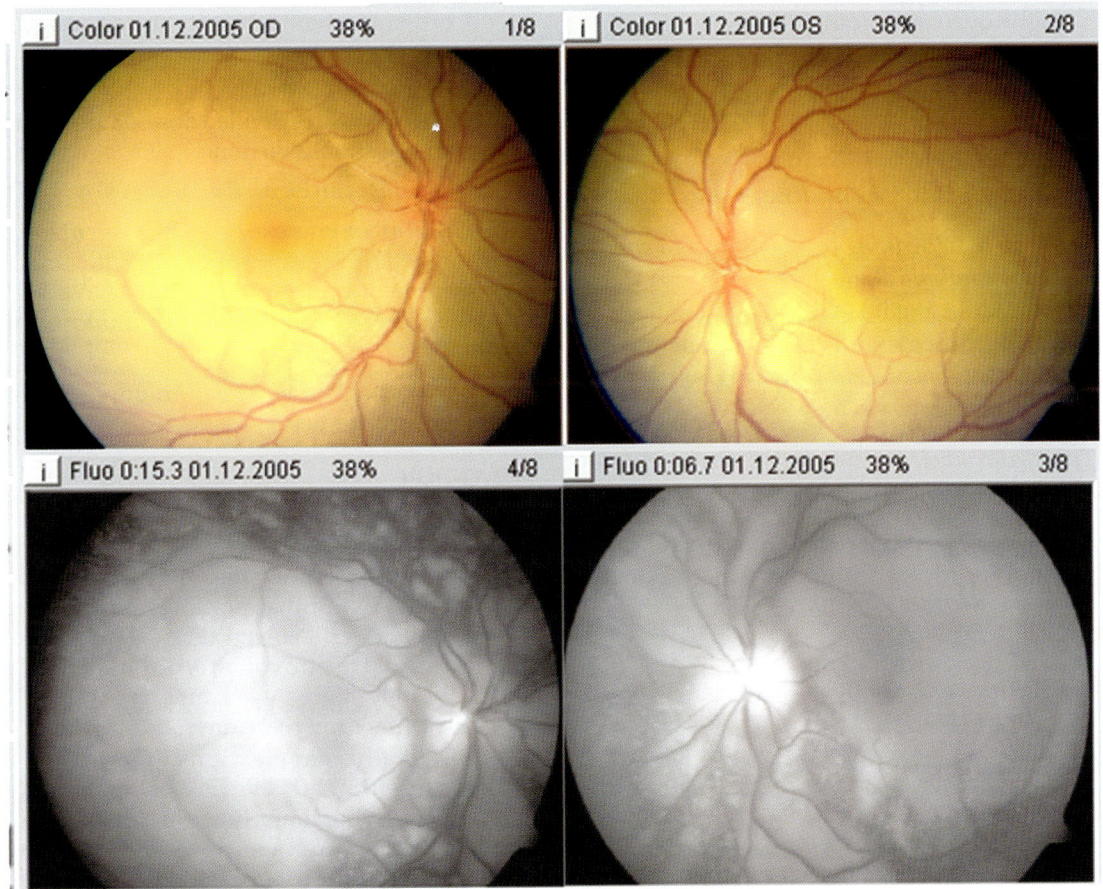

Fig. 8.3 *FFA showing pooling of dye in the late frames under the neurosensory retina suggestive of exudative RD in a case of sympathetic ophthalmitis*

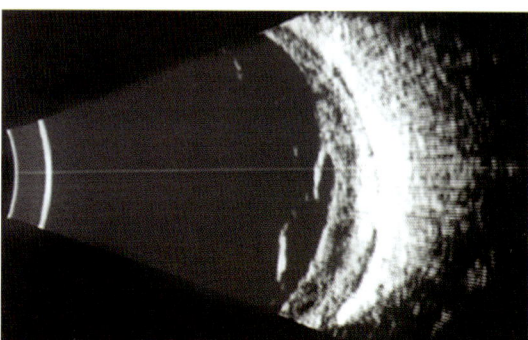

Fig. 8.4 USG B-scan showing choroidal thickening

DIFFERENTIAL DIAGNOSIS

The diagnosis of sympathetic ophthalmia is clinical. Following differential diagnosis of bilateral granulomatous panuveitis must be kept in mind.

• Vogt-Koyanagi-Harada disease

• Sarcoidosis

• Tuberculosis

• Syphilis

• Bilateral phacoanaphylactic uveitis

VKH can have striking resembalance to sympathetic ophthalmia along with presence of Dalen-Fuchs nodule. But it lacks history of antecedent trauma and has presence of extraocular findings, like vitiligo, sensorineural hearing loss, poliosis and meningismus.

Tubercular uveitis can be ruled out by chest X-ray, mantoux and sputum for AFB.

Sarcoid uveitis is ruled out by negative mantoux, elevated angiotensin converting enzyme (ACE) levels, lysozyme and contrast enhanced CT chest.

Syphilitic uveitis should be ruled out by VDRL, RPR, FTA-ABS tests.

Phacoanaphylactic uveitis another entity that should be considered in differential diagnosis. It is characterized by zonal granulomatous inflammation involving lens. However, it is usually unilateral and aspiration of lens material results in recovery.

TREATMENT AND PREVENTION

TREATMENT

Systemic immunosuppressive therapy in the form of oral prednisolone at 1–2 mg/kg bodyweight is the firstline treatment; in very severe inflammatory disease, intravenous methyl prednisolone as pulse therapy may be required followed by oral steroids as long as disease activity persists, followed by slow taper and maintenance therapy with low doses at least for 3–6 months.

Topical steroid drops are given concomitantly with *cycloplegics* to avoid synechia formation.

Cyclosporine can be used, in patients who are intolerant or not responding to steroid therapy at the dose of 5 mg/kg/day and tapered to a maintenance dose of 1 mg/kg/day after signs of clinical improvement. Renal function and blood pressure should be monitored in such patients. It can be used with or without steroid.

Azathioprine has been used at 100 to 150 mg per day in two or three divided doses. Monitoring of blood cells should be done.

Mycophenolate can be used at dosages of 1g BD.

Other useful immunosuppressive agents are chlorambucil, cyclophosphamide and tacrolimus. Daclizumab and infliximab have also been tried in resistant cases and found to be useful.

Note. In resistant cases, use of multiple agents can be advantageous.

PREVENTION

Primary prevention involves early repair of penetrating injury with excision of non-viable uveal tissue. Considering the extremely low risk of sympathetic ophthalmia after penetrating trauma due to well-evolved surgical techniques and administration of steroids; primary enucleation of injured eye is not an acceptable modality of therapy these days.

Theoretically, enucleation done before 2 weeks can eliminate the risk of developing sympathetic ophthalmia, however, in the era of steroids and immunosuppressive therapy primary enucleation is considered extremely rarely; if at all it is performed it has only diagnostic value.

PROGNOSIS

It depends on severity of the inflammation. The more severe is the inflammation the worse the ocular complication and visual outcome. Prompt high dose steroid therapy with immuno-suppressive medication as and when needed, however, can result in vision ≥6/12 in the sympathizing eye in 50% of the cases.

SUMMARY

Sympathetic ophthalmia is a potentially devasta-ting condition. Hence the role of early surgery for trauma and immunosuppressive therapy is of paramount importance for the prevention of the disease. High index of suspicion is required for identification and treatment of the disease early in its course. As of now the treating surgeons are more likely to salvage the injured eye and less likely to suggest enucleation given its favourable response to steroid therapy.

BIBLIOGRAPHY

1. Arevalo JF, Garcia RA, Al-Dhibi HA, Sanchez JG, Suarez-Tata L. Update on sympathetic ophthalmia. Middle East Afr J Ophthalmol. 2012 Jan; 19(1):13–21.

2. BenErza D. sympathetic ophthalmia. In: BenErza, editor. Ocular Inflammation, Basic and Clinical Concepts. London: MartinDunitz Ltd; 1999.

3. Chang GC, Young LH. Sympathetic ophthalmia. Semin Ophthalmol. 2011 Sep; 26(4–5):316–320.

4. Chu XK, Chan C-C. Sympathetic ophthalmia: to the twenty-first century and beyond. J Ophthalmic Inflamm Infect. 2013; 3(1):49.

5. Kilmartin DJ, Dick AD, Forrester JV. Prospective surveillance of sympathetic ophthalmia in UK and Republic of Ireland. Br J Ophthalmol 2000; 84:259–283.

6. Morak GE Jr. Recent advances in sympathetic ophthalmia. Surv Ophthalmol 1979; 24:141–156.

7. Nussenblatt, RB, Whitcup, SM, Palestine AG. Uveitis: fundamentals and clinical practice. Philadelphia: Mosby, 2004.

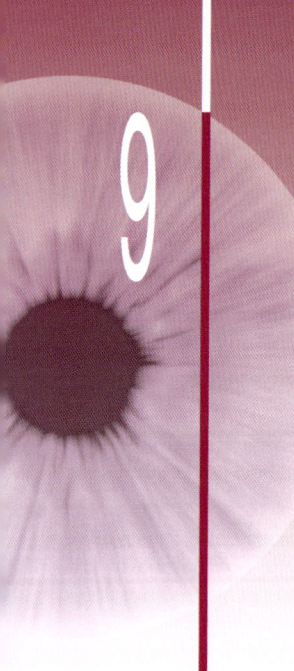

9

POST-TRAUMATIC ENDOPHTHALMITIS

GENERAL CONSIDERATIONS
- Incidence
- Microbial spectrum and risk factors

CLINICAL PROFILE AND MANAGEMENT
- Clinical picture

- Prophylaxis
- Treatment
- Prognosis

Summary

GENERAL CONSIDERATIONS

INCIDENCE

The incidence of endophthalmitis after trauma is 100 times more than after surgery. The reported incidence ranges from 3.1 to 11.9% of open globe injuries in the absence of an IOFB. The incidence in the presence of IOFB ranges from 3.8 to 48.1%, and a still higher incidence is reported in eyes with retained IOFBs contaminated with organic matter from a rural setting. In a study, the occurrence of post-traumatic endophthalmitis was reported in 30% in rural districts in contrast to 11% in urban districts. Post-traumatic endophthalmitis (PTE) comprises approximately 25–30% of all cases of infectious endophthalmitis.

MICROBIAL SPECTRUM AND RISK FACTORS

Microbial spectrum

Post-traumatic endophthalmitis (PTE) can be categorized as culture-independent or culture-positive. The former includes all clinically diagnosed cases of endophthalmitis and the latter includes only culture-positive cases. The overall incidence of culture-independent posttraumatic endophthalmitis is higher than culture-positive endophthalmitis cases. It must be understood that the presence of positive cultures following

open globe trauma is not synonymous with the development of post-traumatic endophthalmitis. Ariyasu et al cultured 30 ruptured globes. Although one-third of these patients had positive anterior chamber fluid cultures, no patient developed endophthalmitis. In our experience, contamination after OGI was seen in 26% cases but only 18% developed endophthalmitis. Similar to postoperative endophthalmitis, two-thirds of the bacteria in PTE are Gram-positive and 10 to 15% are Gram-negative and 15% are fungi. Culture positivity is seen in 38–60% cases of post-traumatic endophthalmitis. In contrast to postoperative endophthalmitis, virulent Bacillus species are the common pathogens in post-traumatic endophthalmitis. Polymicrobial infection is seen in 10–30% cases (Table 9.1).

Table 9.1 *Microbial spectrum of post-traumatic endophthalmitis (Kunimoto, et al, 2007)*

Microbe	South India (%)	West (%)
S. epidermidis	21.2	8–21
S. aureus	4.4	6
Staphylococcal sp	0.9	0
Streptococcal sp	26.5	8–21
Bacillus sp	17.7	17–32
Gram-negative	22.1	11–18
Filamentous fungi	17.7	4–14

126

Risk factors

The risk factors for PTE include rural setting trauma, vegetative matter associated injury, delayed repair after 24 hours, dirty wound, age greater than 50 years, large wound size, location of wound, ocular tissue prolapse, placement of primary intraocular lens (IOL), extent of injury and lens disruption. Thompson and coworkers reported endophthalmitis in 13.6% of 88 ruptured globe cases with lens disruption and in only 0.9% (1 case) of 117 cases with an intact crystalline lens. In their series, when both an IOFB and lens rupture were present, 15.6% of cases developed endophthalmitis. Delayed repair beyond 24 hours is another risk factor for PTE. The risk of PTE was 2.3% versus 15.7%, if the repair was delayed by >24 hours. The sports related injuries, like due to fish hook or homemade bow and arrow are at higher risk of endophthalmitis. Seventy-five per cent of bow and arrow injuries in India develop endophthalmitis. The presence of IOFB leads to two fold increase in relative risk of PTE. Wood IOFBs (18%) may be associated with a statistically higher risk of infectious endophthalmitis as compared to metallic IOFBs (9%).

CLINICAL PROFILE AND MANAGEMENT

CLINICAL PICTURE

The start, course and symptoms of endophthalmitis after trauma are very varied, corresponding to the causative organisms. Symptoms of extreme pain with hypopyon and vitritis indicate an infection until proven otherwise. It is present at initial presentation in 50% cases of post-traumatic endophthalmitis. The peak interval between trauma and endophthalmitis is 3–6 days.

Initial symptoms are usually pain, redness, purulent discharge, photophobia out of proportion to the injury and progressive visual loss with increasing intraocular inflammation.

Clinical signs are lid oedema, ciliary injection corneal clouding, hypopyon, loss of red reflex and vitreous clouding (Fig. 9.1). Retinal periphlebitis is an early sign of endophthalmitis but it may not be discernible due to compromising media opacities.

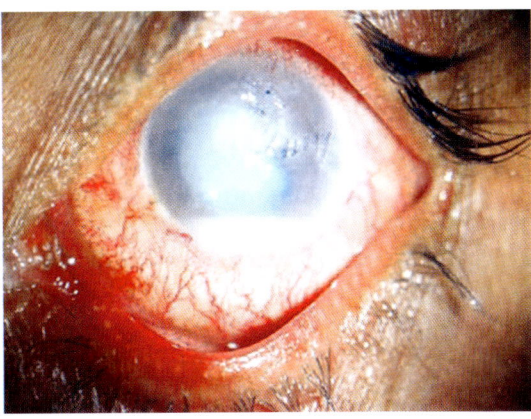

Fig. 9.1 *Clinical photograph of a Zone I injury with corneal clouding and hypopyon and total loss of red reflex suggestive of post-traumatic endophthalmitis*

Bacillus species traumatic endophthalmitis

There is high incidence of *Bacillus species in traumatic endophthalmitis.*

It is characterized by:

- *Rapid onset* (<24 hours) with high risk of progression to panophthalmitis and poor visual outcome.
- *Symptoms.* The patient has very severe pain, chemosis, large hypopyon and rapidly progressive lid oedema and proptosis.
- *Ring-shaped corneal infiltrate* is another characteristic but late sign.
- *Intraocular gas buble* is diagnostic of clostridia but has also been reported in *B. cereus* traumatic endophthalmitis.

Fungal traumatic endophthalmitis

Fungi are causative organism in 10–15% case of PTE. Fungal endophthalmitis usually commences only weeks to months after the injury. Inflammation that progresses slowly following primary repair may be indicative of fungal PTE in India. It is more common if the injury is with vegetative matter or there is soil contamination.

Characteristic signs include fluffy ball opacities and string of pearls in the vitreous. The vitritis is of chronic nature and there may be white infiltrates around the primary wound.

Reactive endophthalmitis

Metallic non-magnetic IOFBs (e.g. copper) can cause non-infectious inflammation, termed reactive endophthalmitis, if left in the eye.

Copper foreign body. A 100% copper IOFB can cause a rapid sterile endophthalmitis-like reaction with hypopyon. Lower per cent copper IOFBs can cause chalcosis that includes chronic uveitis, green discolouration of iris, greenish-brown discolouration of the peripheral cornea (Kayser-Fleischer ring, due to copper deposition in Descemet's membrane) and sunflower cataract. IOFBs containing greater than 85% copper can cause more severe reaction causing vision loss (Chapter 7).

Iron foreign bodies are the most common RIOFBs. These foreign bodies once are retained usually do not cause endophthalmitis since velocity with which they travel and the generated heat make these sterile. However, these are reactive and will cause reactive endophthalmitis. IOFBs with free iron content can cause siderosis; the iron ions interact with the epithelial cells causing cytotoxity with cell degeneration and visual loss (Chapter 7).

Glass, plastic, and porcelain are inert materials that generally are well tolerated in the eye.

Note. However, all IOFBs (inert or non-inert) increase the risk of endophthalmitis because they may be contaminated with infectious material.

Plain radiography and computed tomography scans are used to detect IOFBs. In order to detect small objects by computed tomography, the cut width should be less than 2 mm. B-scan ultrasound may be used to help locate radiolucent foreign bodies, such as glass or plastic. Extreme caution should be taken, if there is any suspicion of an open globe injury. Minimal pressure should be applied during echography, and the probe should be placed on the eyelid and not directly on the ocular surface.

MANAGEMENT

Diagnosis

Any inflammation in a case of trauma more than anticipated should be taken as endophthalmitis.

All PTE cases where the view of the posterior segment is not possible must be subjected to a gentle ultrasound to rule out the presence of intraocular foreign body (high echogenicity with after-shadow) and for the confirmation of endophthalmitis. An echo-free vitreous cavity rules out endophthalmitis whereas mild to moderate echogenicity in the vitreous cavity along with anterior segment signs confirms PTE (Fig. 9.2). It also gives information regarding retinal detachment and other membranes. Ultrasonography may be done after primary repair to evaluate PTE. X-ray orbit can be done pre-operatively to look for intraocular foreign body.

Investigations

Appropriate cultures and stains are required to establish the type of infectious agent in the eye in case the examination reveals serious doubt of endophthalmitis. Otherwise also, it is advisable to obtain vitreous and aqueous samples before initiation of the therapy. The collection of sample is recommended under general anaesthesia, however, in less severe cases of trauma, it may be taken under topical anaesthesia.

Vitreous biopsy should be preferred over a vitreous tap and the sample is collected in an operation room setting with the help of a vitreous cutter without starting the infusion in order to avoid dilution of the sample. If the vitreoretina facility is lacking, then vitreous tap may be taken by needle aspiration with a

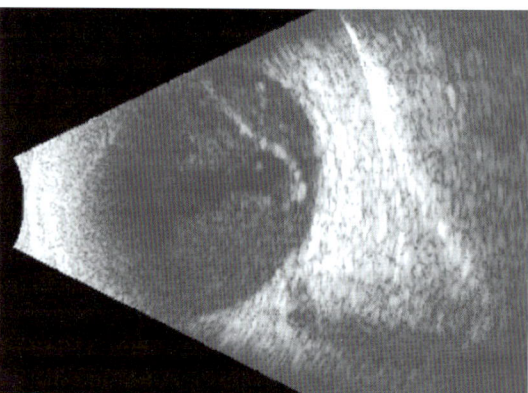

Fig. 9.2 *Multiple moderate to high echogenic point like echoes in the vitreous cavity suggestive of vitreous exudates in endophthalmitis*

22-gauge needle 4 mm from the limbus infero-temporally. Aqueous can be taken, in addition, with an anterior chamber tap with 26gauge needle on a tuberculin syringe aspirating 0.2 ml of aqueous.

Smear examination. The samples should be examined by Gram stain, 20% KOH mount and calcoflour white stain for fungus.

Culture. The samples should be promptly inoculated on fresh, blood agar, chocolate agar and thioglycollate broth and incubated at 37°C. A separate Sabouraud's plate is incubated at room temperature for fungi. All foreign bodies removed from the eye should be submitted to culture and depending upon culture report and sensitivity, the treatment of endophthalmitis may be modified. About 60% of presumptive infectious endophthalmitis are culture-positive. The culture report not only helps in better treatment but can also prognosticate the condition. The prognosis is better with gram positive, however, it is poorer with gram-negative and fungus but grave with with *B. cereus.*

Prophylaxis

At the time of repair, the wound should be properly irrigated to clean any debris on it. Any dead or dirty looking tissue should be sent for cultures. Cultures may be obtained from the wound, conjunctiva, anterior chamber, and/or vitreous which are then inoculated on blood and chocolate agar. Thioglycollate broth and heart-brain infusion are also used as a culture medium, and Gram stain of excised tissue or fluid should be performed. Fungal infection can be detected via Grocott-Gomori methenamine-silver stain, periodic acid–Schiff stain, by culturing on Sabouraud's dextrose, or by potassium hydroxide (KOH) preparation. The aqueous and vitreous samples can be inoculated directly into blood culture bottles.

Systemic antibiotics. After repair, systemic antibiotics in addition to topical with wider organism coverage should be used routinely for prophylaxis against PTE. Quinolones are the preferred intravenous antibiotics since they cross blood–retinal barrier.

In our practice, prophylactic intravenous quinolones are given in trauma cases for at least 5 days. These antibiotics cross the blood–ocular barrier reasonably well and may reach therapeutic levels in the eye. Their entry into the eye is also aided by the weakening of the blood–ocular barrier that results from infection and trauma-induced inflammation.

Prophylactic intravitreal antibiotic injections is debatable. The decision to use these at the time of initial repair depends on whether the patient is a high-risk case for endophthalmitis—provided that the injections can be given safely and reliably into the vitreous cavity. In our experience, prophylactic intravitreal antibiotics in absence of foreign body decreases the incidence of post-traumatic endophthalmitis to negligible. *Subconjunctival steroids* should be considered along with antibiotics at the time of primary surgical repair of a ruptured globe.

Treatment

The principles of management are the same for post-traumatic and acute postoperative endophthalmitis, but the visual outcome is poorer in the former. After the diagnosis of PTE is established, early pars plana vitrectomy is recommended as soon as possible provided the corneal clarity permits. If the same is not possible, immediate intravitreal antibiotics are administered and vitreous biopsy/tap sample is sent for microbiological evaluation and PCR. However, if the facility exists, a PPV may be done with a keratoprosthesis.

Medical treatment

Intravitreal antibiotics given include combination of intravitreal vancomycin (1 mg/0.1 ml) and intravitreal ceftazidime (2.25 mg/0.1 ml) through pars plana (Table 9.2). The type and nature of the injury may guide the choice of antibiotics. For example, Clostridium should be considered, if soil contamination of the wound is present. Fungal infection should be considered, if there is contamination with vegetable matter, however due to high macular toxicity antifungals should be avoided without positive smear or culture proof of fungal endophthalmitis. Results of the culture, if obtained at the initial open globe repair, may also

Table 9.2 *Treatment chart of traumatic endophthalmitis as per the ESCRS guidelines*

Intravitreal injection	Bacterial	Vancomycin 1 mg/0.1 ml
		Ceftazidime 2.25 mg/0.1 ml
	B. cereus	Clindamycin 0.5 mg/0.1 ml
	Fungus	Amphotericin B 5 µg/0.1 ml
		Voriconazole 50 µg/0.1 ml
		Dexamethasone 400 µg/0.1 ml
Systemic therapy	Levofloxacin	100 mg i.v. OD × 5–7 days
	Vancomycin	1 gm i.v. every 12h 5–7 days
	Ceftazidime	1 gm i.v. every 12 h 5–7 days
	Voriconazole	Oral 400 mg BD × 10–15 days
	Fluconazole	Oral 100 mg BD × 10–15 days
Topical therapy	Vancomycin	5% every hour
	Ceftazidime	5% every hour
	Voriconazole	1% every hour
	Amphotericin B	0.1% to 0.3% every hour
	Fluconazole	0.2% every hour
	Miconazole	1% every hour
	Natamycin	5% every hour

direct the choice of antibiotics. For injuries that run a high risk of contamination with Bacillus species (homemade bow and arrow injuries), intravitreal clindamycin (0.5 mg/0.1 ml) should be given (Fig. 9.3).

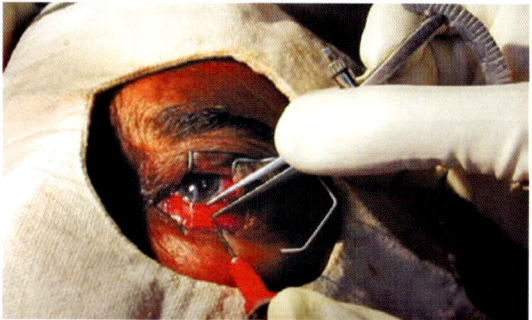

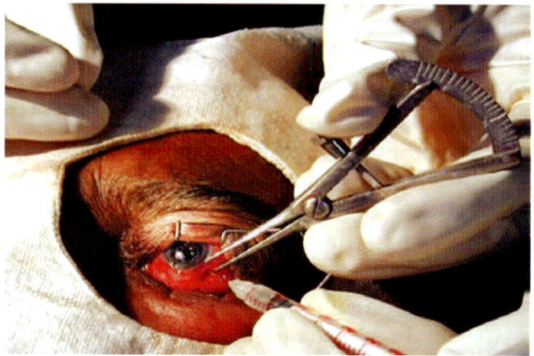

Fig. 9.3 *Vitreous tap and injection with 30 G needle 4 mm from limbus in pseudophakic patient*

Intravitreal dexamethasone of 400 µg in 0.1 ml may be added along with antimicrobial agent. Systemic steroids may also be instituted under close observation in the dosage of 1 mg/kg.

Systemic antibiotics. Systemically, it is preferred to administer the same antibiotics as given intravitreally in order to maintain adequate concentration of the antibiotic even after 48 hours of intravitreal administration. There is no role of oral or intramuscular route, only intravenous route is recommended for antibiotics.

It is advisable to start the intravenous therapy before the primary repair of open globe injury whereas intravitreal injection is given intraoperatively particularly in suspected cases of PTE associated with vegetative injury and soil contamination.

Intensive topical therapy with antibiotics, antifungals, cycloplegics, and steroid should be started on first postoperative day.

Surgical treatment: Vitrectomy

The introduction of advanced and safe vitrectomy machines and improved expertise of vitreoretinal surgical techniques have led to the acceptance of recommendation of early vitrectomy in most cases of suspected traumatic endophthalmitis. So far only core vitrectomy used to be performed; however, performing a more complete vitrectomy consistent with safe intraoperative visualization (proportional PPV, a term coined by Robert Morris) may increase the success rate in restoring/salvaging macular function. Vitrectomy in endophthalmitis is beneficial by debulking the load of inflammatory debris and toxins, allowing better penetration of antimicrobial agent and by removing the scaffold for tractional membranes. Recently, the administration of silicone oil after completion of vitrectomy has been reported to be beneficial not only in reducing the postoperative complications but also in containing the infection and recurrences of endophthalmitis.

PROGNOSIS

The visual prognosis is poorer in post-traumatic endophthalmitis than postoperative endophthalmitis. It is further poorer in geriatric and pediatric age group. However, prognosis of post-traumatic endophthalmitis depends upon the following factors:

- Extent of injury, i.e. involvement of lens and vitreous
- Retention of intraocular foreign body (RIOFB)
- Concurrent retinal detachment
- Virulence and type of organism
- Time lag in the diagnosis and institution of the therapy.
- Availability of vitreoretinal operation room facility.

The prognosis is poorer in PTE because of various reasons. The diagnosis is delayed as signs of endophthalmitis are often masked due to disrupted anatomy, polymicrobial infection is seen in 10–30% cases and more virulent organisms including Bacillus are cultured from 20–40% cases.

Main causes of poor visual outcome after treatment include recurrent/chronic endophthalmitis, macular infarction, optic atrophy, epiretinal membranes and macular oedema.

Although the prognosis in traumatic endophthalmitis has improved in the last two decades but still it is not favourable. Success is defined by many authors as retrieving 3/60 (20/400) or better visual acuity and it has been reported to be 40–50% by most of the series.

SUMMARY

Open globe injury is a grave clinical condition but an association of endophthalmitis is catastrophe. It is a formidable clinical challenge both in diagnosis and management since the signs are often masked due to disrupted anatomy. Availability of vitreoretinal expertise and operating room facility provide a timely intervention thereby containing infection, early removal of RIOFB and restoration of concurrent RD, if any. Thus early diagnosis and prompt treatment helps in improving the visual outcome.

BIBLIOGRAPHY

1. ESCRS reference 2012. Barry Handout. To be added.
2. Kunimoto DY, Das T, Sharma S, et al. Microbiologic spectrum and susceptibility of isolates: Part II. Post-traumatic endophthalmitis. Endophthalmitis research group. Am J Ophthalmol 1999 Aug; 128(2): 242–244.
3. Soheilian M, Rafati N, Mohebbi MR, Yazdani S, Habibabadi HF, Feghhi M, Shahriary HA, Eslamipour J, Piri N, Peyman GA. Traumatic Endophthalmitis Trial Research Group: Prophylaxis of acute post-traumatic bacterial endophthalmitis: a multi-center, randomized clinical trial of intraocular antibiotic injection, report 2. Arch Ophthalmol 2007; 125:460–465.

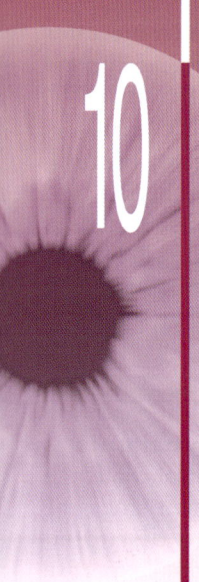

NEURO-OPHTHALMIC TRAUMA

10.1 TRAUMATIC OPTIC NEUROPATHY
- Introduction and applied anatomy
- Epidemiology
- Classification and pathophysiology
- Clinical profile and management

10.2 TRAUMATIC LESIONS OF VISUAL PATHWAY
- Traumatic lesion of chiasma
- Retrochiasmal traumatic lesions

10.3 TRAUMA TO OCULAR MOTOR SYSTEM
- Traumatic lesions of extraocular muscles
- Trauma to ocular motor nerves
- Traumatic central ocular motor dysfunction

10.4 TRAUMA TO TRIGEMINAL AND FACIAL NERVES
- Introduction

- Trauma to trigeminal nerve
- Trauma to facial nerve

10.5 OCULAR MANIFESTATIONS OF HEAD INJURY
Introduction
Ocular manifestations of traumatic brain injury
- Soft tissue signs
- Pupilomotor disorder
- Papilloedema
- Traumatic optic neuropathy and injury to visual pathway
- Disorder of gaze and extraocular movements
- Terson's syndrome
- Ocular disorders in concussive head trauma

10.1 TRAUMATIC OPTIC NEUROPATHY

INTRODUCTION AND APPLIED ANATOMY

INTRODUCTION

Traumatic optic neuropathy refers to any acute insult to the optic nerve secondary to trauma. The optic nerve for all practical purposes is considered an extension of the brain and any injury to this nerve is managed as an injury to the brain. The natural history of traumatic optic neuropathy still remains to be adequately deciphered.

APPLIED ANATOMY

Optic nerve arises as a collection of nerve fibres from the retinal ganglion cells, ultimately acquiring a diameter of 3–4 mm along with its surrounding meningeal sheath. The optic nerve leaves the eye at the optic disc and ends at the level of the optic chiasma where it fuses with the nerve of the opposite side and forms the platform for the cross-over of the nasal fibres (Fig. 10.1.1). The length of the optic nerve measures approximately — 50 mm and is divided anatomically into four portions: *intraocular* (1 mm), *intraorbital* (20–30 mm), *intracanalicular* (5–11 mm) and *intracranial* (7–17 mm).

The optic nerve throughout its tortuous intraorbital course is surrounded by the three meninges which form a protective sheath. This sheath is perforated around 10 mm posterior to the globe by the central retinal artery and vein. Within the confines of the optic canal, the sheath is fused to the periostium of the sphenoid; this is responsible for the relative immobility and rigidity of the optic nerve in the canal.

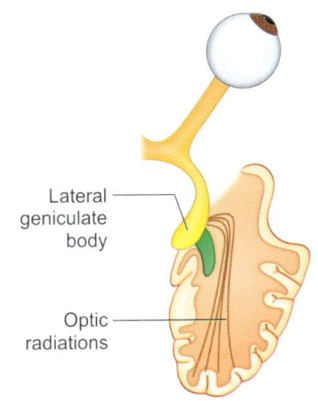

Fig. 10.1.1 *Gross anatomy of optic nerve*

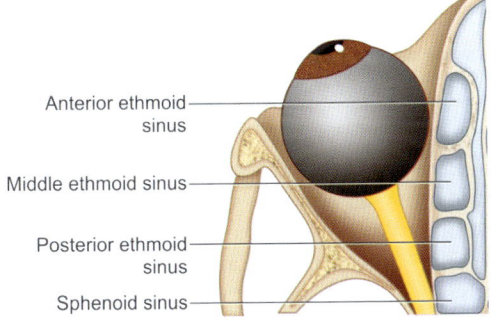

Fig. 10.1.2 *Optic nerve in the orbit and optic nerve canal*

Orbit is a pyramidal space with the optic canal lying at its apex. The optic canal is a perforation in the lesser wing of the sphenoid which serves as a channel for the passage of the optic nerve along with its sheath to the brain and serves as an entrance for the ophthalmic artery into the orbit (Fig. 10.1.2).

EPIDEMIOLOGY

Traumatic optic neuropathy usually occurs in the setting of head injuries mostly as a part of road traffic accidents. Life-threatening injuries which usually occur in such situation take precedence over the management of ocular injury thereby delaying the diagnosis and management of traumatic optic neuropathy. It has been estimated that traumatic optic neuropathy accompanies closed head injuries in about 0.5–5% cases. Majority of cases are seen in males usually in their early thirties. Traumatic optic neuropathy has also been associated with open globe injuries (stab wounds, foreign bodies) or recreational activities (paintball injuries).

CLASSIFICATION AND PATHOPHYSIOLOGY

CLASSIFICATION

Traumatic optic neuropathy may be classified as either anterior or posterior depending upon the site of injury. The mechanism of the trauma classifies the injury as either a direct or indirect injury (Fig. 10.1.3).

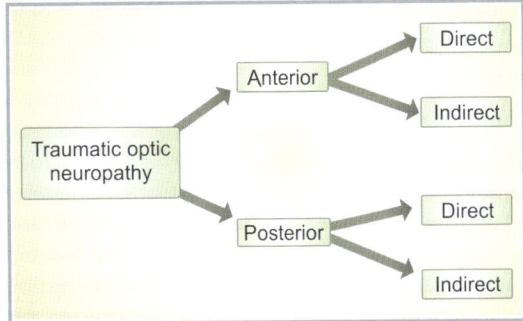

Fig. 10.1.3 *Classification of traumatic optic neuropathy*

PATHOPHYSIOLOGY

Pathophysiology of optic nerve injury is thought to be multifactorial.

Anterior vs posterior traumatic optic neuropathy

Trauma to the anterior part of the optic nerve is associated with injury to the retinal vasculature. Sudden ocular movements at the time of impact may lead to injuries to the anterior optic nerve and at the extreme may lead to optic nerve avulsion (Fig. 10.1.4). Bony pressure in fracture

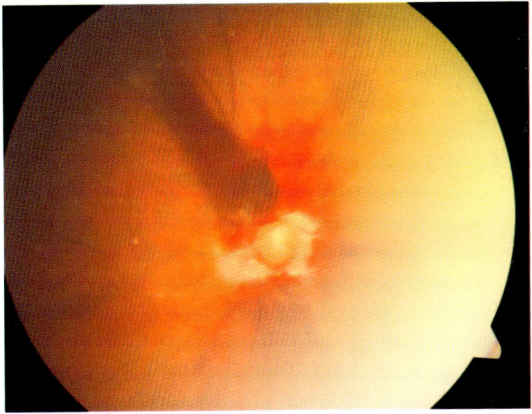

Fig. 10.1.4 *Fundus photograph of a patient with optic nerve avulsion*

of the optic nerve canal, and optic nerve sheath haemorrhage are not uncommonly associated with traumatic optic neuropathy.

Trauma to the anterior part of the optic nerve leads to not only a damage to the axons of the retinal ganglion cells but also to the central retinal artery and vein. Thus a vascular insult also supervenes and may lead to retinal infarcts and haemorrhages, central or branch retinal artery occlusion, central or branch retinal vein occlusion or anterior ischaemic optic neuropathy. Disc oedema is more commonly observed in anterior injuries.

Trauma to the optic nerve posterior to the entry of the central retinal artery and vein usually spares the vascular injury. Axonal injury in the posterior optic nerve does not lead to any acute changes in the optic nerve head, retinal ganglion cells or retinal nerve fibre layer. The fundoscopic evaluation at the time of initial presentation is essentially normal and it is only after a few weeks that the features of axonal injury manifest in the form of optic disc pallor and decreased RNFL thickness.

Direct vs indirect injury

Direct traumatic optic neuropathy is diagnosed when there is a structure either endogenous (bony chip from a fracture site) or exogenous (foreign body) which impinges upon or transcends through the optic nerve. Direct injuries are likely to produce a sudden diminution of vision with less likelihood of recovery, since the injury dissects the axons leading to immediate loss of axonal conduction and a less likelihood of regeneration.

 Direct optic nerve injury results from avulsion, transection, orbital emphysema and haemorrhage while in cases of indirect injury the deformative shearing forces travel along the bony walls to the optic nerve usually at the level of the optic canal.

 The posterior part of the optic nerve is immobile as the sheath of the optic nerve is adherent to the canal wall; furthermore the canal wall itself is non-compliant and thus not able to accommodate oedema or haemorrhage. In this case, any swelling of the optic nerve would produce an effect of compartment syndrome.

Indirect traumatic optic neuropathy is diagnosed when no structural impingement is found to be the cause of traumatic optic neuropathy. Indirect trauma is the forces transmitted to the optic nerve at the time of trauma.

• *Posterior indirect optic neuropathy* is the most common cause of traumatic optic neuropathy with the most common site of injury being the optic canal followed by the intracranial portion of the optic nerve. Despite being the most common cause of traumatic optic neuropathy, posterior indirect injuries usually bear the most favourable prognosis with spontaneous visual improvement also occurring at a variable time after the initial insult.

Primary versus secondary optic nerve injuries

A concept of primary and secondary injuries has been proposed.

Primary injury results in mechanical shearing of the optic nerve axons with disturbance in the microcirculation. The mechanical stress on the retinal ganglion cells is an irreversible process with subsequent cellular degeneration.

Secondary injury results in damage to the retinal ganglion cells subsequent to the initial trauma. The vascular ischaemia and the over-added trauma to the optic nerve leads to oedema of the nerve within the confines of the optic canal. As mentioned above, the compartmental syndrome that results leads to a further diminished blood supply to the remaining retinal ganglion cells, ultimately causing cell death. It is due to this secondary injury that in around 10% of the cases, the symptoms of optic nerve injury appears as a delayed complication.

CLINICAL PROFILE AND MANAGEMENT

CLINICAL PROFILE

Diagnosis of traumatic optic neuropathy is essentially clinical with a history supportive of trauma to the head or the face. A careful history should be elucidated since the nature of trauma may at times be trivial. In most cases, patients usually present with other life-threatening injuries which need a more urgent management as a part of road traffic accidents or falls. The diagnosis of traumatic optic neuropathy in these cases can thus be delayed. Clinical features of traumatic optic neuropathy are:

Unilateral or bilateral ocular involvement. Traumatic optic neuropathy is usually unilateral but intracranial injury can lead to involvement of the optic chiasma thereby causing a bilateral injury.

Relative afferent pupillary defect. A relative afferent pupillary defect can be detected in cases of optic neuropathy with the help of a swinging flash-light test. Quantification of the defect can be carried out with the help of neutral density filters. An RAPD would be present in all cases except those that are bilaterally symmetrical. An RAPD defect later than 2.1 log units when measured with neutral density filter in unilateral cases is indicative of a poor prognosis.

Variable loss of visual acuity. Patients may present with a visual acuity ranging from normal to no light perception. Majority of the patients (40 to 60%) present with a visual loss of light perception or worse. As mentioned previously, direct injuries produce a more profound immediate diminished vision with a less likelihood of recovery. Although the prognosis is better in cases of indirect injury, a high degree of clinical vigilance must be maintained as patients may present with a delayed visual loss.

Impairment of colour vision. Trauma to the optic nerve leads to a red green colour deficiency as noted on screening with Ishihara isochromatic plates.

Variable visual field defects. No visualfield loss pattern is characteristic of traumatic optic neuropathy. Visual field defects in patients presenting with poor initial visual acuity should be documented by confrontation test. Although a central scotoma is characteristic, field defects may occur in the form of nerve fibre bundle defects, paracentral scotomas or generalized constriction and depression of the visual field.

Fundoscopy. The appearance of the fundus depends on the anatomical site of the trauma.

- *In case of anterior injuries* with involvement of the retinal vasculature, there is optic disc swelling and surrounding retinal haemorrhages.
- *Optic nerve avulsion* (Fig. 10.1.4) may occur in some cases.

- As the site of injury moves posteriorly, the fundus takes on a more normal appearance.
- *Optic atrophy* usually takes about six weeks to set in:

DIAGNOSTIC TESTS

Neuroimaging studies

Imaging modalities take on an important role in the assessment of a patient with traumatic optic neuropathy. CT scan over MRI is the preferred imaging modality in the emergency setting. The radiologist should be instructed to use smaller cuts to better image the course of the optic nerve. The imaging would delineate the skeleton framework of the orbit and would indicate the presence of any displaced fragment impinging upon the optic nerve. In majority of the cases (indirect injury), imaging studies typically demonstrate no abnormality in the visual pathway. A fracture of the orbital walls may at times be associated.

Visual evoked potentials (VEP)

VEP can be helpful to document the presence of traumatic optic neuropathy in patients who were otherwise non-compliant or unresponsive. The use of VEP in the emergency setting is questionable, however, it can be used to document recovery and for serial evaluations when clinical parameters are equivocal. Flash VEP with an amplitude within 50% of the normal points towards a favourable outcome in cases of optic neuropathy.

Retinal nerve fibre layer imaging

Serial evaluations of the RNFL thickness by OCT can be used to monitor axonal loss following the initial trauma.

TREATMENT

Management of traumatic optic neuropathy remains controversial because of lack of evidence-based guidelines. The main treatment options in current use are:
- Systemic steroids of varying dose, duration and mode of administration,
- Surgical decompression of the optic canal,
- Combination of steroids and surgery, and
- Observation alone.

Steroids in traumatic optic neuropathy

For all practical purposes, the optic nerve is considered an extension of the central nervous system and hence trauma to the nerve is managed according to the lines of trauma to the CNS. Steroids have been used in the management of traumatic optic neuropathy since early 1980s as they were thought to exert a neuroprotective effect following trauma.[1] Very high dose corticosteroids have antioxidant properties and they limit free-radical induced lipid peroxidation following injury. This rational was strengthened following the results of the *National Acute Spinal Cord Injury Study (NASCIS-II)*[2], a multicentre, randomized, double-blind, placebo-controlled study of patients with acute spinal cord injury. Patients were treated with an initial bolus dose of 30 mg/kg of methylprednisolone followed by an infusion of 5.4 mg/kg/hr of the same for 24 hours. It was seen that patients receiving steroids within the first 8 hours of their injury had significant improvement in both sensory and motor functions compared to placebo treated patients or those who were treated after 8 hours.

In NASCIS-III[3], it was established that treatment should be continued for 24 hours, if initiated within 3 hours after injury and for 48 hours if initiated within 3–8 hours. The controversies surrounding NASCIS are that optic nerve is a predominantly "white matter" tract and differs histologically from the spinal cord in both its cellular environment and organization and, therefore, extrapolating data from spinal cord injury to traumatic optic neuropathy remains biologically questionable.

Corticosteroid Randomisation after Significant Head Injury (CRASH)[4] trial another major study, condemns steroid use in traumatic optic neuropathy. The study found a greater risk of death in patients with head injury who were treated with high-dose corticosteroids. Though the cause of increased death in patients with traumatic optic neuropathy with coexisting head injury remains unknown, the trial suggests that steroids must be given with caution in this subgroup.

There have been various other studies looking at the role of steroids in traumatic optic neuro-pathy but the comparison of these studies is difficult because of the varying range of steroid regimens used in terms of dose, duration and mode of administration and also the differential follow up times in the treatment groups.

Yu and Griffiths suggest that traumatic optic neuropathy presenting more than 8 hours after the initial insult should not be treated with steroids, though treatment within the 8 hour window still remains controversial.

International Optic Nerve Trauma Study[5] results published in 1999 concluded that neither corticosteroids nor optic canal surgery should be considered the standard of care in the management of traumatic optic neuropathy.

Surgical options

Several retrospective case studies have advocated that early decompression of the optic canal via intracranial, transethmoidal, endonasal approaches improves functional outcome in traumatic optic neuropathy. However, there are several limitations, comparison among these studies is difficult because of the wide variety of surgical interventions and injury mechanisms. Other limitations include the tendency to operate on patients with no light perception, concomitant use of high dose steroids and inherent difficulty in defining improvement when the first assessment is made at the bedside and the final assessment in the clinic.

Surgical decompression has been advocated only in cases with demonstrable bony lesions impinging on the optic nerve in conscious patients. Decompression is not advocated in situations wherein the bony fragments are more likely to transect the RGC axons resulting in irreversible injury. In cases of optic nerve sheath haemorrhage, the haematoma can be drained by a sheath fenestration. Orbital haemorrhage, as in retrobulbar haemorrhage, can be managed via a lateral canthotomy with subsequent drainage.

Observation

A visual recovery rate of 40–60% has been reported for indirect traumatic optic neuropathy cases managed conservatively. There exists no robust data to prove that steroids provide any benefit over conservative treatment. It is widely speculated that the final visual acuity achieved is the same in both the conservative approach and with the use of steroids; steroids only hasten the rate at which the final visual acuity is approached.

Therefore, in cases wherein the patient is not willing to give consent for steroids, an unconscious patient or a paediatric patient even conservative management with observation of the patient is a viable option.

Future options

Megadose steroids providing no proven benefit in the management of traumatic optic neuropathy have paved the way for further research into the subject. Neuroprotection or more specifically axoprotection is the aim for the latest research projects. Hypothermia, progesterone, FK-506 and other neuroprotective factors, such as ciliary neurotrophic factor, have been tried in various studies to some benefit, however, further research is still warranted to prove their efficacy beyond doubt.

PROGNOSIS AND CONCLUSION

Prognosis

Studies have shown an association between the presenting visual acuity and the final visual acuity. Fifty per cent of patients with traumatic optic neuropathy can have some improvement in vision; although the gain is in most cases minimal. Patients presenting with no light perception at presentation are likely to have little or no recovery in vision. Other factors which indicate a poor prognosis include loss of consciousness at the time of trauma, no vision gain at 48 hours following trauma and a diminished amplitude on visually evoked potential (VEP). Some studies have shown that orbital fractures are associated with a poor outcome. The presence of orbital fracture may imply a greater transmission of force to the optic canal and hence more trauma to the optic nerve. Transection of the optic nerve, partial or complete, as seen in cases of direct injuries has a poor prognosis and no intervention is found to be of proven benefit.

Conclusion

Traumatic optic neuropathy commonly occurring as a part of polytrauma presents with a masquerade of systemic injuries which can make the diagnosis difficult. Proper history taking and an in-depth examination are essential to arrive at a diagnosis. A big question mark, however, looms upon the treatment protocol to be followed in these cases. Till further research provides any concrete evidence of benefit, steroids remain the backbone of management; however, not without their side effects. It has been suggested that the use of megadose steroids should be limited to patients who present within 8 hours of the initial insult. Surgery has been found to be beneficial only in cases of direct injury. Even though a certain amount of vision gain does occur spontaneously, the final outlook remains guarded both with and without therapy.

REFERENCES

1. Maegele M. Reversal of isolated unilateral optic nerve edema with concomitant visual impairment following blunt trauma: a case report. J Med Case Reports 2008; 2:50.
2. Bracken MB, Shepard MJ, Collins WF, Holford TR, Young W, Baskin DS, et al. A randomized, controlled trial of methylprednisolone or naloxone in the treatment of acute spinal cord injury. Results of the Second National Acute Spinal Cord Injury Study. N Engl J Med 1990; 322: 1405–1411.
3. Bracken MB, Shepard MJ, Holford TR, Leo-Summers L, Aldrich EF, Fazi M, et al. Administration of methylprednisolone for 24 or 48 hours or tirilazad mesylate for 48 hours in the treatment of acute spinal cord injury. Results of the Third National Acute Spinal Cord Injury Randomized Controlled Trial. JAMA 77: 1597–1604, 1997.
4. Yates D1, Farrell B, Teasdale G, Sandercock P, Roberts I. Corticosteroids in head injury—the CRASH trial. J Accid Emerg Med 1999; 16:83–84.
5. Levin LA1, Beck RW, Joseph MP, Seiff S, Kraker R. The treatment of traumatic optic neuropathy: the International Optic Nerve Trauma Study. Ophthalmology. 1999; 106:1268–1277.

10.2 TRAUMATIC LESIONS OF VISUAL PATHWAY

Traumatic lesions of visual pathway other than optic neuropathy include:
- Chiasmal traumatic lesions
- Retrochiasmal traumatic lesions

TRAUMATIC LESIONS OF CHIASMA

ETIOPATHOGENESIS

Chiasmal trauma, like traumatic optic neuropathy, may be either direct or indirect

Direct traumatic chiasmal neuropathy

Direct traumatic chiasmal neuropathy is associated with penetrating head injury. Such lesions are extremely rare, since accidental penetration of the cranial cavity that injures the chiasma is also apt to injure the major blood vessels and lead to death.

Indirect traumatic chiasmal neuropathies

Indirect traumatic chiasmal neuropathies are associated with closed head injuries. Though rare in general, such injuries are comparatively more common than the direct chiasmal injuries.

Exact mechanism leading to indirect traumatic chiasmal neuropathy is not identified. Possible mechanisms include:
- *Tears or axonal disruption* associated with contusion or cranial bone fracture may play a role in same cases
- *Vascular pathogenesis,* as with posterior indirect optic neuropathy, may also be responsible in many cases.

CLINICAL PROFILE

Features of chiasmal lesion are often recognized late, as most such patients are unconcious following severe head injury. These can be described as below.

Chiasmal syndrome

Chiasmal syndrome refers to the set of signs and symptoms associated with lesions of optic chiasma. Chiasmal syndrome has been classified into three types:

I. *Anterior chiasmal syndrome* is produced by lesions that affect the ipsilateral optic nerve fibres and the contralateral inferonasal fibres located in the Wilbrand knee; typically producing the so-called junctional scotoma.

II. *Middle chiasmal syndrome* is produced by lesion involving the decussating fibres in the body of chiasma typically producing bitemporal hemianopia. Rarely the middle lesions can affect the uncrossed temporal fibres and produce nasal or binasal hemianopia.

III. *Posterior chiasmal syndrome* is produced by lesions affecting the caudal fibres in chiasma. Characteristic features are as below:
- *Paracentral bitemporal field defects* occur because macular fibres cross more posteriorly in the chiasma and are damaged in the posterior chiasmal lesions.
- *Visual acuity and colour vision* may be preserved as temporal macular fibres are not damaged.
- *Homonymous hemianopia* on the contralateral side may occur when posterior chiasmal lesions involve the optic tract.

Clinical features

Chiasmal syndrome is characterized by following clinical features:

I. Symptoms

1. *Visual loss.* Visual loss, especially of unexplained etiology should be suspected of a chiasmal syndrome and should warrant MRI of the brain. In some cases, visual field defects may be present with normal visual acuity.

2. *Headache* may sometimes be associated with pituitary tumours and is usually due to stretching of meninges.

3. *Diplopia* may occur due to:
- *Misalignment of two eyes* occurring as a result of III, IV or VI cranial nerves due to extension of lesion into either or both cavernous sinuses.
- *Hemifield slide phenomenon* refers to diplopia in the absence of ocular misalignment seen in patients with bitemporal hemianopia. It occurs due to vertical slide of eyes in the absence of binocular area of overlapping or interlocking visual field.

4. *Photophobia* may be complained by some patients. Possibly it occurs due to hyper-sensitivity of trigeminal in patients with para-sellar tumours.

5. *Postfixation blindness,* i.e. an area of blind-ness immediately beyond the point of fixation during near vision fixation. This occurs because of the fact that when eyes converge the area beyond the point of regard falls within the bitemporal hemianopic area.

6. *Difficulty in depth perception,* near work, or precision task may be encountered by many patients.

II. Signs

1. *RAPD* is usually present in patients with asymmetric or unilateral visual loss.

2. *Acquired colour vision defects.* Acquired dyschromatopsia in one or both eyes may be noted in patients with chiasmal syndrome.

3. *Optic disc changes* include:
- *Optic disc pallor* may be seen in patients with partial optic atrophy. A characteristic band atrophy of the optic disc is produced in patients with bitemporal hemianopia.
- *Papilledema,* i.e. disc oedema, though unusual, may be seen in some patients due to raised intracranial pressure especially with cranio-pharyngioma.

4. *Visual field defects.* Depending upon the location of lesion, following field defects can occur in chiasmal disorders:
- Junctional scotoma,
- Monocular temporal hemianopic defect,
- Bitemporal hemianopia,
- Homonymous hemianopia, and
- Binasal visual field defects.

i. *Junctional scotoma* refers to a combination of central scotoma in one eye and temporal hemianopic defect in the other eye (Figs 10.2.1[2]

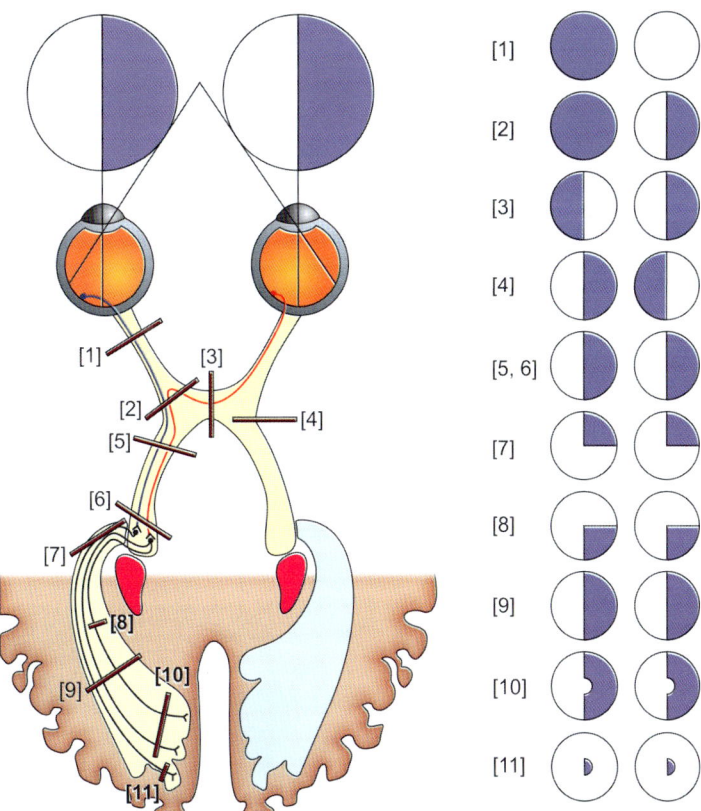

Fig. 10.2.1 *Lesions of the visual pathways at the level of : [1] optic nerve; [2] proximal part of optic nerve; [3] central chiasma; [4] lateral chiasma (both sides); [5] optic tract; [6] geniculate body; [7] part of optic radiations in temporal lobe; [8] part of optic radiations in parietal lobe; [9] optic radiations; [10] visual cortex sparing the macula; [11] visual cortex, only macula*

and 10.2.2). Location of lesion in such cases is at the junction of optic nerve and chiasma on the side of scotoma (Figs 10.2.1[2]).

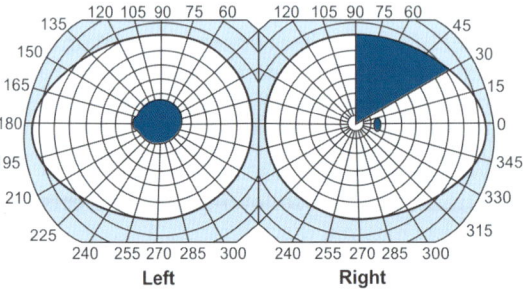

Fig. 10.2.2 *Junctional scotoma; pattern of field defects*

ii. *Monocular temporal hemianopic visual field defects* with no visual field loss in the contra-lateral eye (Fig. 10.2.3) can occur when the lesion involves only the crossing visual fibres at the anterior angle of the optic chiasma.

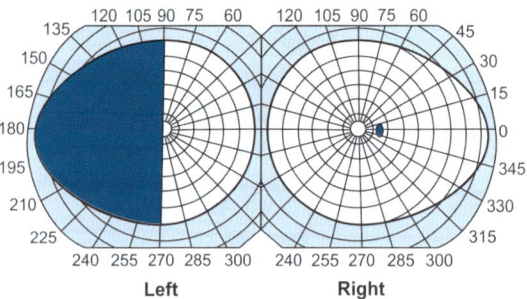

Fig. 10.2.3 *Monocular temporal hemianopic defect*

iii. *Bitemporal hemianopia* (Fig. 10.1.1[3]) typically obeying the vertical meridian is a classical field defect noted in patients with sagittal (central) lesions of chiasma. The visual field defect may be complete or incomplete (Fig. 10.2.4). In many

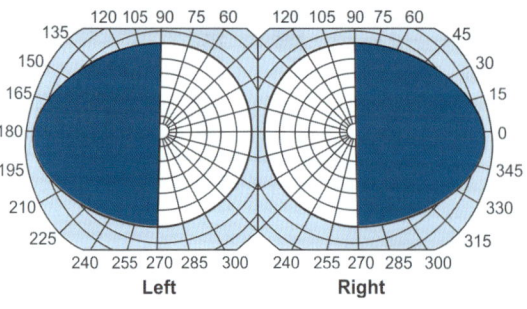

Fig. 10.2.4 *Bitemporal hemianopia.*

cases, pure bitemporal hemianopic field may not occur. A central bitemporal field defect (Fig. 10.2.5) may occur in patients with prefixed chiasma or posterior trauma because macular fibres are located posteriorly.

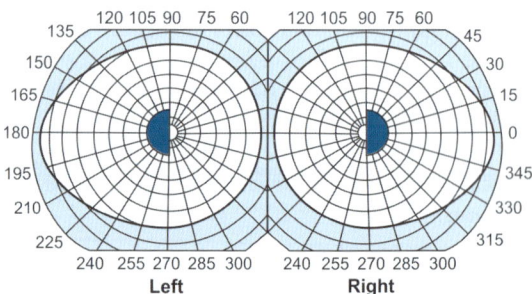

Fig. 10.2.5 *Central bitemporal hemianopia*

- *Bitemporal hemianopic paralysis of pupillary reflex* is almost always associated with bitemporal hemianopic defects.

- *Partial descending optic atrophy* is usually produced by central chiasmal lesions.

iv. *Homonymous hemianopia,* usually incongruous (Fig. 10.2.6), may occur due to involvement of optic tract in parasellar lesions.

- Circumstances in which parasellar chiasmal lesions produce homonymous hemianopia include:

  - Prefixed optic chiasma, and
  - Posteriorly directed traumatic lesions

- *Optic tract syndrome* is the term used when homonymous hemianopia is associated with a central scotoma and relative afferent pupillary defect (RAPD) on the side of lesion.

v. *Binasal visual field defects* (Fig. 10.2.1[4]) are seen in patients with lateral chiasmal lesions. In

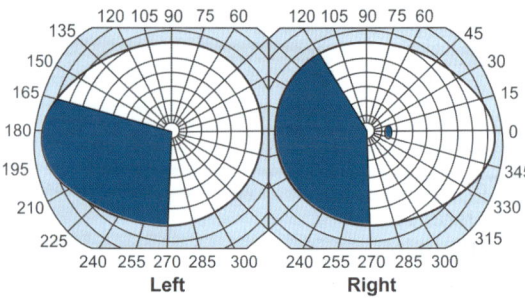

Fig. 10.2.6 *Incongruous homonymous hemianopia*

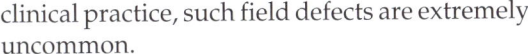

clinical practice, such field defects are extremely uncommon.

- *Binasal hemianopic paralysis of pupillary reflex* is usually associated with binasal hemi-anopia.
- *Partial (temporal) descending optic atrophy* is usually produced by lateral chiasmal lesions.

5. *Other ocular features* which may occur in patients with chiasmal syndrome include:

- *Ocular misalignment* due to involvement of III, IV or VI cranial nerve due to extension of trauma into the cavernous sinus.
- *See-saw nystagmus* is also reported to occur in patients with parasellar trauma.

ROLE OF OPHTHALMOLOGIST

Role of ophthalmologist is primarily to identify and document the visual deficits.

RETROCHIASMAL TRAUMATIC LESIONS

ETIOPATHOGENESIS

Similar to traumatic chiasmal lesions, the retro-chiasmal lesions may also occur as:

1. Direct traumatic retrochiasmal lesions, and
2. Indirect traumatic retrochiasmal lesions

GENERAL CONSIDERATIONS

Neuroimaging is considered superior to the clinical examination in detecting, localizing and characterizing acute traumatic retrochiasmal lesion in contrast to the situation in acute traumatic optic neuropathy and acute chiasmal neuropathy.

Retrochiasmal lesions include:

- Lesions of optic tract,
- Lesions of lateral geniculate nucleus,
- Lesions of optic radiations,
  – Temporal lobe lesions, and
  – Parietal lobe lesions
- Lesions of occipital lobe

Contralateral homonymous hemianopias of different forms (depending upon site of lesion) without loss of visual acuity is the predominant visual field defect of all the retrochiasmal lesions.

- *Incomplete homonymous hemianopia* can be congruous or incongruous. Congruous homonymous hemianopias are identical in shape, size, depth and slope of the margins. The congruousity of field defects increases from optic tracts to occipital cortex. This is because of the fact that as the visual fibres travel toward occipital lobe the corresponding retinal points lie adjacent to one another and hence visual field defects due to posterior lesions are more congruous. Thus, depending upon the incongruousity of field defect, the site of lesion can be localized.
- *Complete homonymous hemianopia* cannot be categorized into congruous versus incongruous and then it is not possible to localize the site of lesion. In such cases, the clinician must rely on other symptoms and signs of neurological disease or on neuroimaging.

Homonymous visual field defects in intracranial trauma versus in vascular lesions

In intracranial trauma, irrespective of the location, the homonymous visual field defects are characterized by:

- Slow progression
- Progression occurs from periphery to centre
- Defects appear early for coloured objects than for black and white objects
- After surgical decompression, the recovery progresses from centre towards periphery.

In vascular lesions, such as haemorrhage or infarction, the homonymous visual field defects are characterized by:

- Sudden onset with rapid progression, and
- Recovery occurs from centre towards periphery.

LESIONS OF OPTIC TRACT

The set of clinical features produced by lesions of optic tract are referred as 'optic tract syndrome', which are of two types: type I and type II.

Optic tract syndrome type I

Etiology

Optic tract syndrome type I caused by a large compressive mass lesion that involves the optic tract, optic chiasma and even the optic nerve can also occur due to trauma to these structures.

Characteristic features

Optic tract syndrome type I is characterized by following set of signs:

- *Visual acuity* is decreased ipsilaterally.
- *Hemianopia.* Contralateral incongruous homonymous hemianopia (Fig. 10.2.6), since nerve fibres of corresponding retinal points from two eyes do not lie adjacent to each other in the optic tracts.
- *Pupillary reflex* defects may be any of the following:
  - *Ipsilateral RAPD,* i.e. relative afferent pupillary defect
  - *Wernicke's hemianopic pupil,* i.e. pupillary reflex is present when light is shown to normal halves of retinae and absent when shown to blind halves of retinae.
- *Optic disc changes* include bowtie atrophy on the side contralateral to the side of lesion (the side with temporal field defect) and temporal pallor on the ipsilateral side.

Optic tract syndrome type II

Etiology

Optic tract syndrome type II resulting from intrinsic lesions of optic tract produced by conditions, like: demyelinating diseases, and infarction; can also occur following trauma.

Characteristic features

- *Visual acuity* is usually intact
- *Pupillary reflex defects* may be:
  - RAPD on the side opposite to lesion
  - Wernicke's hemianopic pupil
- *Homonymous hemianopia* is complete or nearly so (Figs 10.2.1[5] and 10.2.7)
- *Optic disc changes* are similar to optic tract syndrome type I

LESIONS OF LATERAL GENICULATE NUCLEUS

Lesions of lateral geniculate nucleus (LGN) are extremely rare. Characteristic features include:

Field defects of following types may occur:

- *Homonymous hemianopia* is incongruous similar to OTS type I (Fig. 10.2.6)
- *Homonymous horizontal sectoranopia* nearly congruous (Fig. 10.2.8), associated with sectorial optic atrophy may occur due to posterior choroidal artery infarction
- *Hourglass-shaped visual field defects* due to infarction of anterior choroidal artery supplying ventral nucleus or *hourglass-preserved visual field defects* due to infarction of posterior choroidal artery supplying the dorsal nucleus may occur with bilateral LGN involvement.

Pupillary reflexes are normal.

Optic disc pallor may occur.

LESIONS OF OPTIC RADIATIONS

Temporal lobe lesions

Causes

Temporal lobe lesions may occur due to mechanical effects or vascular occlusions following trauma.

Visual features

Anterior temporal lobe lesions involving Meyer's loop, formed by anteroinferior sweeping of the inferior fibres of optic radiations (Fig. 10.2.9A), produce midperipheral and peripheral contralateral homonymous superior quadrantopia (pie-in-the-sky field defect) (Figs 10.2.1[7] and 10.2.9B).

More extensive temporal lobe lesions produce a homonymous hemianopia, but the field defect will be denser superiorly (Fig. 10.2.10).

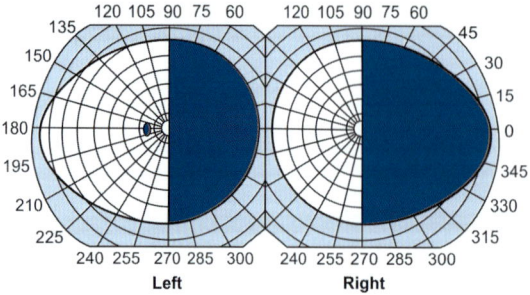

Fig. 10.2.7 *Complete homonymous hemianopia*

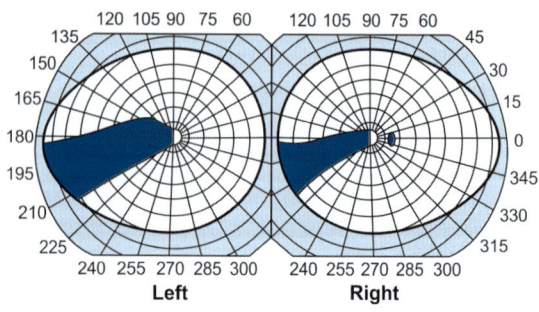

Fig. 10.2.8 *Homonymous horizontal sectoranopia*

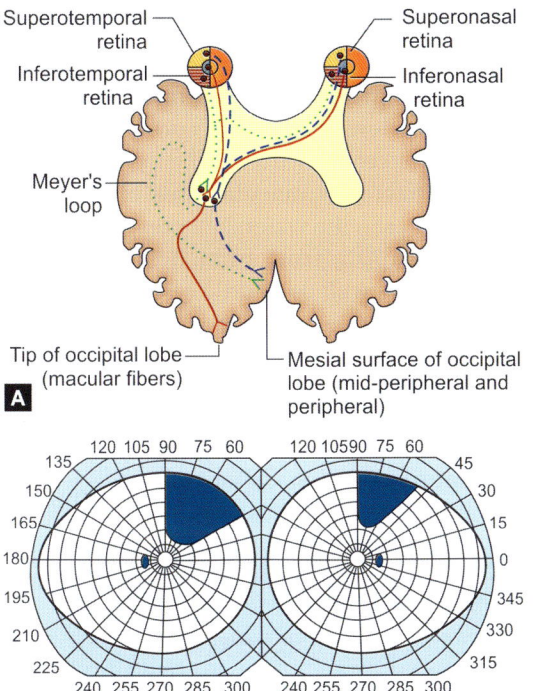

Fig. 10.2.9 *Anterior temporal lobe lesion involving inferior fibres of optic radiations forming Meyer's loop (A) and producing homonymous superior quadrantopia (B)*

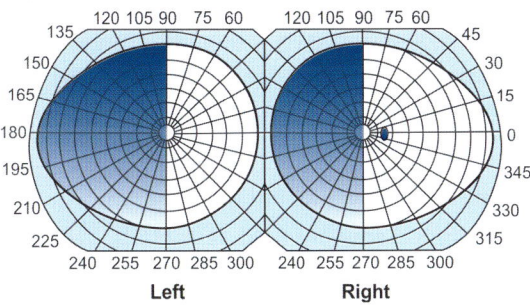

Fig. 10.2.10 *Homonymous hemianopia denser superiorly produced by extensively temporal lobe lesions*

Systemic features

Systemic features of temporal lobe lesions which may be associated with visual fields include:

- Headache
- Auditory hallucinations or illusions
- Memory disturbances
- Language disturbances, when dominant temporal lobe is involved
- Mood, emotion and behaviour changes

- Uncinate fits characterized by aura of unusual taste or smell followed by abnormal motor activity of the mouth and lips.

Parietal lobe lesions

Visual field defects

- *Inferior quadrantic hemianopia,* i.e. pie-in-the-floor (Figs 10.2.1[8] and 10.2.11) occurs initially in the lesions of parietal lobe (containing superior fibres of optic radiations).
- *Homonymous hemianopia denser inferiorly* (Fig. 10.2.12) occurs with further extension of lesion.

Neuro-ophthalmic features

Neuro-ophthalmic features seen in parietal lobe traumatic lesions include:

- *Spasticity of conjugate gaze,* i.e. tonic deviation of eyes to the side opposite a parietal lesion during an attempt to produce Bell's phenomenon (i.e. during forced lid closure).
- *Asymmetric optokinetic nystagmus,* i.e. evoked nystagmus is dampened when stimuli are moved in the direction of the involved parietal lobe.
- *Deficient pursuit eye movements* to the side of lesion.

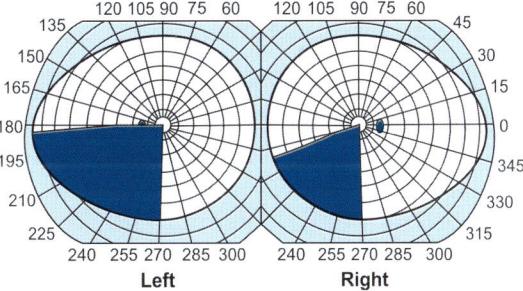

Fig. 10.2.11 *Inferior quadrantic hemianopia (pie-in-the-floor) produced by parietal lobe lesions involving superior fibres of optic radiations*

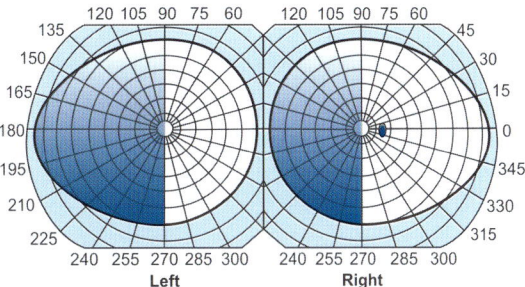

Fig. 10.2.12 *Homonymous hemianopia denser inferiorly produced by parietal lobe lesions*

Neurologic features

Neurologic features associated with parietal lobe lesion include:

- *Impairment* of complex sensory integration.
- *Neglect of contralateral space and inattention* may occur in patients with non-dominant parietal lobe lesions.
- *Gerstmann syndrome* characterized by contralateral homonymous hemianopia, finger agnosia, right-left confusion, agraphia, and acaculia may occur in lesions involving dominant parietal lobe.

LESIONS OF VISUAL CORTEX

Characteristic features of visual cortex lesions can be described as:

- Visual field defects, and
- Other manifestations of occipital lobe lesions

Visual field defects in occipital lobe lesions

Visual field defects in unilateral occipital lobe lesions

Different types of visual field defects occurring in occipital lobe lesions with their characteristic features are described below.

Central homonymous hemianopia

Central homonymous hemianopia is characterized by only loss of central halves of field of vision. Such field defects are exquisitely congruous (Figs 10.2.1[11] and 10.2.13).

Sites of lines include trauma affecting tip of occipital lobe.

Macular sparing homonymous hemianopia

- *True macular sparing homonymous hemianopia* is seen in patients with traumatic obstruction of blood flow to the visual cortex through the posterior cerebral artery. This occurs because of the fact that macular area of the visual cortex lies in the watershed area, i.e. has dual blood supply from branches of posterior cerebral as well as middle cerebral arteries.
- *Macular sparing is labelled* when at least 5° of macular field is spared in both eyes on the side of hemianopia (Figs 10.2.1[10] and 10.2.14).
- *False macular sparing* may sometimes be produced by an artefact of testing as a result of shifting fixation. Patient may shift fixation, anticipating the appearance of the test object.

Homonymous hemianopia with sparing of temporal crescent

- *Temporal crescent of visual field* in each eye is produced by the nasal crescent of retina for which there is no corresponding visual points in the other eye (Fig. 10.2.15).
- *Homonymous hemianopia with sparing of temporal crescent* (Fig. 10.2.16) is characteristic of occipital lobe lesion since this is the only site where the temporal crescent field fibres are separated from the other nasal retina fibres of the contralateral eye. Because of sparing of temporal crescent of field in one eye, the homonymous hemianopia appears incongruous.

Temporal crescent field defect

- Temporal crescent field defect (Fig. 10.2.17) is produced due to lesion involving that area of visual cortex (Fig. 10.2.15C) which represents the nasal crescent of retina (Fig. 10.2.15B) for

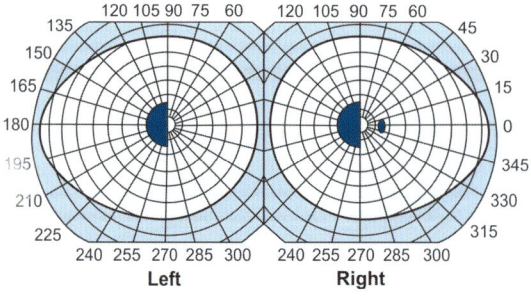

Fig. 10.2.13 *Central homonymous hemianopia seen in occipital lobe lesions*

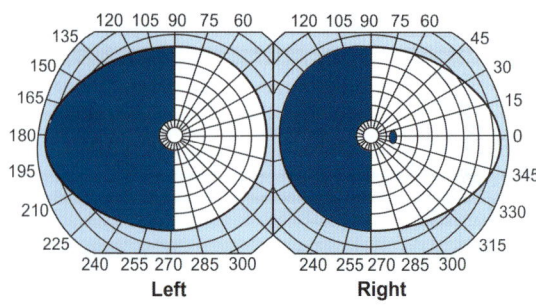

Fig. 10.2.14 *Macular sparing homonymous hemianopia*

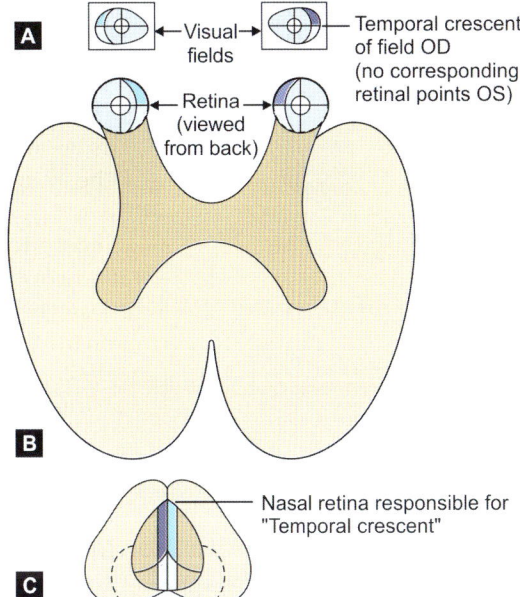

Fig. 10.2.15 *Temporal crescent of visual field (A), corresponding to crescent of extreme nasal retina (B), is projected to contralateral visual cortex (anterior mesial surface) (C)*

which there is no corresponding visual points on the contralateral retina. Therefore, this is the only area of the visual cortex which produces unilateral visual field defect. Representation of the temporal crescent occupies less than 10% of total surface area of striate cortex.

- Temporal crescent field defect (Fig. 10.2.17) has its widest extent in the horizontal meridian and extends from 60° to 90°. It is important to note that standard automated static perimetry programmes fail to detect this field defect because it is further in the peripheral field than these tests measure.

Visual field defects in bilateral occipital lobe lesions

In bilateral occipital lobe lesions, following field defects may occur:

1. *Bilateral homonymous hemianopia with macular sparing* produces a picture of ring scotoma (Fig. 10.2.18). Such field defects need to be differentiated from:

- Glaucomatous field defect
- Hysterical and malingering defects
- Field defects due to optic disc drusen
- Field defects in post-papilledemic optic atrophy
- Field defects in retinitis pigmentosa

Note. In all the above conditions except hysteria and malingering, the typical fundus picture helps in making the diagnosis. Differentiation from hysteria and malingering requires visual field testing at the tangent screen at 1 and 2 metres (Fig. 10.2.19).

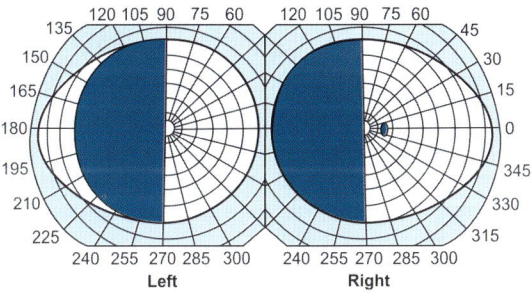

Fig. 10.2.16 *Left homonymous hemianopia with sparing of the temporal crescent of the left eye*

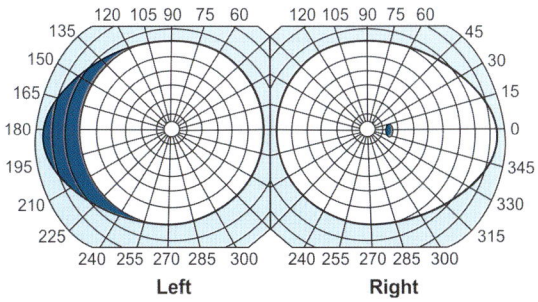

Fig. 10.2.17 *Temporal crescent field defect*

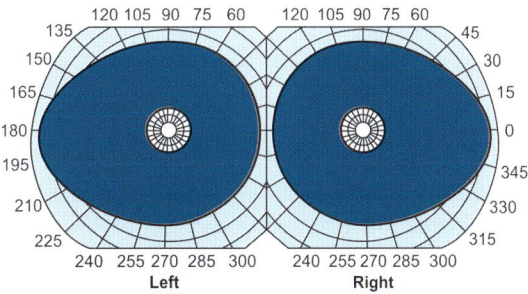

Fig. 10.2.18 *Bilateral homonymous hemianopia producing a picture of ring scotoma*

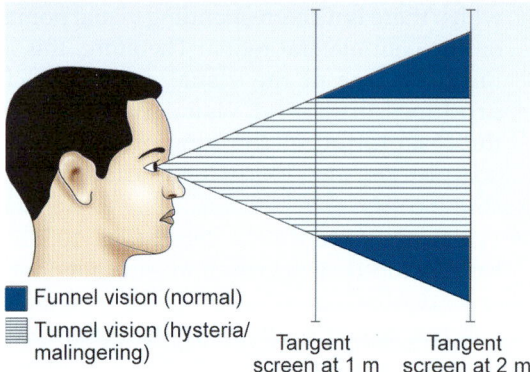

Funnel vision (normal)
Tunnel vision (hysteria/ malingering)
Tangent screen at 1 m   Tangent screen at 2 m

Fig. 10.2.19 *Normal funnel vision versus tunnel vision seen in hysteria/malingering depicted on tangent screen at 1 and 2 metres*

2. *Bilateral central homonymous hemianopia* presents like bilateral central scotoma (Fig. 10.2.20).

3. *Bilateral homonymous quadrantic defects* (usually inferior) present as inferior altitudinal defects (Fig. 10.2.21).

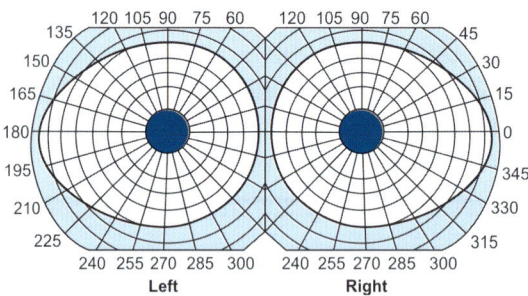

Fig. 10.2.20 *Bilateral central homonymous hemianopia*

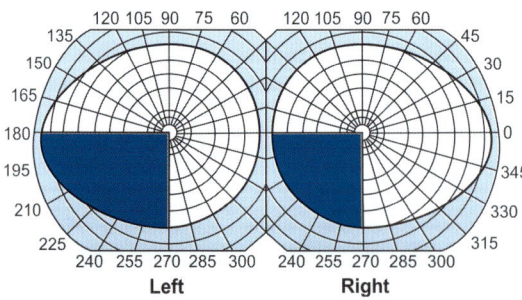

Fig. 10.2.21 *Bilateral homonymous quadrantic defects*

4. *Checker board field defects* or *crossed quadrantopia* (Fig. 10.2.22) is produced by lesions which affect the superior occipital lobe above the calcarine fissure on one side and the inferior occipital lobe below the calcarine fissure on the other side.

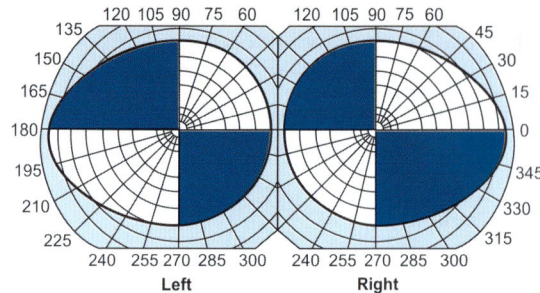

Fig. 10.2.22 *Checker-board field defects (crossed quadrantopia)*

Other manifestations of occipital lobe lesions

Manifestations of occipital lobe lesions other than the visual field defects include:

1. **Cortical blindness** can occur in bilateral occipital lobe lesions.

2. **Dyschromatopsia.** Bilateral occipital lobe lesions can also produce acquired colour vision defects, i.e. dyschromatopsia.

3. **Visual hallucinations** seen in occipital lobe lesions are unformed, while hallucinations seen in temporal lobe lesions are formed.

4. **Palinopsia** refers to persistent or recurrent perception of a visual image after removal of the stimulus.

- It is typically seen following parietal or occipital lobe lesions in the non-dominant hemisphere.
- Palinopsia is usually associated with homonymous hemianopia.

5. **Visual allesthesia** is characterized by transposition of visual stimuli from one hemifield to another. It is known to occur most commonly with parieto-occipital lesions.

6. **Polyopia** (perceiving multiple images of a visual stimulus) associated with occipital lobe lesions does not resolve by closing either eye or with pinhole.

BIBLIOGRAPHY

1. Foroozan, R. Chiasmal Syndromes. CurrOpin Ophthalmol 2003; 14:325–331.
2. Horton JC. Wilbrand's knee of the primate optic chiasm is an artifact of monocular enucleation. Trans Am Ophthalmol Soc. 1997; 95:579–609.
3. Lee, A. Optic chiasmal disorders. Accessed February 1, 2007.
4. Lee, JH, Tobias, S, Kwon, JT, Sade, B, Kosmorsky, G. Wilbrand's knee: does it exist? SurgNeurol 2006 Jul: 66(1):11–7; discussion 17.

10.3 TRAUMA TO OCULAR MOTOR SYSTEM

Trauma to ocular motor system may manifest as:

- Traumatic lesions of extraocular muscles
- Trauma to ocular motor nerves
- Traumatic gaze palsies
- Traumatic lesions of trigeminal nerve
- Traumatic lesions of facial nerve

TRAUMATIC LESIONS OF EXTRAOCULAR MUSCLES

Traumatic lesions of extraocular muscles, which may result in partial or complete loss of function of one or more than one muscle include:

- Contusion of extraocular muscles
- Traumatic laceration and disinsertion
- Entrapment of muscle
- Intramuscular and muscular sheath hemorrhage

CONTUSION OF EXTRAOCULAR MUSCLES

- *Contusion of extraocular muscle* may occur following blunt trauma to the eye and orbit.
- *Dysfunction of muscle* may occur due to traumatic inflammation.
- *Contused extraocular muscle* usually regains normal function within a few days. Systemic steroids or NSAIDs may be useful in such cases. To avoid annoying diplopia during the recovery period, occlusion may be advised. As a whole, prognosis is good in such cases and surgery is rarely required.

LACERATION AND DISINSERTION

Laceration and disinsertion may occur following penetrating orbital trauma or iatrogenic following surgical trauma as in excision of pterigium, limbal dermoid removal, squint surgery or buckling procedure for retinal detachment.

Diagnostic ultrasound, EMG or CT scan may be required.

Surgically reattachment of the disinherited muscle is required.

ENTRAPMENT OF EXTRAOCULAR MUSCLE

Entrapment of extraocular muscles may occur following blow-out-fractures.

- *Inferior rectus entrapment* following blow-out-fracture of the orbital floor may produce a picture of double elevator palsy.
- *Medial rectus entrapment* following medial wall fracture may produce an apparent Duane's retraction syndrome.
- *Forced duction test* helps in distinguishing restrictive from paretic extraocular muscle dysfunction.
- *Diagnostic* CT (Fig. 10.3.1) or MRI scan of the orbit is required.
- *Surgical treatment.* After conservative management, release of entrapped muscle and repair of orbital wall, is indicated in patients with intractable diplopia.

INTRAMUSCULAR OR MUSCLE SHEATH HAEMORRHAGE

Blunt trauma to extraocular muscles may some times result in intramuscular or muscle sheath haemorrhage. The involved muscle becomes swollen and shows dyfunction in the form of inability to contract and relax properly and may manifest as diplopia.

Conservative management in the form of cold compresses and anti-inflammatory drugs and rest to the eyeball is all that is required in most cases.

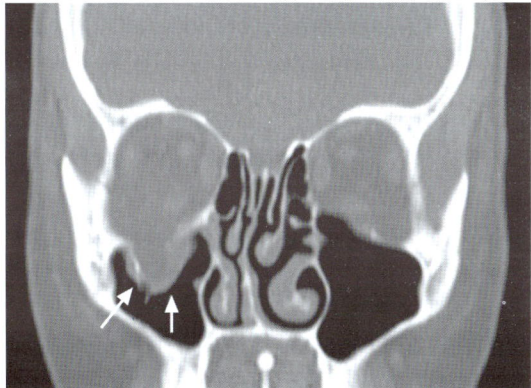

Fig. 10.3.1 *CT scan of orbit: Axial view depicting fracture floor of the orbit with herniation of the orbital contents*

TRAUMA TO OCULAR MOTOR NERVES

Trauma to ocular motor nerves comprises isolated total or partial paresis of 3rd, or 4th, or 6th cranial nerve or a combined involvement of more than one nerve. It has been observed that:

- *Sixth cranial nerve palsy* is the commest occurrence in trauma followed by fourth and third nerve palsy.

- *Fourth cranial nerve palsy* occurs most commonly due to trauma as compared to its other causes.

- *Third cranial nerve palsy* usually follows more severe trauma, than sixth and fourth nerve, respectively. It is important to note that most of the time the traumatic paresis of ocular motor nerves is associated with skull fracture and or loss of consciousness. Therefore, when ocular motor nerve paresis occurs with minor head trauma, one must investigate to rule out basal skull tumours, such as meningioma or chordoma.

- *Incidence of traumatic ocular motor nerve palsies* reported by various workers in patients with head injury is as below:

  – Rucker(1966): 13.9%

  – Rush(1981): 19.7%

  – Shukla (2002): 2.8%

Comparative incidence of involvement of 3rd, 4th and 6th cranial nerve palsy reported by Rucker (1966) and Shukla (2002) is as below:

Nerve involved	Rucker	Shukla
	Number of cases (%)	
Isolated 6th	55 (39.56)	11(24.44)
Isolated 3rd	34(24.46)	29(64.45)
Isolated 4th	23(16.54)	0.5(11.11)
3rd and 4th nerves	09(6.47)	—
3rd and 6th nerves	09(6.47)	—
3rd, 4th and 6th nerves	08 (5.75)	—
4th and 6th nerves	01 (0.72)	—
Total	139(100)	45(100)

TRAUMATIC THIRD NERVE PALSY

Modes of trauma

1. **Direct third nerve injury** following a severe trauma may occur by following mechanisms:

- *Fasicular lesions* may very rarely occur in severe head trauma.

- *Basilar part of the nerve* involved by shearing forces in the midbrain, i.e. there occurs avulsion of the rootlets.

- *Intracavernous part* may be involved along with other nerves due to carotid–cavernous fistula.

- *Orbital part* may be contused at the level of superior orbital fissure.

2. **Indirect third nerve injury** occurs in patients with extradural haematomas cerebral haemorrhage or cerebral oedema. Such lesions may cause tentorial pressure with downward herniation of the temporal lobe. This compress the third nerve as it passes over the tentorial edge (Fig. 10.3.2). Initially there occurs fixed dilated pupil, which is followed by a total third nerve palsy. The palsy may be accompanied by other ocular motor abnormalities including nystagmus, Skewe deviation, vertical gaze paresis and internuclear ophthalmoplegia, because of intrinsic brainstem injury.

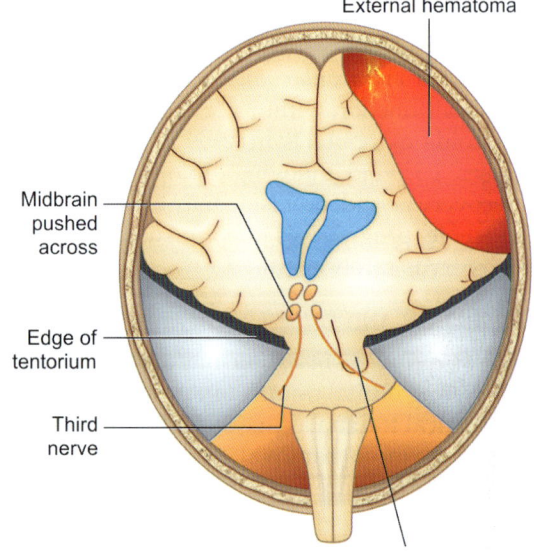

Fig. 10.3.2 *Mechanism of third nerve palsy in extradural haematoma*

Clinical features

A complete and total third nerve palsy is of common occurrence in trauma. Clinical features of complete third nerve palsy (Fig. 10.3.3) include the following:

1. *Ptosis* due to paralysis of the LPS muscle.
2. *Deviation.* Eyeball is turned down, out and slightly intorted due to unopposed action of the lateral rectus and superior oblique muscles.
3. *Ocular movements* are restricted due to paralysis of the muscles as follows:
   - Adduction—due to medial rectus
   - Elevation—due to superior rectus and inferior oblique
   - Depression—due to inferior rectus
   - Extorsion—due to inferior rectus and inferior oblique
4. *Pupil* is fixed and dilated due to paralysis of the sphincter pupillae muscle.
5. Accommodation is completely lost due to paralysis of the ciliary muscle.
6. *Crossed diplopia*, elicited on manually raising the eyelid, occurs due to paralytic divergent squint.

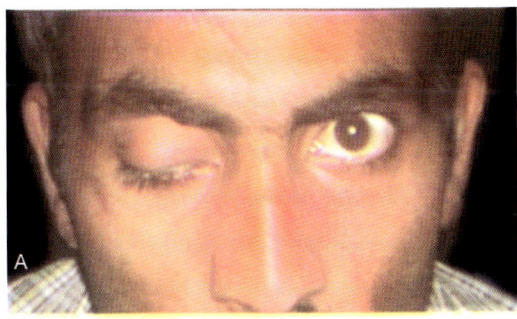
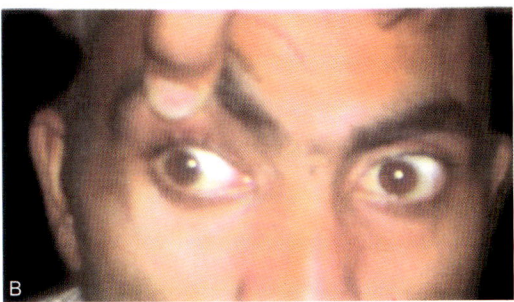

Fig. 10.3.3 *A patients with third cranial nerve paralysis showing (A) ptosis; (B) divergent squint*

7. *Head posture.* If the pupillary area is uncovered, head takes a posture consistent with the directions of actions of the paralysed muscles, i.e. head is turned on the opposite side, tilted towards the same side and chin is slightly raised.

TRAUMATIC FOURTH NERVE PALSY

Modes of trauma

Trauma is the most common cause (34%) of fourth nerve palsy.

- *Traumatic avulsion* of the nerve from the posterior aspect of midbrain is a common mode. It frequently causes bilateral trochlear nerve palsy due to an impact in the area of anterior medullary velum, where the two nerve decussate.
- *Traumatic contusion against the tentorium* is another mode. It is reported that a blow to one side of the forehead leads to contrecoup forces directed against the contralateral posterior midbrain at the tentorium.
- *Trauma to superior oblique tendon* is also a common cause of restriction of the movements of superior oblique muscle.

Clinical features

Features of fourth nerve palsy are:

1. *Abnormal head posture.* To avoid diplopia head takes a posture towards the action of superior oblique muscle, i.e. face is slightly turned to the opposite side, chin is depressed and head is tilted towards the opposite shoulder (Fig. 10.3.4A).
2. *Hyperdeviation.* The involved eye is higher as a result of the weakness of the superior oblique muscle (Fig. 10.3.4L). This becomes more obvious when the head is tilted towards ipsilateral shoulder (Bielschowsky's head tilt test Fig. 10.3.4K).
3. *Ocular movements.* Depression is limited in adduction. Extorsion is also limited (Fig. 10.3.4).
4. *Diplopia.* Homonymous vertical diplopia occurs on looking downwards. Usually, vision is single so long as the eyes look above the horizontal plane. Diplopia is especially noticed by the patient when coming down the stairs.

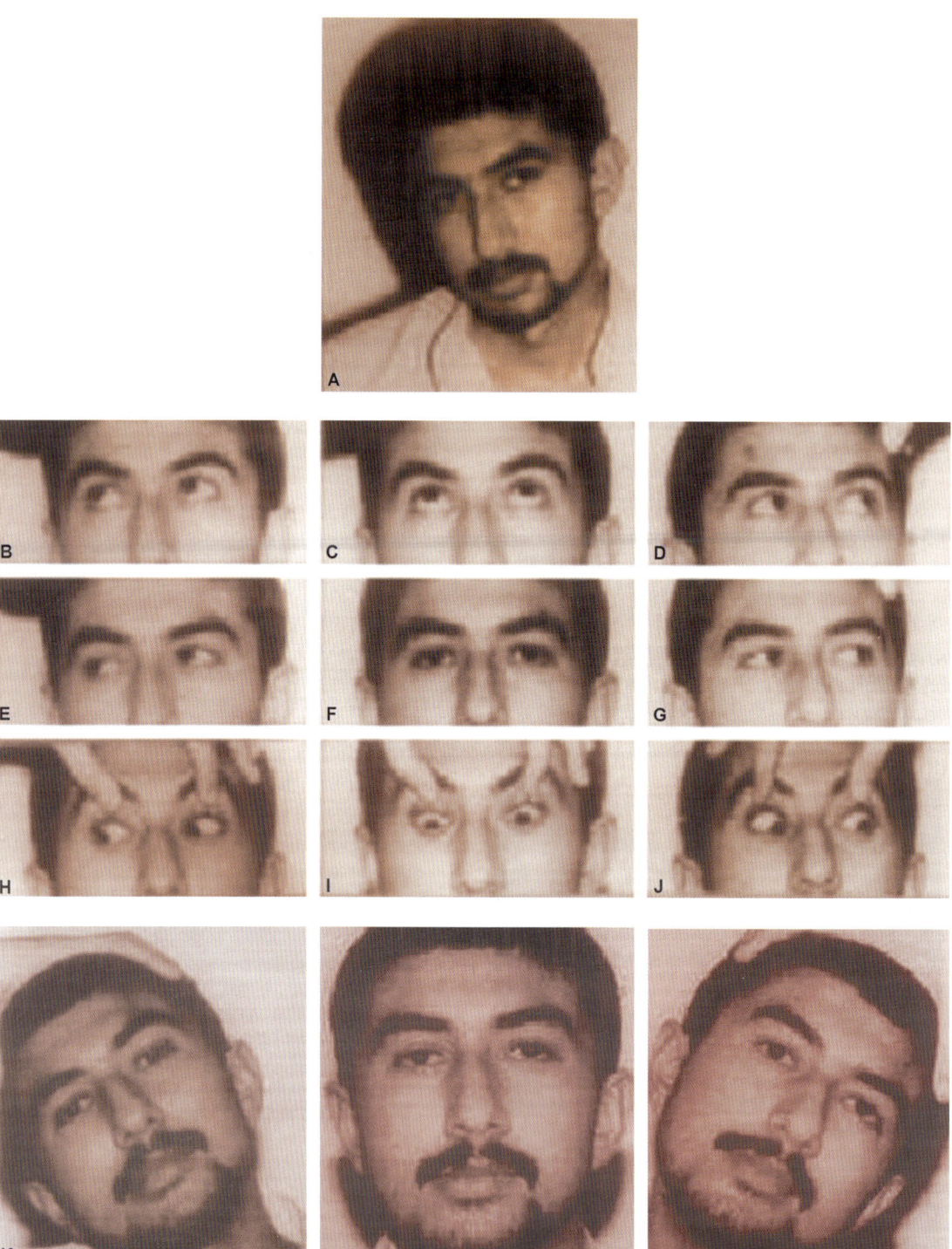

Fig. 10.3.4. *Left superior oblique palsy. A, Abnormal head posture, note head is tilted to the right shoulder, face is slightly turned to the right and chin is slightly depressed. B to J, Eyeballs in nine positions of gaze, note left hypertropia (F) which increases on right gaze (E). Also note left hypertropia (K) which increases on tilting the head to the left shoulder (M) and no change in hypertropia on tilting the head to the right shoulder (L). (Courtesy: Dr Kanwar Mohan)*

TRAUMATIC SIXTH NERVE PALSY

Sixth cranial nerve palsy is the commonest occurrence in trauma followed by 4th and 3rd nerve palsy. It is usually associated with more severe trauma than that causing 4th nerve palsy and the extent of trauma is such that it is usually associated with loss of counciousness.

Modes of trauma

Avulsion of nerve from the pons is the commenst site and occurs due to sheering forces in blunt trauma.

Injury to nerve due to acceleration—deceleration forces may occur at following sites:
- Petroclinoid ligament,
- Superior orbital fissure, and
- Where the nerve crosses the anterior inferior cerebellar artery.

Injury to the sixth nerve at the petrous tip occurs in crush injuries of the head. Trigeminal nerve is also involved along with sixth nerve in much cases.

Strangulation of sixth nerve by branches of basilar artery due to hyperextension of cervical spine with or without fracture of cervical vertebrae may be associated with acute or delayed palsy.

Clinical features

Clinical features in an isolated 6th nerve palsy are as follows:

1. *Incomitant esotropia* occurs in the involved eye (Fig. 10.3.5A) due to unopposed action of the medial rectus muscle. The esotropia increases in gaze towards the paretic lateral rectus muscle (Fig. 10.3.5B) and patient becomes orthotropic in the opposite gaze (Fig. 10.3.5C). When tested with cover test, secondary deviation in the uninvolved eye is larger than the primary deviation.

2. *Abnormal head posture* is frequently associated with incomitant esotropia. Face is turned towards the action of the paralysed lateral rectus.

3. *Diplopia* may not be a problem in visually immature children. However, visually mature old patients have an uncrossed horizontal diplopia with maximal image separation at distance and to the side of involvement (Fig. 10.3.6).

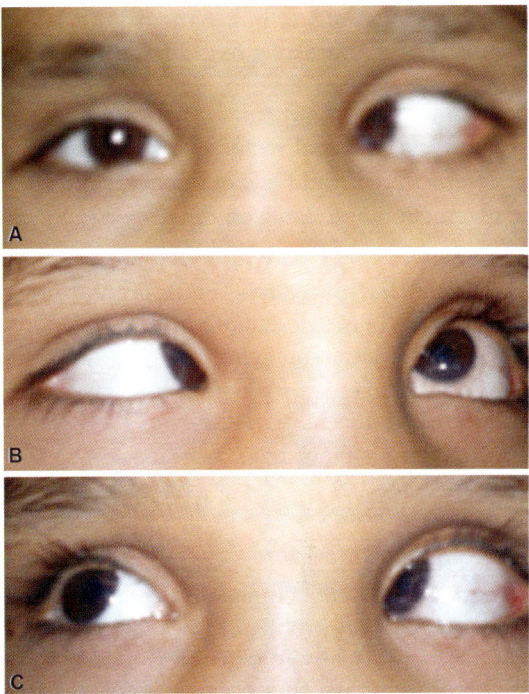

Fig. 10.3.5 *A patient with left lateral rectus palsy having left esotropia in primary gaze* (A) *which increases in left lateral gaze* (B) *and becomes orthotropic in right gaze* (C)

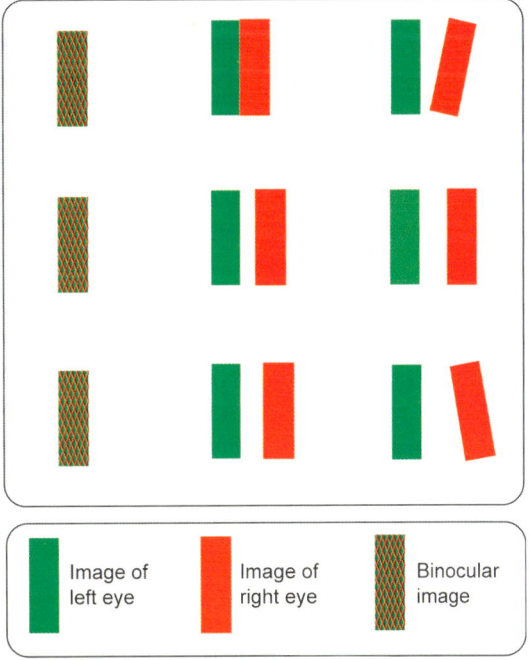

▌ Image of left eye	▌ Image of right eye	▨ Binocular image

Fig. 10.3.6 *Diplopia chart of a patient with right lateral rectus palsy*

4. *Ocular movements* in a patient with lateral rectus muscle paralysis (e.g. of right eye) are affected as below:

- Abduction in right eye is limited due to paralysis of lateral rectus muscle.
- Overaction of right eye on levoversion.
- Overaction of left eye on dextroversion.
- Underaction of left eye on levoversion.

5. *Differential diagnosis.* Sixth cranial nerve palsy should be differentiated from:

1. Duane's retraction syndrome.
2. Congenital esotropia with crossed fixation – pseudoabducens paralysis.
3. Nystagmus blockage syndrome.

Management

I. Treatment of the cause

The diagnosis of 6th cranial nerve palsy as such does not pose any problem. However, etiological diagnosis especially in cases of isolated lateral rectus muscle palsy may not be possible in many a cases. A careful history should be taken to define antecedent infections, head trauma, or other possible inciting factors for sixth nerve paresis. Neurological evaluation with computerized tomography or magnetic resonance imaging is indicated, when neurological signs or symptoms are present. After an exhaustive investigative work-up, if some cause is found and when treatable, appropriate measures should be taken; which by and large are the domain of neurophysicians and/or neurosurgeons.

II. Conservative measures

A wait and watch for a minimum period of 6–8 months is must, when self-improvement is expected, especially in idiopathic cases and cases with benign palsies. Following conservative measures may be useful during this period:

1. *Measures to expedite recovery from palsy are:*
i. *Vitamin B-complex* may be used as a neurotonic.
ii. *Systemic steroids* may hasten the recovery in patients with non-specific inflammations.

2. *Measures to prevent amblyopia and relieve diplopia.* The main aim of conservative measures while waiting for spontaneous recovery is to provide relief from diplopia and additionally in children to prevent amblyopia and preserve binocular vision. Following measures may be useful:

i. *Alternate patching* relieves diplopia, prevents amblyopia and also prevents medial rectus contracture.
ii. *Botulinum toxin* injection into the antagonist medial rectus causes its paralysis and is thus useful for a temporary alignment of the eyes in the primary position. Such injections are also useful in preventing the contracture of the medial rectus muscle, while the patient is observed for several months prior to surgical intervention.
iii. *Fresnel press-on prisms* are useful to correct the diplopia in primary position.

Note. A spontaneous resolution of the sixth nerve paresis, sometimes occurs, making the surgery unneccessary. Hess screen charting (Fig.10.3.7) is useful for a meticulous follow-up of the patients during this wating period.

III. Surgical treatment

Surgery is indicated, when spontaneous resolution does not take place after 6 months or more of follow-up and after exclusion of the intracranial lesions.

Aim of surgical treatment is to provide a useful field of binocular single vision and to eliminate the abnormal head posture. Following surgical measures have been recommended by the experienced surgeons:

1. *Recess-resect operation.* A large recession of the antagonist medial rectus with resection of the lateral rectus muscle is often a successful first operation in most patients with incomplete paralysis. This procedure often provides a useful field of binocular single vision and eliminates the abnormal head posture. In case a mild paresis is still present, *weakening of the contralateral medial rectus muscle* with or without Faden procedure may be considered as a second operation.

Adjustable suture surgery may be helpful for final adjustments in co-operative patients with paralytic squint.

2. *Muscle transposition procedures* recommended for a complete paralysis of lateral rectus muscle.

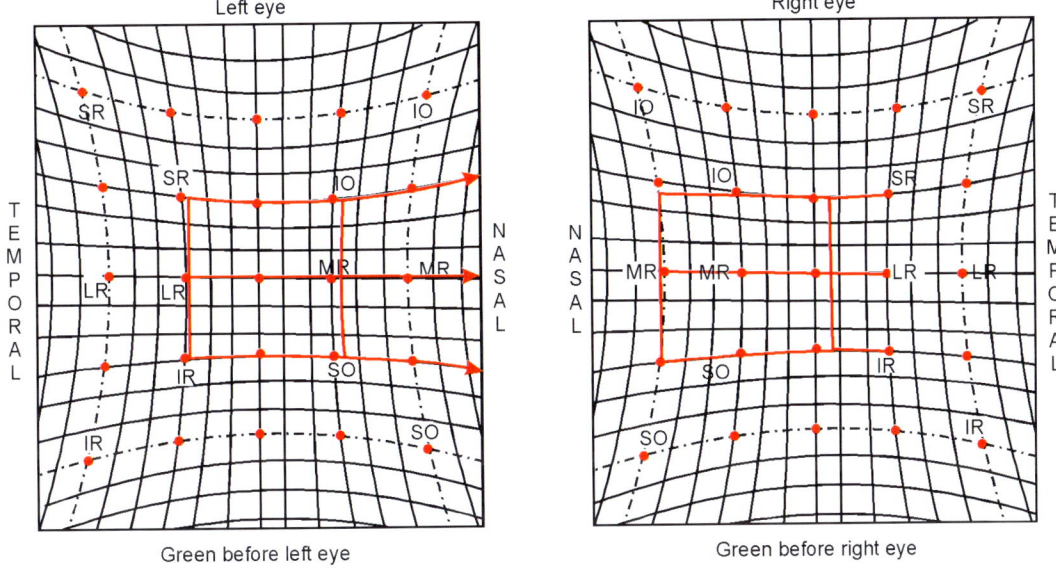

Left eye — Green before left eye

Right eye — Green before right eye

Fig. 10.3.7 *Hess chart of a patient with paralysis of right lateral rectus muscle*

Medial rectus recession should also be combined especially, when there is medial rectus contracture. Forced duction test is useful in discovering MR contracture.

i. *Jensen's procedure* combined with the medial rectus recession is useful by balancing the partially active forces. In the Jensen's procedure, the superior rectus, inferior rectus muscles and the paralysed lateral rectus muscle are split for 8–10 mm from their insertion backwards with the help of a muscle hook. Then the superior half of the lateral rectus is united with the lateral half of the superior rectus and the inferior half of the lateral rectus with the lateral half of inferior rectus with the help of a non-absorable suture (e.g. 5–0 Mersilene). The knot should be tied near the equator (Fig. 10.3.8).

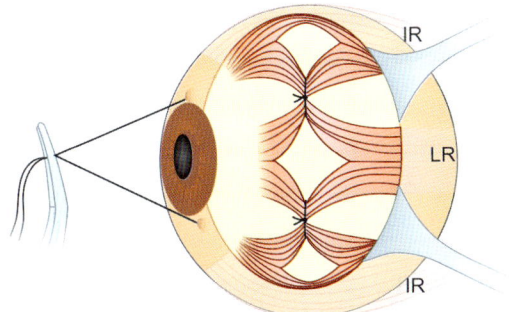

Fig. 10.3.8 *Jensen's procedure for lateral rectus palsy*

ii. *Hummelscheim operation.* In this procedure, after spliting the superior and inferior recti, their lateral halves are disinserted and sutured to the tendon of lateral rectus muscle. This operation is rarely done nowadays and is thus mainly of historical interest.

iii. *Berens and Girard procedure.* In this procedure, the full inferior and superior rectus tendons are disinserted and sutured with the tendon of lateral rectus at its insertion. This procedure combined with a recession of the medial rectus is recommended by von Noorden in children with complete paralysis of sixth cranial nerve.

TRAUMATIC PALSY OF COMBINED THIRD, FOURTH, AND SIXTH CRANIAL NERVES

Causes

Causes of combined third, fourth, and sixth cranial nerves include:

1. *Penetrating injuries* involving the orbit and superior orbital fissure.
2. *Traumatic carotid-cavernous fistula* may be associated with either isolated or combined palsy of third, fourth and sixth cranial nerves.

Clinical features

1. *Features of paralysis of ocular motor nerves.*
2. *Other clinical features* of traumatic carotid-cavernous fistula include: headache, pulsatile proptosis, and asymptomatic bruit.

TRAUMATIC CENTRAL OCULAR MOTOR DYSFUNCTION

Head trauma may be associated with almost all types of central ocular motor dysfunction.

OCULAR MOTOR SIGNS IN COMA

Careful elicitation of ocular motor signs in a comatosed patients is essential for planning management and predicting prognosis in patients with head trauma. The common examination includes observing:

- Lid closure and opening response;
- Positions of eyeballs,
- Eye movements on passive head turn, and
- Caloric test

Observing lid closure and opening response

Lid closure in a comatosed patient indicates normal function of lower pons. Slow closure of eyelids, often they have been opened passively, is typical in stupor and coma.

Lid opening. Elevator muscle function can be determined in a comatose patients by passively making the patients upright with normal function the eyelids will open reflexly for a period of time.

Observing position of eyeballs

- *Transient deviation* in downgaze or upgaze and roving eye movement are common in comatose patients.
- *Forced downgaze deviation* suggests thalamic or subthalamic lesions in the form of haemorrhage or infraction.
- *Forced upgaze deviation* is suggestive of hypoxic injury to the brain.

Eye movements on passive head turn

Observation of eye movements on passive head turn test gives following clues:

- *Full conjugate horizontal movement* on passive head turning excludes brainstem lesion.
- *No eye movements,* in the absence of paralytic drugs, suggest a major brainstem lesions.
- *Inability of eyes to move on one side* suggests a unilateral lesions in pontine centre.
- *Lack of adduction of one eye* is suggestive of either third nerve palsy or internuclear-ophthalmoplegia.

- *Lack of abduction* of one eye indicates sixth nerve palsy.

Caloric test

Caloric test is based on the fact that a jerk nystagmus is induced when tympanic membrane is stimulated by either cold or warm water.

Normal response is as below:

- *With cold water stimulation* of one ear, there occurs contralateral jerk nystagmus, i.e. slow phase towards the direction of stimulated ear, followed by a rapid phase in contralateral direction.
- *With warm water stimaulation,* a reverse response is seen, i.e. rapid phase is towards the stimulated ear.

It can be remembered by the mnemonic 'COWS' (Cold–opposite, Warm–same)

Abnormal response is seen in patients with abnormal labyrinth in one side.

No caloric response in patients with head injury is suggestive of high morbidity and mortality.

TRAUMATIC LOCALIZED CENTRAL OCULAR MOTOR DYSFUNCTION

Traumatic localized central ocular motor dysfunction includes:

- Traumatic gaze palsy
- Traumatic internuclear ophthalmoplegia, and
- Post-head trauma nystagmus and other supranuclear disorders of eye movement.

Traumatic gaze palsies

Horizontal gaze palsy

Horizontal conjugate gaze paralysis refers to equal paralysis of same sided horizontal movement in both eyes, i.e. either levoversion or dextroversion is deficient or defective.

Site of lesion

As described earlier, the frontal lobe is connected with the mesencephalon through the frontomesencephalic pathway. This pathway descends into the internal capsule and is thought to cross completely at the level of fourth nerve nucleus (Figs 10.3.9 to 10.3.11). It is primarily involved in the saccadic eye movement system.

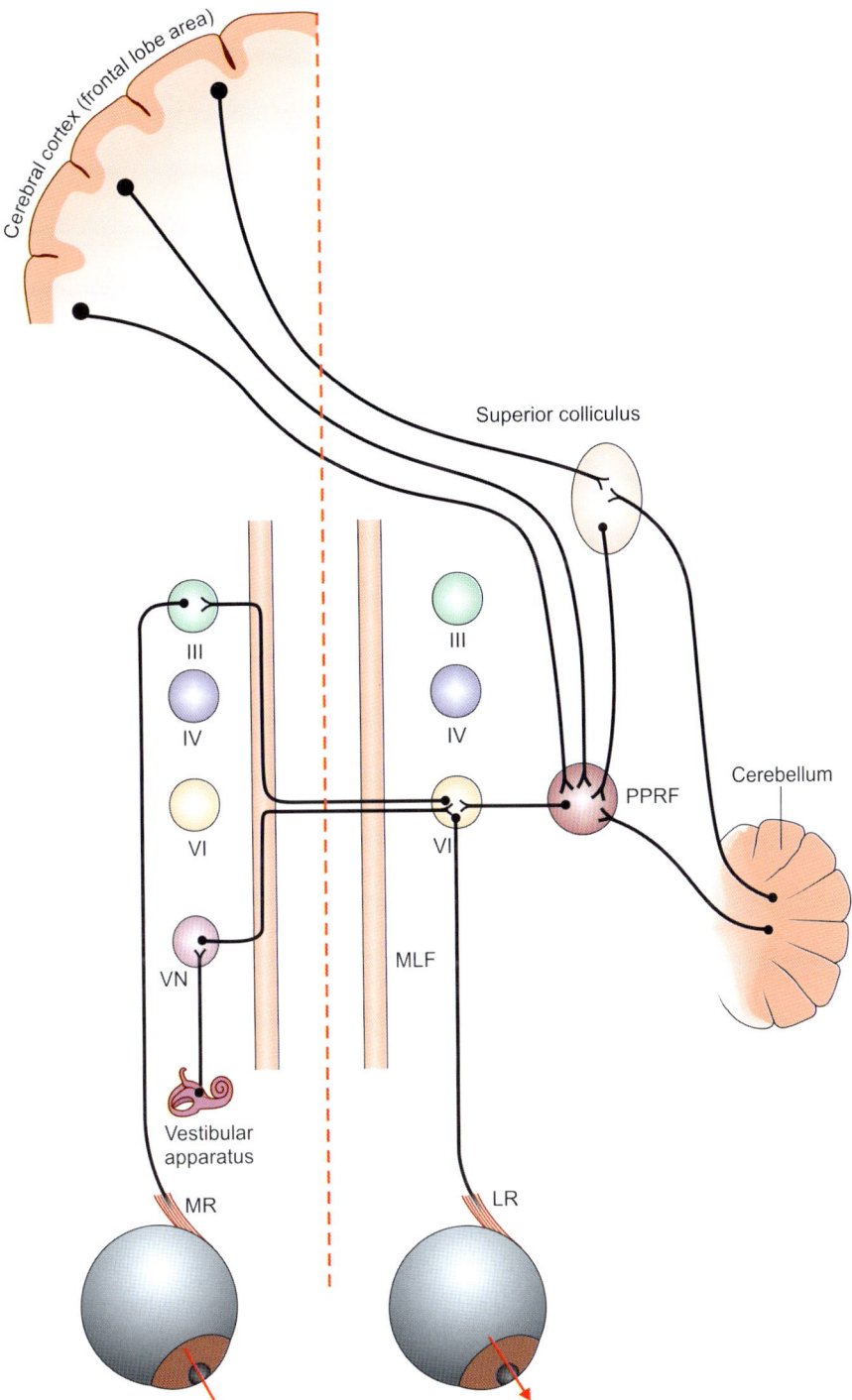

Fig. 10.3.9 *Pathway for horizontal gaze saccadic eye movements. The horizontal gaze centre (present in PPRF) is connected with ipsilateral lateral rectus muscle (LR) and with abducens internuclear neurons whose axons cross the midline and travel in the medial longitudinal fasciculus (MLF) of the opposite side to that part of the nucleus of IIIrd nerve which innervates the medial rectus muscle*

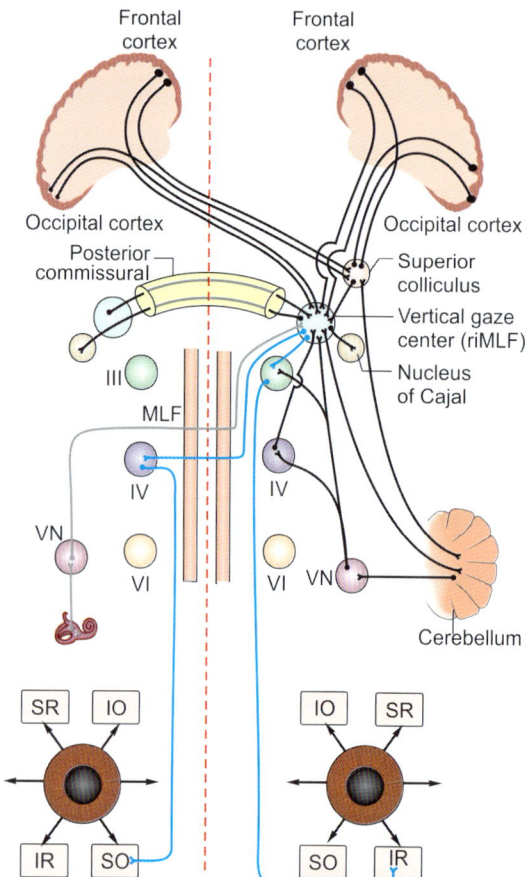

Fig. 10.3.10 *Pathway for vertical gaze (downgaze) saccadic eye movements*

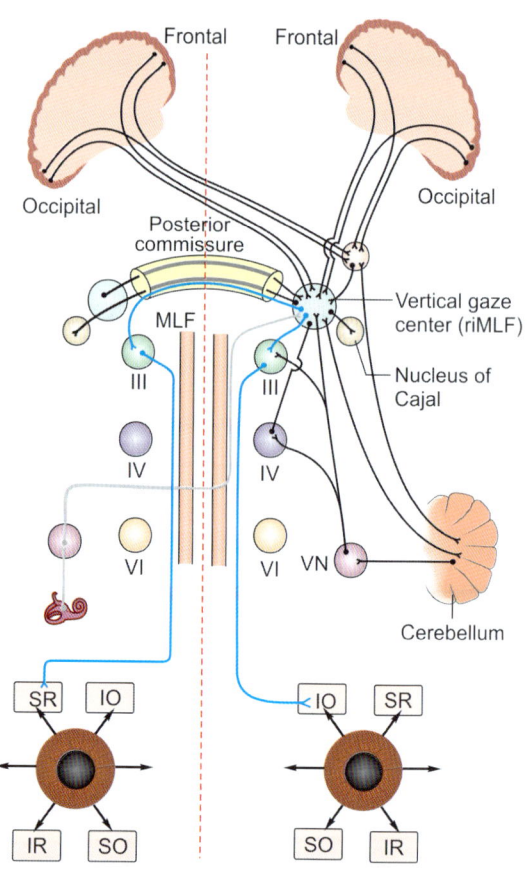

Fig. 10.3.11 *Pathway for vertical gaze (upgaze) saccadic eye movements*

A destructive lesion in the cortical centre or frontomesencephalic pathway above decussation (Fig. 10.3.12A) produces defects in conjugate gaze to the opposite side. Lesions below the decussation (Fig. 10.3.12B) produce defects in conjugate gaze to the same side as the lesion. Lesions involving 6th nerve nucleus (1 in Fig. 10.3.13) and PPRF (2 in Fig. 10.3.13) can also produce horizontal gaze palsy on the same side. It is important to note that since the area of the frontal lobe concerned with horizontal eye movements is so large, small lesions of the frontal lobe rarely affect conjugate horizontal gaze.

Efferent fibres from the occipital lobe connecting the mesencephalon from the occipitoparietomesencephalic pathway. This pathway also crosses to the opposite side at the level of 4th nerve nucleus. Lesions involving this pathway will also produce conjugate movements to the opposite side or same side depending upon the site of lesions similar to frontal lobe lesions. However, the conjugate paralysis caused by lesions of occipitoparietal pathway is of lesser magnitude than that caused by lesions involving the frontal voluntary system.

Clinical features

As described above, when the frontomesencephalic tract is interrupted by a lesion above the crossing, there is a deficit of rapid eye movements to the opposite side; thus the right-sided lesion will affect:

1. Saccades to the left.
2. The fast phase of the optokinetic nystagmus, when it is to the left.

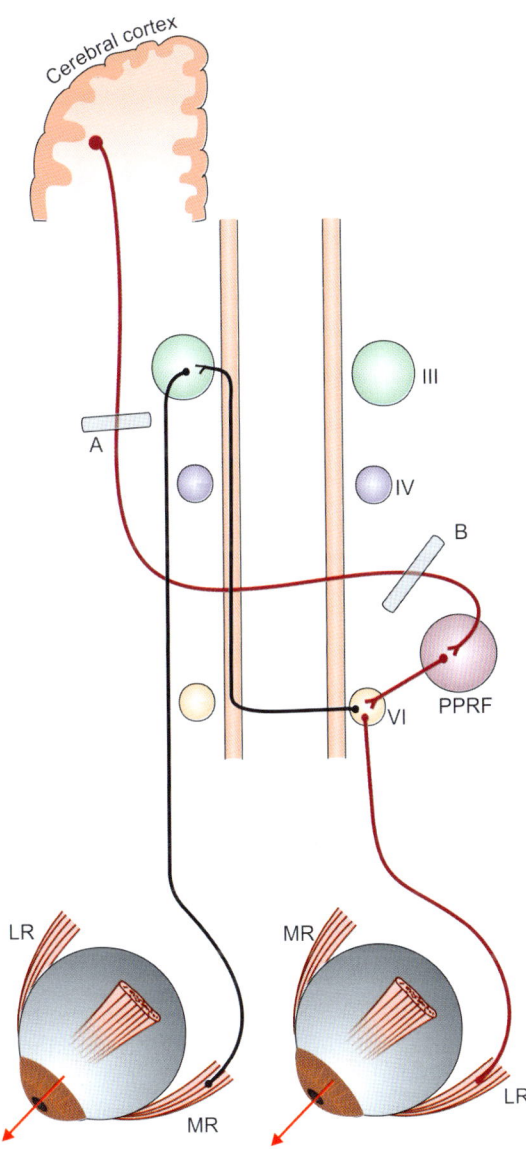

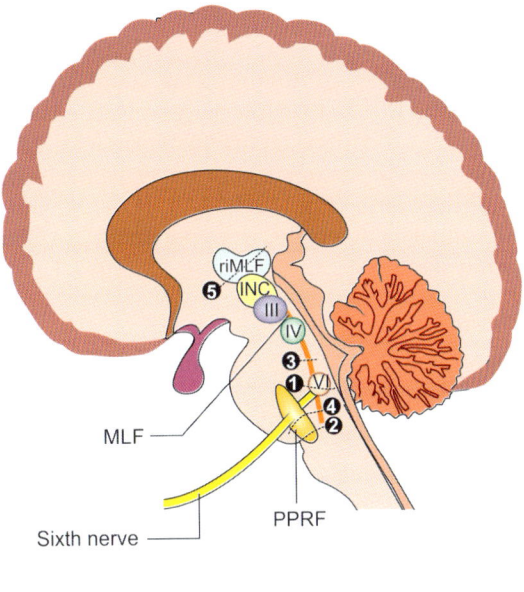

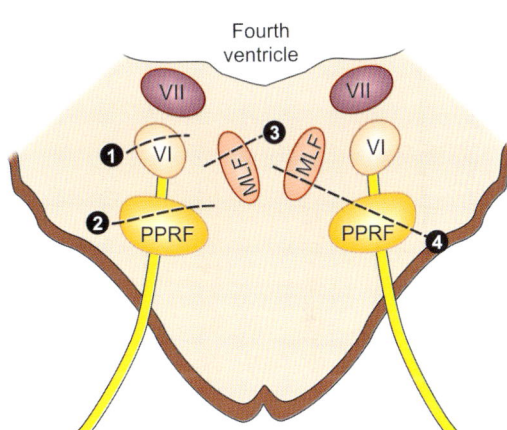

Fig. 10.3.13 *Site of lesions producing supranuclear disorders. Horizontal gaze palsy may result from lesion involving 6th nerve nucleus (1) and PPRF (2); Internuclear ophthalmoplegia results from a lesion of medial longitudinal fasciculus (3), one-and-a-half syndrome results from a lesion involving both the MLF and PPRF (4); and vertical gaze palsy may result from a lesion involving riMLF (5)*

Fig. 10.3.12 *Site of lesions producing conjugate paralysis to the opposite side (A) and the same side (B)*

3. The fast phase of caloric or vestibular nystagmus when it is to the left.
4. On looking to the left, there may be a gaze paretic nystagmus with the fast phase to the left with varying amplitude and rhythm.
5. Gaze paralysis and conjugate deviations caused by hemispheric lesions are usually transient, probably due to compensation from the contralateral uninvolved hemi-sphere. While, paralysis resulting from lesions in the brainstem are less marked but last as long as the lesion exists since no compensation of function occurs.
6. Lesions causing gaze paralysis (e.g. infarction, and haemorrhages and tumours) also produce severe neurologic signs, such as hemiplegia and thus the eye signs, are usually overshadowed.

Traumatic internuclear ophthalmoplegia

Internuclear ophthalmoplegia (INO) results from a lesion of the medial longitudinal fasciculus (MLF) that interrupts fibres passing from the subcortical centre for horizontal gaze of one side to the nucleus of the third nerve on the other side (Fig. 10.3.14A). It is the only supranuclear defect that does not result in a gaze paralysis.

Clinical features

Unilateral INO. A patient with unilateral INO on version movements will exhibit:

- *Exotropia* in the involved side (Fig. 10.3.15A).
- *Limitation of adduction* on the involved side (Fig. 10.3.15B).

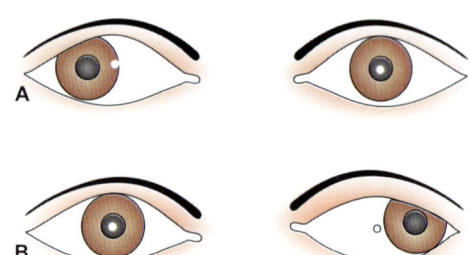

Fig. 10.3.15 *Diagrammatic depiction of right internuclear ophthalmoplegia. Note right exotropia in primary position (A) and limitation of adduction in the right eye with normal abduction in the left eye (B)*

- *Normal abduction* of the opposite eye (Fig. 10.3.15B).
- *Nystagmus* is associated with abduction of the opposite side. Nystagmus in INO is a secondary response to the weakness of adduction and not caused directly by the central defect.
- *Convergence* is normal in many patients and thus both eyes adduct normally to fixate a near object.
- *Skew deviation* of some degree may be noted with the eye ipsilateral to the lesion slightly higher than the other.

Bilateral INO is more frequent than unilateral INO. Depending upon the site of lesion, other cranial nuclei and convergence mechanism may also be involved.

Differential diagnosis

1. ***Isolated medial rectus palsy*** needs to be differentiated from the INO.

2. ***Pseudointernuclear ophthalmoplegia*** should be distinguished from the true INO. Pseudo-INO, i.e. a condition characterized by limitation of adduction and nystagmus of the abducting eye caused by lesions other than lesions of MLF, such as:

- That occurring due to myasthenia gravis
- That following recession and retroequatorial posterior fixation of both medial rectus muscles.

Treatment

Unfortunately, still there is no effective treatment for INO.

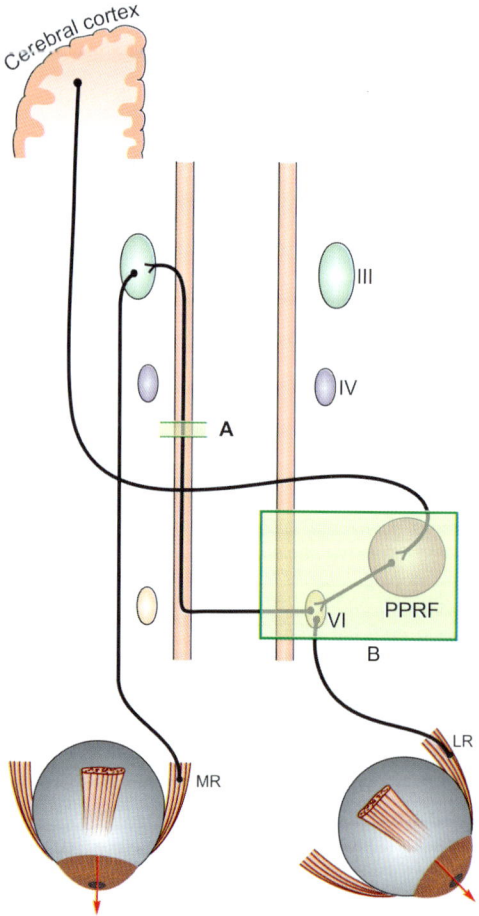

Fig. 10.3.14 *Site of lesion: A, producing internuclear ophthalmoplegia; B, producing gaze palsy plus INO*

ONE-AND-A-HALF SYNDROME

One-and-a-half syndrome (paralytic pontine exotropia) consists of a unilateral internuclear ophthalmoplegia and a contralateral-horizontal gaze palsy.

Etiology

An extensive caudal lesion in the pons can affect resulting in a palsy of both medial rectus muscles and one lateral rectus (i.e. gaze palsy plus INO) (Fig. 10.3.14B and 4 in Fig. 10.3.13). Causes include demyelination, vascular, tumour and inflammation.

Features

The main clinical and diagnostic features are as follows: The only remaining horizontal movement is abduction by the unaffected lateral rectus, which is associated with the typical abducting nystagmus. When the patient attempts to fixate with this eye in the primary position, the nystagmus will reduce or cease. There is, therefore, a palsy of conjugate gaze on one side and an INO on looking to the other side. A marked compensatory head posture may be adopted to achieve fixation with the preferred eye. Although complete 'one-and-a-half' synd-romes are rare, partial or incomplete syndromes are more common. These can be diagnosed on clinical assessment. A Hess chart is useful in monitoring the condition. However, care must be taken in its interpretation, as synergist muscles are affected in patients with lesions involving the horizontal gaze centre as well as the MLF (partial one-and-a-half syndrome). Since the basis of the Hess chart is a comparison of action of synergistic muscles, the test is comparing abnormal with abnormal and, if viewed in isolation, the gaze palsy element may be missed.

Nystagmus and supranuclear disorders of eye movements

Nystagmus

- *Horizontal nystagmus with low frequency and large amplitude* is suggestive of injury to the paramedian pontine gaze nuclei.
- *Horizontal nystagmus with high frequency and small amplitude* is suggestive of injury to horizontal vestibular nucleus.

- See-saw nystagmus is suggestive of injury to subthalamic structures on one side, e.g. traumatic chiasmal syndrome.
  Injury to pontomedullary junction following hyperextension head injury.
- *Latent nystagmus* may become manifest after injury to one eye.

Other supranuclear disorders of ocular motility associated with head injury

- *Ocular bobbing*, i.e. intermittent downward and upward movements of the eyes, is suggestive of lower brainstem injury particulary bilateral pontine horizontal gaze centres.
- *Ping-pong gaze*, i.e. cyclic alternate horizontal deviation of the eyes is suggestive of bilateral cerebral hemispheric damage.
- *Opsoclonus refers* to random, rapid or saccadic movements in many directions, may rarely be associated with severe head trauma.
- *Ocular flatter, dysmetria, lateropulsion, rebound nystagmus, and upbeat nystagmus*, may be associated with cerebral injury.

BIBLIOGRAPHY

1. Elston JS. Traumatic third nerve palsy. Br J Ophthalmol 1984; 68:538–43.
2. Eyster EF, Hoyt WF, Wilson CB. Oculomotor palsy from minor head trauma. JAMA 1972; 220:1083–6.
3. Heinz J. Cranial nerve avulsion and other neural injuries. Med J Aust 1969; 2:1246–9.
4. Miller NR. The oculomotor nerves. CurrOpin Neurol 1996; 9:21–5.
5. Muthu P, Pritty P. Mild head injury with isolated third nerve palsy. Emerg Med J2001; 18:310–1.
6. Nagaseki Y, Shimizu T, Kakizawa T, et al. Primary internal ophthalmoplegia due to head injury. ActaNeurochir 1989; 97:117–22.
7. Saad N. Lee J. The role of botulinum toxin in third nerve palsy. Aust N Z J Ophthalmol 1992; 20:121–7.
8. Solomons NB, Solomon DJ, DeVilliers JC. Direct traumatic third nerve palsy. S Afr Med J 1980; 58:109–111. Memon MY, Paine KWE. Direct injury of the oculomotor nerve in craniocerebral trauma. J Neurosurg 1971; 35:461–4.
9. Tiffin PAC, MacEwen CJ, Craig EA, et al. Acquired palsy of the oculomotor, trochlear and abducens nerves. Eye 1996; 10:377–84.

10.4 TRAUMA TO TRIGEMINAL AND FACIAL NERVES

INTRODUCTION

Trigeminal (5th cranial nerve) and facial (7th cranial nerve) are two other important cranial nerves related to the eye. A brief account of trauma to these nerves is given below briefly.

TRAUMA TO TRIGEMINAL NERVE

Trauma may involve Gasserian ganglion, trigeminal nerve trunks or peripheral branches.

Trauma to Gassarian ganglion and/or main trunk

I. *Penetrating injury to skull* (gunshot) may involve Gassarian ganglion and can cause ocular and facial anaesthesia. There may also be associated injury to 3rd, 4th or 6th nerve.

II. *Crush injuries of skull* may also involve Gassarian ganglion or its branches. In such cases, 6th nerve is also frequently involved. There may occur involvement of 3rd and 4th nerves as well thus causing complete unilateral ophthalmoplegia.

Trauma to infraorbital nerve

Infraorbital nerve involvement frequently occurs in patients with orbital floor fractures. It is associated with facial anaesthesia and other features of orbital floor fracture, such as initial proptosis, periorbital oedema followed soon by enophthalmos and mechanical ptosis.

Clinically applied aspect

Corneal sensations must be checked in each and every case of face and head trauma.

Corneal complications. If corneal anaesthesia is missed, rapidly there may occur corneal epithelial defects and ulcer (neuroparalytic ulcer). This is most critical when there is concomitant facial nerve palsy predisposing to exposure keratitis as well.

Measures to prevent corneal complications include patching, lid suturing or tarsorrhaphy along with frequent use of lubricants.

TRAUMA TO FACIAL NERVE

Facial nerve palsy is frequently associated with head and face trauma. Lesions may be supranuclear or infranuclear.

Supranuclear lesions

In *supranuclear lesions* of the facial nerve (usually a part of the hemiplegia), only the lower part of the *contralateral face* is paralysed. The upper part (frontalis and part of orbicularis oculi) escapes due to its bilateral representation in the cerebral cortex. At this level, cerebrovascular accidents and trauma are the most likely causes.

Infranuclear lesions

Infranuclear lesions, i.e. the peripheral facial nerve injury which has a good prognosis, results from fracture of the petrous potion of the temporal bone.

Features of infranuclear lesions of facial nerve are (Fig. 10.4.1):
- Whole of the face of the ipsilateral side is paralysed, abolishing both voluntary and emotional movements.
- The face becomes asymmetrical and is drawn up to the normal side.
- The affected side is motionless. Wrinkles disappear from the forehead.

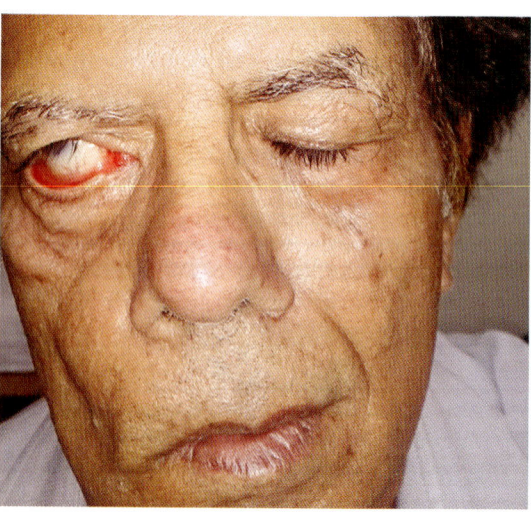

Fig. 10.4.1: *Infranuclear right facial nerve palsy*

- The eye cannot be closed (lagophthalmos).
- Any attempt to smile draws the mouth to the normal side.
- During mastication, food accumulates between the teeth and the cheek.
- Articulation of labialis is impaired.
- The lesions found distal to the chorda tympani produce isolated facial palsy. In lesions proximal to the geniculate ganglion, the palsy is associated with loss of taste sensations on the anterior two-thirds of the tongue and diminished salivation.
- A lesion proximal to the nerve to stapedius is associated with an additional complaint of ipsilateral hyperacusis.
- *Ramsay-Hunt syndrome* occurs due to herpes zoster infection of the geniculate ganglion of the facial nerve. It is characterized by the lower motor neuron type of facial palsy associated with severe pain in the ear and vesicles near the ear.
- *Lesions at the level of pons* result in the involvement of both the abducent and the facial nerves.
- *Lesions at the cerebellopontine angle* result in the involvement of both the facial and auditory nerves.

Clinically applied aspects

- *Early recognition and management of facial nerve* is important to prevent sight-threatening corneal complications.

- *Measures to prevent corneal complications* are similar to as described for trigeminal nerve injury.

BIBLIOGRAPHY

1. Blum Andrew S. and Seward B. Rutkove, eds. The Clinical Neurophysiology Primer. Humana Press Inc. Totowa, New Jersey. 2007.

2. Daube, Jasper, ed. Clinical Neurophysiology. F.A. Davis Company, Philadelphia. 1996.

3. Dumitru, Daniel, Anthony Amato and MachielZwarts. Electrodiagnostic Medicine, 2nd Ed. Hanley and Belfus, Philadalephia. 2002.

4. Hughes, Richard AC. "Diseases of the Fifth Cranial Nerve." Peripheral Neuropathy. Ed. Dyck, Peter J. and P. K. Thomas. 4th Ed. Elsevier Saunders. Philadelphia. 2005.

5. Kimura, Jun. Electrodiagnosis in Diseases of Nerve and Muscle: Principles and Practice. 3rd Ed. Oxford University Press, New York. 2001.

6. Klein, Caroline M. "Diseases of the Seventh Cranial Nerve." Peripheral Neuropathy. Ed. Dyck, Peter J and PK. Thomas. 4th Ed. Elsevier Saunders. Philadelphia. 2005.

7. Oh, Shin. Clinical Electromyography: Nerve Conduction Studies. 2nd Ed. Williams and Wilkins, Baltimore. 1993.

8. Preston, David and Barbara Shapiro. Electromyography and Neuromuscular Disorders; Clinical Electrophysiologic Correlations. 2nd Ed. Elsevier, Philadelphia. 2005

10.5 OCULAR MANIFESTATIONS OF HEAD INJURY

INTRODUCTION

Head injury basically traumatic brain injury (TBI) is recognized as a major cause of morbidity and mortality worldwide. Because more than half of cranial nerves are linked to the eye and with a significant proportion of circuits in the brain involved in vision many aspects of the visual system are vulnerable to moderate, severe, or mild TBI. Evident so, examination of the integrity of the visual system helps in both screen and monitor the recovery of patients with head injury. The ocular manifestations of TBI can be broadly classified as below:

- Soft tissue signs
- Pupillomotor disorders
- Papilloedema
- Traumatic optic neuropathy and injury to visual pathway
- Disorders of gaze and extraocular movement
- Terson's syndrome
- Ocular disorders in concussive head trauma

OCULAR MANIFESTATIONS OF TRAUMATIC BRAIN INJURY

I. SOFT TISSUE SIGNS

Periorbital ecchymosis known as *Raccoon eyes* or *Panda eyes* (Fig. 10.5.1) is the most important ocular soft tissue sign. When bilateral it is highly suggestive of a skull base fracture, with a positive predictive value of 85%.

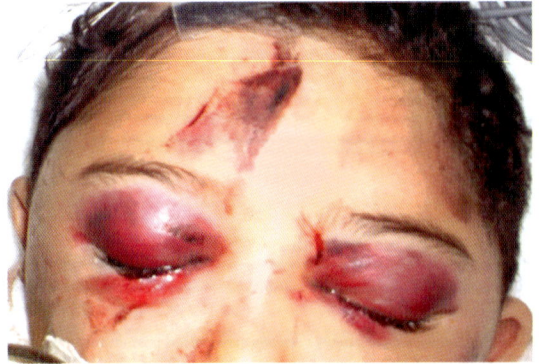

Fig. 10.5.1 *Periorbital ecchymosis in a patient with head injury*

Battle's sign, an ecchymosis behind the ear and fracture of the anterior cranial fossa, may also accompany it.

II. PUPILLOMOTOR DISORDERS

Involvement of the pupil is an important sign of presence of structural brain lesion in contrast to metabolic brain lesions (encephalopathy) in which the pupil is generally spared. Pupillary signs observed in head injury are as below:

1. *Hutchinson's pupil:* It is characterized by initial ipsilateral miosis followed by dilatation with no light reflex due to raised intracranial pressure (ICP). If the ICP continues to rise further, similar changes ensue on the contralateral side. Named after Sir Jonathan Hutchinson, it can occur due to concussion injury to the brain and is associated with extradural haemorrhage and unconsciousness. It consists of three stages:

- *Stage 1.* In it, the parasympathetic pupillomotor fibres on the side of injury are irritated, leading to constriction of pupil on that side (Fig. 10.5.2A).
- *Stage 2.* In it, the parasympathetic fibres on the side of injury are paralyzed, leading to dilatation of pupil. The fibres on the opposite oculomotor nerve are irritated, leading to constriction on opposite side (Fig. 10.5.2B).
- *Stage 3.* In it, the parasympathetic fibres on both sides are paralyzed—leading to bilateral pupillary dilatation (Fig. 10.5.2C). Pupils become fixed and are an indication of immediate cerebral decompression.

2. **Unilateral miosis:** Unilateral miosis in a patient with head injury occurs due to injury to the ipsilateral hypothalamus leading to preganglionic Horner's pupil.

3. *Bilateral miosis:* Bilateral miosis occurs in intrinsic pontine lesions or from external compression due to cerebellar or posterior fossa haemorrhage. Pathomechanism involves disruption of sympathetic fibres descending through the pons. Since bilateral miosis can also occur in metabolic encephalopathy and opioid poisoning, its comitant presence should be ruled out.

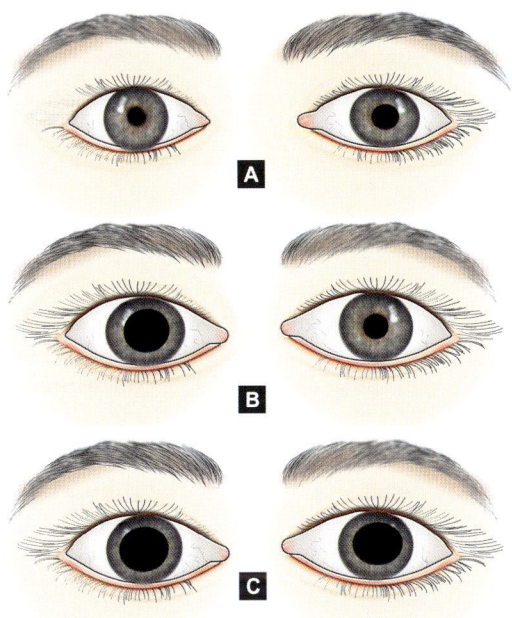

Fig. 10.5.2 *Hutchinson's pupil seen in case of cerebral compression consists of 3 stages:*
A. Stage 1: Pupil of the side of injury contract due to irritation of oculomotor nerve
Pupil on other side—normal
B. Stage 2: Pupil of the injured side becomes dilated due to paralysis of oculomotor nerve
Pupil of other side—contracts
C. Stage 3: Pupils of both sides dilated, no reaction to light

4. ***Midbrain pupil:*** A midbrain pupil is 4–5 mm in diameter, irregular and non-reactive. Although not very common after traumatic brain injury, it occurs due to a posterior fossa haemorrhage compressing the dorsal midbrain. There is varying degree of dysfunction of both sympathetic descending fibres and tectal parasympathetic fibres. There is a tug of war between controls of these two pathways. Midbrain pupil accompanied by Light-near dissociation, vertical gaze palsy, convergence retraction nystagmus, impairment of vergence movements and lid retraction is known as *Perinaud syndrome.*

III. PAPILLOEDEMA

Papilloedema is an important non-invasive marker of raised ICP in patients of traumatic brain injury. Depending upon the severity of raised intracranial pressure, it may vary from mild to severe stages of papilloedema are shown in Figs 10.5.3 to 10.5.6. Based on the time at which it appears after head injury, it can be classified as below:

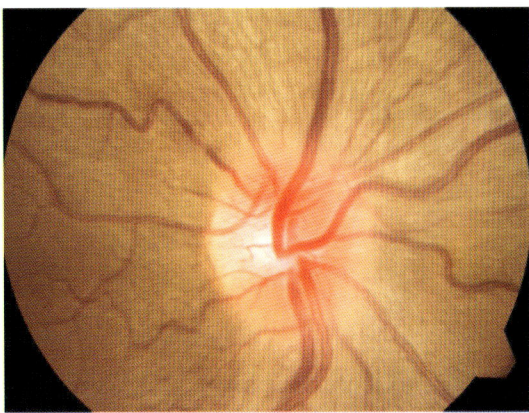

Fig. 10.5.3 *Early papilloedema*

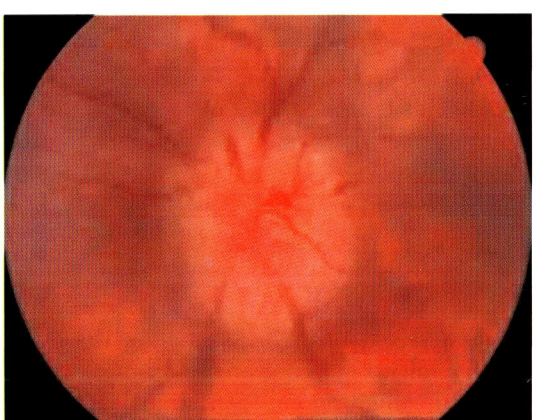

Fig. 10.5.4 *Established stage of papilloedema*

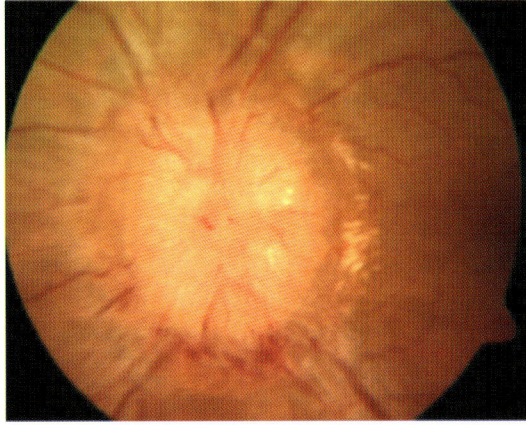

Fig. 10.5.5 *Chronic stage of papilloedema*

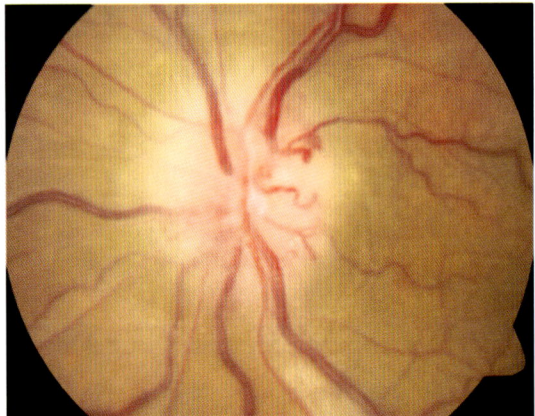

Fig. 10.5.6 *Atrophic stage of papilloedema*

First week papilloedema: Papilloedema occurring in the first week of head injury occurs due to sudden, severe (40–60 mm Hg) rise of intracranial tension which forces the cerebrospinal fluid in the subarachnoid space around the optic nerves and causes axoplasmic stasis. This is caused by a mass effect, such as subdural haematoma, extradural haematoma, intracerebral haemorrhage or contused brain. Paradoxically patients with ICP >60 mm Hg at presentation do not develop papilloedema since most of them do not survive beyond 72 hours of injury.

Second week papilloedema: Papilloedema developing in the second week occurs in patients with sustained moderate rise in ICP due to etiologies listed in week one (20–40 mm Hg). Additionally, subarachnoid haemorrhage, intraventicular haemorrhage, tissue oedema around a focal cerebral contusion, expanding extradural haematoma and a diffuse axonal injury may cause rise in ICP at this stage. Hence especially in cases of cerebral contusion and extradural haematoma, it is prudent to watch out for papilloedema later even if ruled out in initial examination.

Third week papilloedema: Delayed papilloedema occurs from impaired CSF absorption as in resolving subarachnoid haemorrhage or increased production as in ventriculitis and meningitis in patients with compound fractures of cribriform plate or the mastoid bone causing a non-communicating hydrocephalus.

IV. TRAUMATIC OPTIC NEUROPATHY AND INJURY TO VISUAL PATHWAY

Traumatic optic neuropathies: Traumatic optic neuropathy is reported to occur on 0.5–8% of cases of head injury. In most cases, the trauma force is not inflicted directly to the nerve but to the brow area of the face, which is transmitted to the intracanalicular portion of optic nerve. The details have been covered in Chapter 10.1.

Chiasmal and visual pathway injury: Injury to the chiasma is rare and is associated with frontal blows and midline basilar skull fractures. The details have been covered in Chapter 10.2.

V. DISORDERS OF GAZE AND EXTRAOCULAR MOVEMENT

Akin to pupillary involvement disorders of extraocular movement are more common in structural brain lesions than metabolic causes.

The involvement can occur at three 3 levels. Supranuclear, internuclear and infranuclear. In all non-comatose, cooperative patients, an attempt should be made to look for extraocular movements in all directions. In comatose patients, oculocephalic (*Doll's eye testing*) should be done after ruling out injury to cervical spine.

Supranuclear lesions cause conjugate ocular deviations. A horizontal conjugate deviation occurs due to a ipsilateral frontal lobe – putamen lesion or a contralateral pontine or cerebellar haemorrhage. If the eyes are deviated downwards (*up gaze palsy*), it indicates thalamic injury. The details of individual nerve palsies have been discussed in Chapter 10.3.

VI. TERSON'S SYNDROME

It is defined as intraocular subhyloid haemorrhage associated with subarachnoid haemorrhage (SAH), intracerebral haemorrhage or traumatic brain injury. The details have been covered in Chapter 6.3.

VII. OCULAR DISORDERS IN CONCUSSIVE HEAD TRAUMA

Concussion injury to the brain represents mild head trauma. Most of the abnormalities are localized to dysfunction of frontal and temporal cortices. There are abnormalities in saccades anti-saccades with prolonged saccadic latencies, high directional errors and poor spatial accuracy. Memory guided saccades and self-paced saccades may also be involved. There can also be impairment of convergence, accommodation and reduced reading speed.

BIBLIOGRAPHY

1. Ventura RE, Balcer LJ, Galetta SL. The neuro-ophthalmology of head trauma. Lancet Neurol. 2014 Oct; 13(10):1006–1016.

2. Kumaran AM, Sundar G, Chye LT. Traumatic optic neuropathy: a review. Craniomaxillofac Trauma Reconstr. 2015 Mar; 8(1):31–41.

3. Yu-Wai-Man P, Griffiths PG. Steroids for traumatic optic neuropathy. Cochrane Database Syst Rev. 2013 Jun 17; 6.

4. Wirtsch after JD, Rizzo FJ, Smiley BC. Optic nerve axoplasm and papilledema. Surv Ophthalmol. 1975 Nov-Dec; 20(3):157–189.

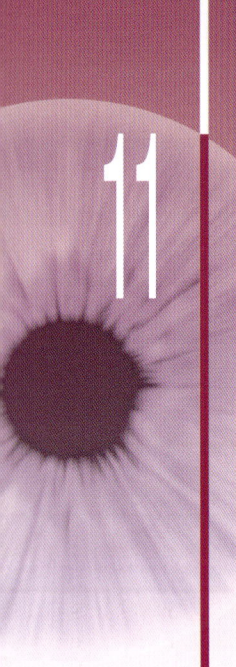

11 EYELID AND LACRIMAL SYSTEM TRAUMA

EYELID TRAUMA

GENERAL CONSIDERATIONS

INTRODUCTION

Trauma to eyelids and lacrimal apparatus can occur in a variety of ways and often in complex combinations. In order to manage the problems presented by trauma to the eyelid effectively, the ophthalmologist needs to have not only a thorough insight of its anatomy, but also an indepth knowledge of general approaches to trauma repair. Lacrimal system trauma might need an immediate repair using microsurgical techniques. Such a trauma may have associated injury to bony structures forming orbit or soft tissue within the orbit. Hence exhaustive evaluation of such trauma after taking meticulous history regarding its mode, type and time since injury is must.

EPIDEMIOLOGY

Eyelid trauma is most commonly seen after road traffic accidents followed by assault injuries. It is more commonly seen in males (male: female ratio being 6.3:1) and is more prevalent in 3rd decade of life (30%). The most common presentation is in the form of laceration (36%) followed by abrasion/bruises (7%) and avulsion (10%).

PATHOPHYSIOLOGY AND TYPES OF EYELID INJURIES

Trauma to an eyelid can occur by blunt forces or sharp objects, like knife. Eyelid injuries may be in the form of:

1. *Abrasions*: Removal of superficial or all the layers of epidermis and sometimes involve even superficial layer of dermis. Abrasions are caused by rubbing or friction against rough surface.

2. *Contusions*: Blunt trauma to the eyelid results in effusion of blood in lid tissues.

3. *Lacerations*: These are caused by blunt trauma which crushes and stretches the tissues resulting in lid tears/ruptures. Lid lacerations are caused by blows from blunt objects, fall on hard surface, road traffic accidents, etc.

4. *Incised lid wounds*: These are clean cut lid injuries caused by sharp objects like knife, sword, scissors, etc.

5. *Puncture wound*: These are produced when a narrow pointed object pierces the lid, e.g. knife, arrow, needle, screw driver, etc.

6. *Firearm injuries* can result in mixture of injuries.

Blunt injury to eyelid is typically associated with swelling around eyes leading to eyelid oedema and ecchymosis (Fig. 11.1). Ecchymosis results due to breakage of small capillaries and extravasation of blood in the surrounding tissues. Eyelids are devoid of subcutaneous fat, hence there is easy seepage of fluid and blood in eyelids leading to ecchymosis, commonly known as "black eye". It is unilateral in most of the cases, however, it may be bilateral (called as "*raccoon eyes*"). The presence of raccoon eyes should not be overlooked. It might be the only sign of basilar skull fracture.

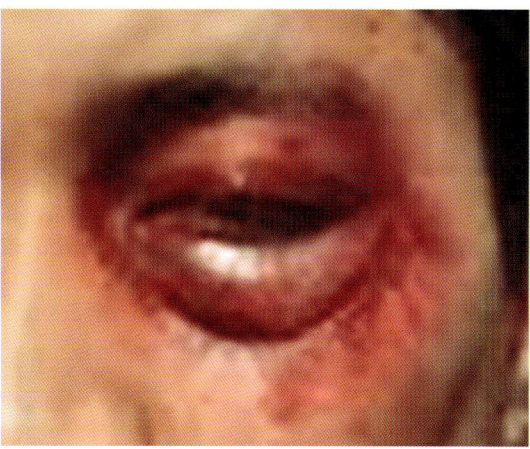

Fig. 11.1 *Traumatic eyelid oedema and ecchymosis*

Direct trauma by sharp objects commonly leads to eyelid laceration. The laceration can involve the lid margin at times (Fig. 11.2). Along with this, the canthal tendon may get injured in the form of avulsion or laceration. It results mainly from horizontal traction on eyelid which leads to avulsion of eyelid at its weakest point, the canthal tendons. The lid laceration can be associated with an entry of foreign body inside eye and hence imaging modalities form an important aspect while evaluating such injuries.

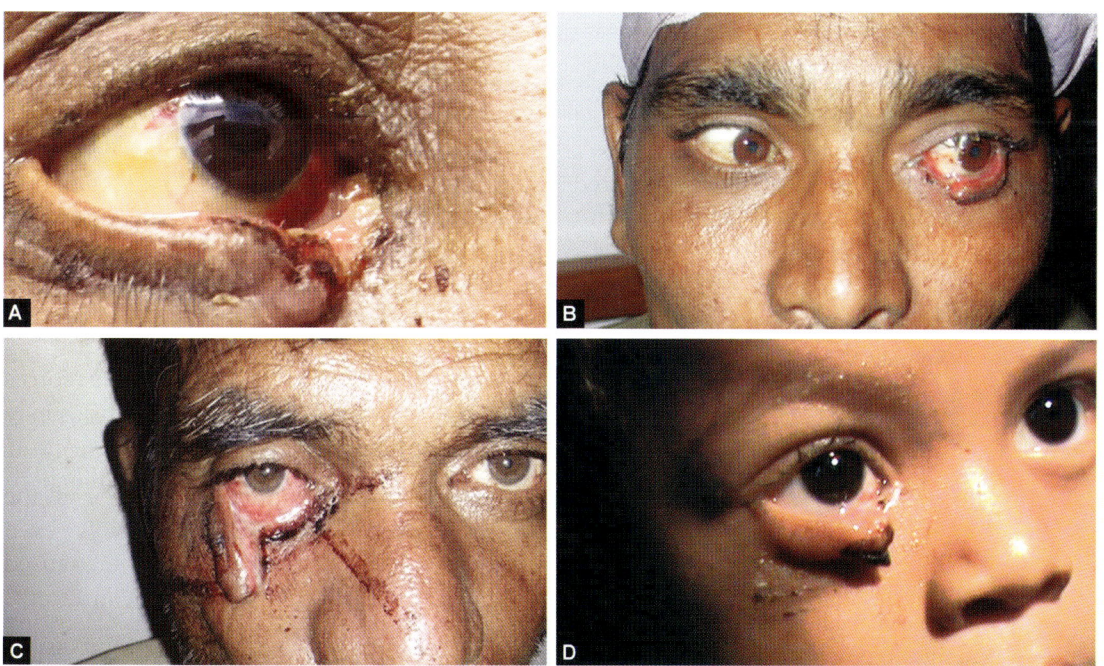

Fig. 11.2A to D: *Lid lacerations: A to D, involving the lid margin*

EVALUATION OF EYELID TRAUMA

It is important to thoroughly evaluate a case of eyelid trauma since frequently it is associated with ocular and systemic injuries.

Before attempting the repair of eyelid trauma, thorough systemic and ocular evaluations must be performed and other significant trauma-related problems, like vitals should be maintained. Following scheme should be considered while evaluating an eyelid trauma case.

HISTORY

Taking meticulous history becomes an important part of evaluation. Essential questions include the time and nature of the injury or accident in order to help define the extent and type of injury, whether safety glasses were worn, any possibility of foreign bodies, such as contact lenses being involved. In case of chemical injury, history pertaining to the type and concentrations should be noted. High energy fluid explosions can inject foreign bodies into the orbit without causing apparent entry sites and may cause tissue necrosis out of proportion to the apparent injury. If the injury is from a dog bite, the type of dog (pet/stray) must be inquired. Such a dog needs to be kept under observation for 10 days. The status of tetanus toxoid vaccination must be inquired. If possible, the condition of the eyes and eyelids before injury should be documented by previous photographs, such as a driver's license. Past medical history should be inquired which can give clues regarding suitability for anaesthesia, current medications and allergies.

OCULAR EXAMINATION

Examination of eyeball

Complete anterior as well as posterior segment examination is mandatory, since major and minor eyelid trauma may be concealing various ocular involvements, like microscopic hyphaema, angle recession, traumatic uveitis, traumatic cataract, vitreous haemorrhage and retinal detachment. The possibility of ruptured globe must always be kept in mind and application of any inadvertent pressure should be avoided, hence care must be taken while opening the oedematous eyelids.

After excluding the anterior and posterior segment lesions, a detailed note of corrected visual acuity, pupillary reactions, intraocular pressure (unless the globe rupture is associated) must be made.

Lid trauma examination

Lid trauma examination should include both nerve as well as muscle evaluation.

- *Sensory nerve function* can be distorted by injury and tissue swelling. Absolute numbness in the typical distribution of a periocular nerve (supraorbital, supratrochlear, infratrochlear, infraorbital, lacrimal or zygomaticofacial) should raise suspicions of nerve transection.
- *Examination of facial nerve* is mandatory as injury to this nerve will affect overall health of the eye.
- *Good eyelid closure* indicates healthy orbicularis oculi muscle. Eyelid swelling can mask good levator function, but the presence of a crease and some lid function despite swelling usually indicates an intact levator. If the levator muscle is injured, traumatic ptosis is anticipated.
- *Wound should be carefully looked for viability* or loss of tissues. Any loss of tissue should be noted. If large pieces of tissues, hair-bearing part of lid are missing, wound should be carefully looked for any piece of tissue that can be used as graft.
- *Lacerations involving eyelid margin* or canaliculus should receive a special attention.
- *Assessment of attachment of lid* to orbital margin and canthal tendon integrity are important as these structures are easily repaired while doing primary repair.

Neurosurgical examination

Neurosurgical examination by an expert is a must in order to rule out an element of head injury before proceeding for ocular examination.

LABORATORY AND IMAGING STUDIES

Laboratory studies

- *Routine investigations*, like Hb, BT, CT, urine analysis, and blood sugar, should be ordered in all cases.

- *Blood alcohol level estimation* may be done whenever required.
- *HIV or hepatitis serology* should be performed when the risk of transmission is aprehanded.

Imaging studies

Lid and adnexal injuries with significant bony tenderness or obvious deformity warrant imaging to evaluate for *fractures*.

Plain X-ray films of the orbit, including Water, Caldwell, and lateral views or even panoramic X-ray images may be useful in the evaluation of fracture or to rule out the presence of foreign body.

   Depending on the size and lead content, the glass foreign bodies may or may not be seen on radiography. Further, wood foreign bodies can be difficult to detect but may appear isodense with orbital fat.

Computed tomography (CT) scans are very useful in lid/orbital trauma. Three-dimensional (3-D) reconstructions can be made for a more detailed analysis. CT scan provides following information:

- Confirm or reveal foreign bodies.
- A retrobulbar haemorrhage,
- A globe rupture, or
- An orbital fracture.

Orbital MRI should be obtained after ruling out metallic foreign body, when an orbital wooden foreign body is suspected which is not seen on CT scan and for the assessment of tissue injuries.

SURGICAL REPAIR

GENERAL PRINCIPLES

- *Early primary repair.* Ideally eyelids should be repaired within 12–24 hrs after injury.
- *Delayed repair.* Although repair of lid lacerations may have to be delayed do to various reasons, however, early repair allows better corneal protection, less tissue oedema, and better wound decontamination. In uncooperative, inebriated patients, repair can be delayed until the patient is out of the effect of alcohol. Further, in severe trauma, delay in eyelid repair is acceptable while more life-threatening injuries are dealt with, but it is important to ensure that the globe is protected from inadvertent pressure in the presence of open globe injury. The drying of cornea is prevented by adequate corneal lubrication till the eyelids are repaired. Patch the wound in proper anatomic alignment. Administer appropriate systemic antibiotics.

- *Copious irrigation* of the wound with saline is must before starting any repair.
- *Dirt, particles, foreign bodies*, fibrin clots should be removed.
- *Appropriate haemostasis* and meticulous handling of the tissue helps in achieving good repair.
- *Try to save or retrieve all lid tissue.* The ocular adnexa has a good blood supply, and even ischemic-appearing tissue often heals.

Principles of reconstruction of tissue loss/lid defect

- Incisions should be parallel to wrinkle lines.
- Always keep the knife perpendicular to skin surface.
- Eliminate all tension from wound edges by generous undermining.
- Certain suture techniques, such as the far-near-near-far technique, help relieve superficial wound tension.
- Do not leave any dead space.
- Ensure complete haemostasis before closing the wound.
- Wound closure should be performed meticulously in 2/3 layers. Ensure eversion of wound edges to avoid postoperative notching by (i) taking wider amount of tissue deeper from skin edges, (ii) vertical mattress sutures, (iii) 2–3 layered closure. There should not be any overlapping of wound edges.
- Maximize horizontal tension and minimize vertical tension; for repair of lower lid wounds.
- The incisions should be vertically oriented to avoid scleral show and ectropion of lower lid.
- Small, superficial defects (<5 mm) or <1 cm in the medial canthal region may be left to heal by granulation (secondary intention).
- Eyelid-margin involvement or extensive tissue loss, however, mandate primary repair.
- Reconstruct either anterior or posterior lamella with graft, but not both because the graft on a graft, mostly fails.

- Maintain sufficient anatomical canthal fixation.

- Try to achieve proper matching of tissues. Narrow the defect as much as possible before sizing a graft to reduce the final size of the graft.

- Larger defects producing severe corneal exposure should be closed either by skin grafts or preferably by flaps.

- There are many techniques available, however, choose the technique which is simplest and most comfortable for you.

- Light dressing is done in the presence of flaps and pressure dressing should be for skin grafts.

Principles for repair of anterior lamellar defects

- Direct skin closure, where possible.

- Skin flaps, e.g. local myocutaneous advancement flap, rotational flap, transposition flaps, OZ plasty, bilobed flaps, etc. may be require.

- Superficial tissue loss which are multiple, appear infected or presented late may be best left to heal by granulation.

- Skin grafting in acute setting frequently predisposes to infection.

- *Skin edges* should be accurately apposed as the wound margin has a tendency to evert. Lid skin sutures can be removed within 4–5 days, however, sutures in other periorbital skin and lid margin are removed in 10–12 days.

- *Maturation of scar* takes around 6–12 months.

- *Management techniques* differ depending upon the involvement of lid margin in the laceration.

Principles for repair of posterior lamellar defects

Any of the following may be required: Posterior lamellar grafts, free conjunctival autograft from contralateral eye, free tarsoconjunctival graft, oral mucosa graft, scleral graft, fascia lata graft, composite eyelid graft, palatal muco-perichondrium graft, auricular cartilage graft, posterior lamellar flaps, or Hughes tarso-conjunctival flap.

TECHNIQUES OF LID REPAIR

A. ANTERIOR LAMELLAR DEFECTS NOT INVOLVING LID MARGIN

Primary closure with undermining

Primary closure can be performed, if redundant skin exists adjacent to the defect. Meticulous closure without tension is attempted. If required, undermining of the surrounding skin is done to release the skin for adequate closure.

As eyelid skin has extensive blood supply, even apparently necrotic eyelid skin survives after repair. Preservation of tissue should be done by avoiding unnecessary excision. However, the necrosed tissue should be excised and wound edges should be freshened before suturing (Fig. 11.3).

Myocutaneous flaps

Myocutaneous flaps in the periocular area are formed of skin and orbicularis muscle that is dissected off the underlying orbital septum and stretched into position over the anterior lamellar defect.

Because myocutaneous flap uses tissue adjacent to defect, the match for colour and texture is good. Since this flap brings its own blood supply, bare bones or free grafts can be covered (Fig. 11.4).

Free skin grafts

Free skin grafts are harvested from a donor site and transferred to fill an anterior lamellar defect. Vascular supply to the free graft must be provided by recipient site for the graft to survive.

Full thickness skin graft (FTSG) employs entire thickness of epidermis and dermis harvested from donor site. Upper eyelid skin is the best choice for reconstruction of eyelid defects. Other sites for harvesting FTSG include retroauricular or preauricular skin, supraclavicular skin and upper inner arm skin.

Split thickness skin graft (STSG) is seldom used in eyelid reconstruction. It is useful when a large area of skin need to be covered and no myocutaneous flap can be mobilized. With STSG, the colour, texture and thickness are often poor match for eyelid skin.

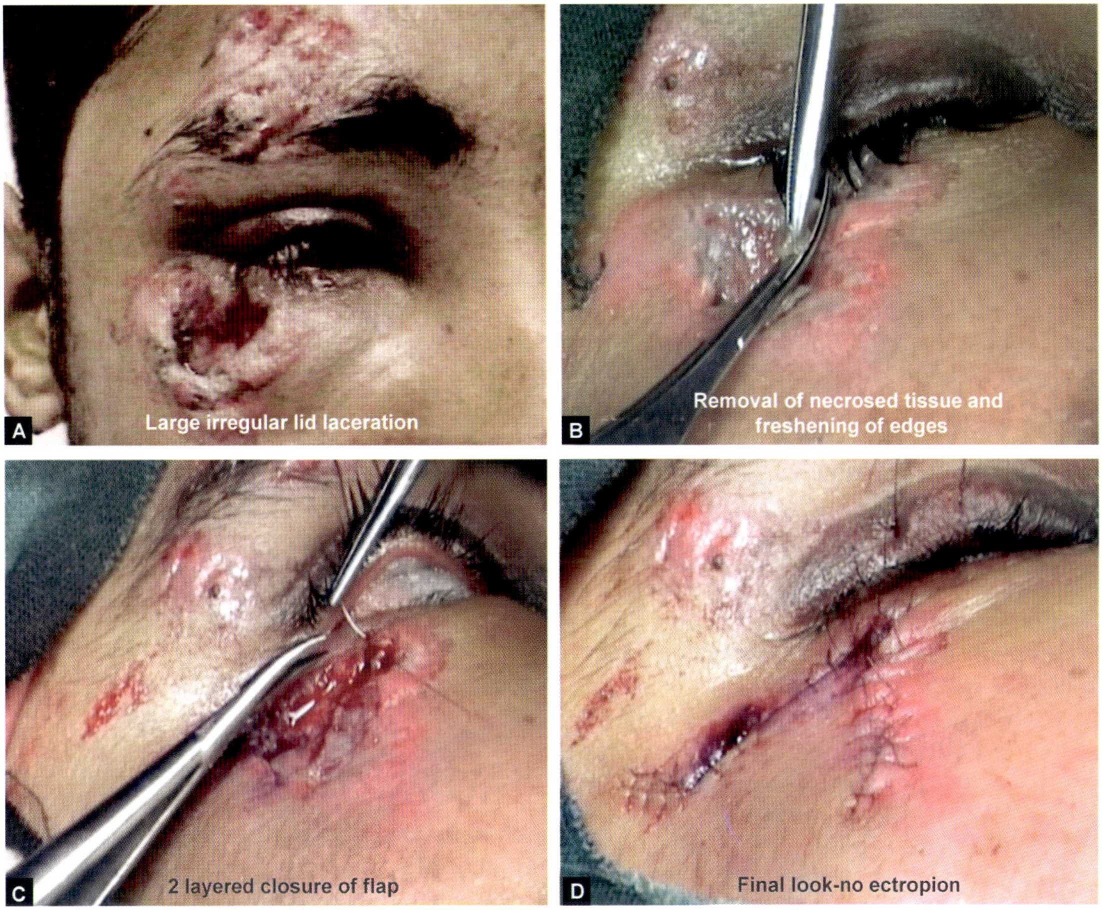

Fig. 11.3 *(A) Simple laceration not involving lid margin; (B) Excision of necrosed tissue; (C) Suturing of wound edges; (D) Final look after suturing*

i. Partial thickness lacerations

These may involve only skin and orbicularis oculi but deeper tissue injury involving orbital septum, preaponeurotic and nasal fat pad, levator aponeurosis or capsulopalpebral fascia may be associated.

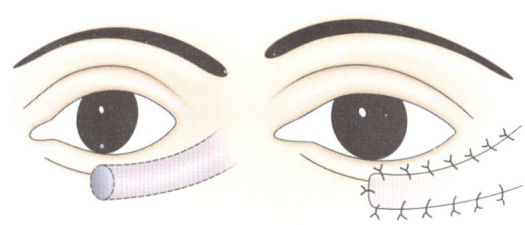

Fig. 11.4 *Myocutaneous advancement flap*

B. REPAIR OF LACERATIONS INVOLVING LID MARGIN

These can be either: partial thickness or full thickness.

- *Defects in the eyelid retractors* can be sutured with 6–0 vicryl interrupted or horizontal mattress sutures.
- *Orbital fat* if exposed must be repositioned if viable, non-viable tissue, however, can be excised.
- *Defects in the orbital septum* can be left open to avoid formation of cicatricial eyelid retraction.
- *Orbicularis* may be closed with buried interrupted 6–0 vicryl sutures.

- *Placement of subcutaneous sutures* is important to avoid postoperative subcutaneous scar or wound dehiscence.
- *Skin* is later sutured with interrupted monofilament 5–0 silk or polypropylene sutures.

Partial thickness lacerations involving only tarsus, conjunctiva and Muller's muscle are sutured with interrupted 6–0 vicryl sutures.

Partial thickness lacerations parallel to lid margin are repaired by directly suturing them with 5–0 silk and sutures are removed after 1 week.

ii. Full thickness lacerations

The repair of full thickness lacerations should begin with the repair of margin.

- *Vertical mattress suture* (6–0 silk) can be placed through the lid and tarsus using grey line as landmark followed by placement of second vertical mattress suture through lid margin posterior to ciliary line (Fig. 11.5A). Approximation of lid margin is assessed to assure adequate apposition. The sutures are left untied and associated partial thickness lacerations of conjunctiva and lower lid retractors if any are repaired.

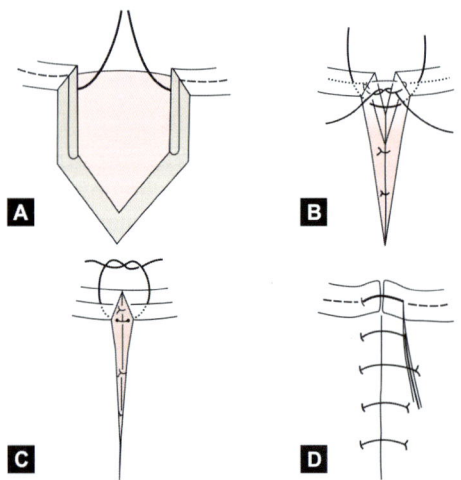

Fig. 11.5 *Repair of full thickness laceration by direct closure (diagrammatic): (A) Placement of vertical mattress suture through tarsus; (B) Interrupted sutures through anterior half of tarsus; (C) Tightening the lid margin suture; (D) Placement of skin and orbicular suture*

- *Repair of tarsus.* Multiple interrupted 6–0 vicryl sutures are placed in the anterior half of the tarsus avoiding conjunctival penetration (Fig. 11.5B).
- *Repair of levator aponeurosis and lower lid retractors,* if required, is then undertaken.
- *Marginal sutures are then tightened* and tied after approximating the wound edges properly (Fig. 11.5C). The ends of these sutures are kept buried underneath the *skin sutures* at the end to avoid rubbing of cornea by these sutures (Fig. 11.5D).

Note. It is of utmost importance to suture the lid margin in a methodic manner as mentioned above otherwise the inadvertent repair is likely to result in lid notching manifesting not only as a cosmetic blemish but disturbs the functional smearing of the tear film as well. In addition to notching, it can also cuase trichiasis. Hence these defects should be repaired by proper re-approximation of the eyelid margin.

C. REPAIR OF CANTHAL TENDON INJURIES

i. Lateral canthal tendon injury

It is generally associated with the laceration of lateral one-third of lid. The lateral canthal tendon anchors lateral canthus to periosteum posterior to lateral orbital rim.

Injury is repaired by placing double-armed horizontal non-absorbable mattress sutures through lateral border of tarsal plate in a half-thickness pattern. Each suture is then passed through the periorbita internal to lateral orbital rim. To achieve satisfactory posterior curvature of the lids, each suture is placed approximately 2 mm posterior to orbital rim (Fig. 11.6).

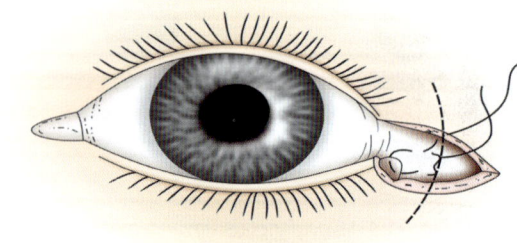

Fig. 11.6 *Repair of lateral canthal tendon injury by placing horizontal mattress suture through lateral aspect of tarsal plate and through periosteum internal to orbital rim*

ii. Medial canthal tendon injury

Medial canthal tendon avulsion should be suspected when there is rounding of the medial canthal angle and acquired telecanthus. Attention to the posterior portion of the tendon's attachment to the posterior lacrimal crest is critical.

Treatment of medial canthal avulsions depends upon the nature of avulsion.

- *If the upper or lower limb is avulsed* but posterior attachment of the tendon is intact the avulsed limb may be sutured to its stump or to the periosteum overlying the anterior lacrimal crest (Fig. 11.7).
- *If the entire tendon, including the posterior portion is avulsed* but there is no naso-orbital fracture, the avulsed tendon should be wired through small drill holes in ipsilateral posterior lacrimal crest.
- *If the entire tendon is avulsed* and there is naso-orbital fracture, transnasal wiring or plating is necessary after reduction of fracture.

D. EYELID INJURIES WITH TISSUE LOSS

Full thickness eyelid defects with tissue loss is classified depending on horizontal extent of defect into:
- Small defects (<1/3)
- Medium defects (1/3 to 1/2)
- Large defects (>1/2)

Repair of small defects (< 1/3 of horizontal length)

Direct closure

If either the upper or lower eyelid has sustained a full-thickness injury that results in less than one-third loss of tissue including the eyelid margin, the repair can generally be closed primarily. In older patients, because of increased eyelid laxity, primary closure of both the uppr and lower eyelids may be accomplished for injuries that have up to 40% tissue loss. However, it is often necessary to freshen up the eyelid margins prior to reconstruction. Direct closure carried out as described above for eyelid margin repair (Fig. 11.8).

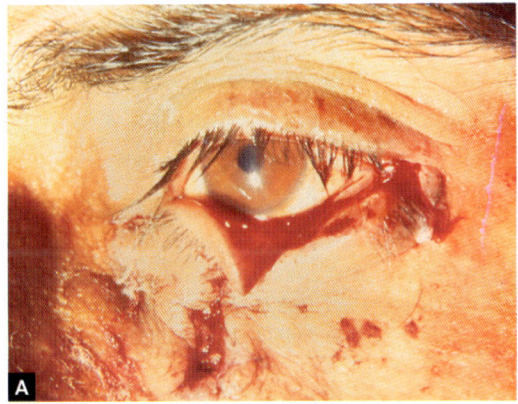

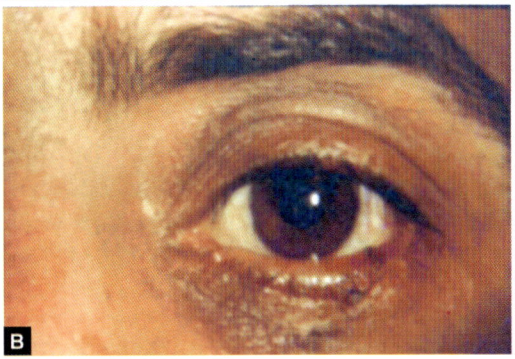

Fig. 11.8 *Clinical photographs of a patient pre- (A) and post- (B) direct closure of the eyelid defect*

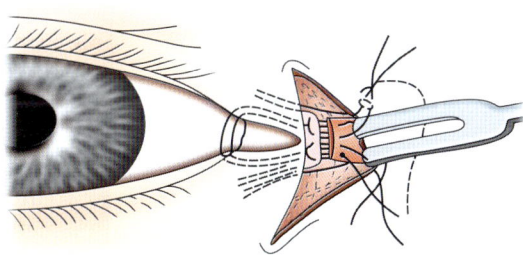

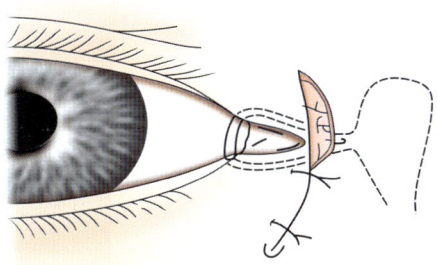

Fig. 11.7 *After intubation of the canaliculi repair of medial canthal, avulsion is done with mattress suture of non-absorbable material*

Lateral canthotomy and cantholysis

When direct closure is attempted, additional horizontal lengthening is provided by lateral canthotomy and cantholysis. In lateral canthotomy, horizontal limb of Y-shaped lateral canthal ligament is incised. For cantholysis, inferior or superior crus of lateral canthal tendon is incised and separated from the bony attachment and lid mobilized. Technique is particularly useful to prevent suturing under tension where laxity of tissue is less (Figs 11.9 and 11.10).

Repair of moderate defects (up to 1/2 of horizontal length)

In old patients or patients with lax skin, mobilization of eyelid with lateral canthotomy and cantholysis as described above can be done to cover defects up to 50% of lid length.

Tenzel semicircular flap

It is useful for reconstruction of up to 50% lid defects. It can be used for both upper lid and lower lid defects when some tarsus remains on either side of the defect.

A high-arched semicircular flap of skin and orbicularis muscle is rotated from lateral canthus after lateral cantholysis. The flap has vertical diameter (approximately 22 mm) more than horizontal diameter (approximately 18 mm). For upper lid defects, the semicircle extends inferior and for lower lid, the semicircle extends superiorly. After undermining of the tissue, the lid is pulled medially and direct closure of wound margins carried out. New lateral canthus created by suturing part of the new lid with intact limb of lateral canthal tendon (Figs 11.11 and 11.12).

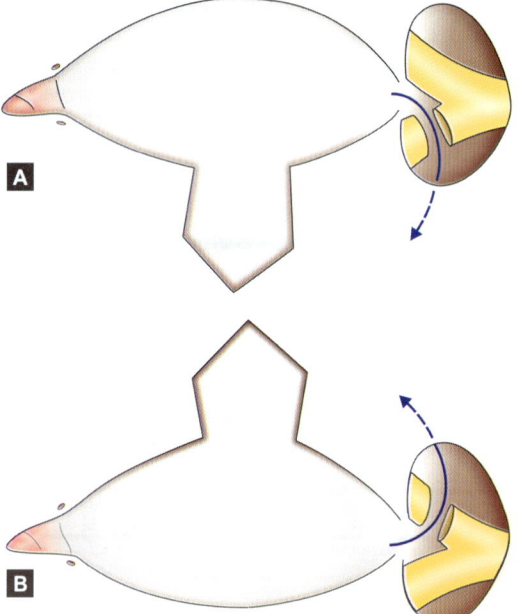

Fig. 11.9 *Closure of eyelid defect with the help of lateral canthoplasty (Diagrammatic): (A) Lower eyelid defect; (B) Upper eyelid defect*

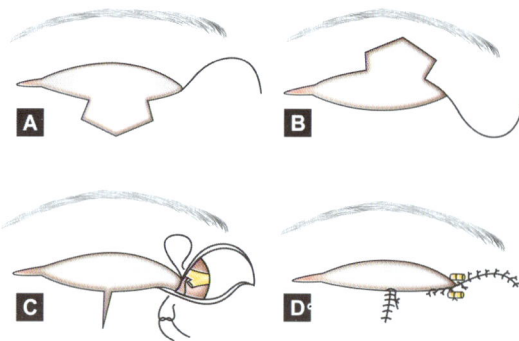

Fig. 11.11 *Closure of eyelid defect with Tenzel's semi-circular flap (diagrammatic depiction)*

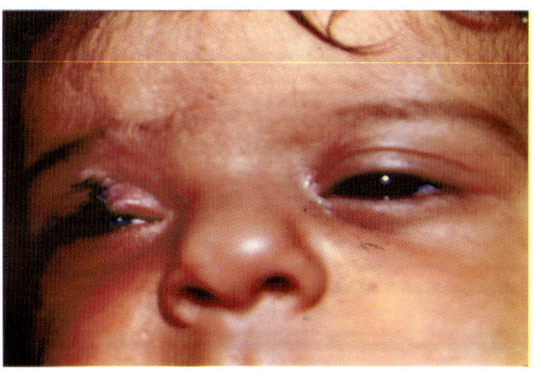

Fig. 11.10 *Clinical photograph of patient repaired with lateral canthoplasty*

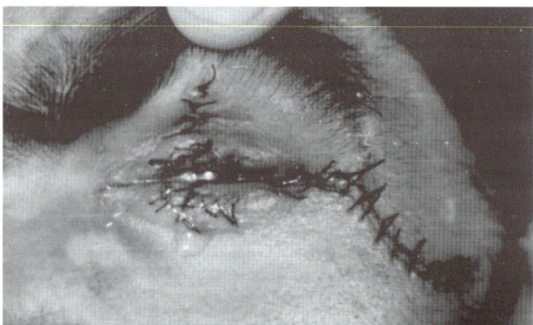

Fig. 11.12 *Clinical photograph of a patient with closure of eyelid defect with Tenzel's semicircular flap*

Repair of large defects (>½ of horizontal length)

Cutler-Beard bridge technique

Cutler-Beard procedure is done in two stages. In first stage, after measuring the upper eyelid defect, a three-sided inverted U-shaped incision is marked on the lower eyelid, about 5 mm below lid margin. After giving full thickness incision, the lower lid flap is pulled under the bridge of lower lid and sutured in layers to the upper lid defect. Since this flap is devoid of tarsus, autogenous cartilage from ear can be used. Separation of the flap is done 6 weeks to 3 months later as second stage surgery. After cutting the flap, lid margin of newly formed upper eyelid is sutured with conjunctiva covering the free margin (Figs 11.13 and 11.14).

Originally described for reconstruction of the upper lid, this technique can be used for reconstruction of the lower lid defect also, a procedure known as *reverse Cutler-Beard* (Fig. 11.15).

Bigger defects involving the lateral canthus, more than half of the upper eyelid and the lateral one-third of lower eyelid can be repaired by *extended Cutler-Beard approach* (Fig. 11.16).

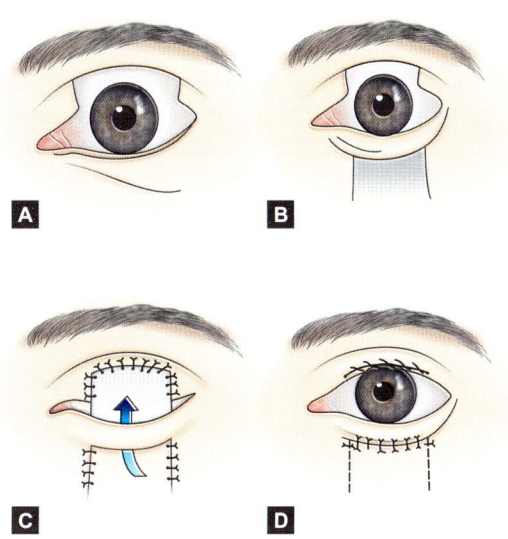

Fig. 11.13 *Closure of eyelid defect with Cutler-Beard approach (Diagrammatic)*

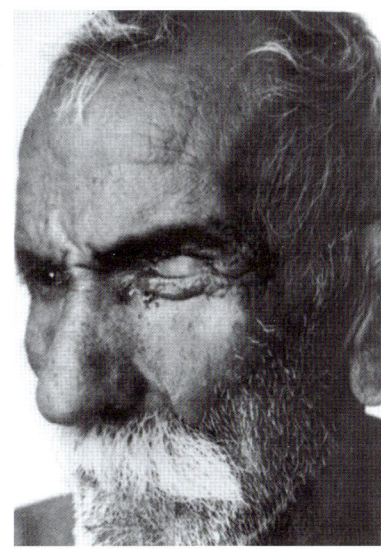

Fig. 11.14 *Clinical photograph of a patient repaired with Cutler-Beard approach*

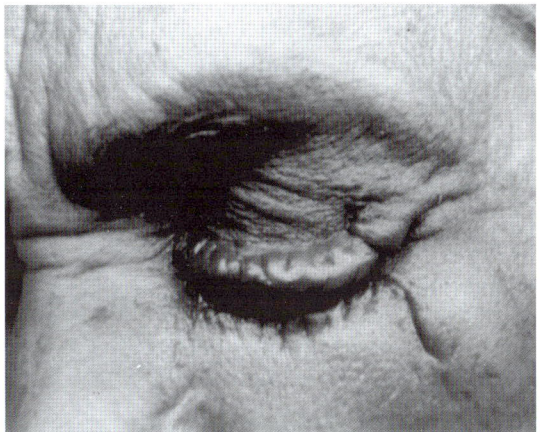

Fig. 11.15 *Clinical photograph of a patient repaired with reverse Cutler-Beard approach*

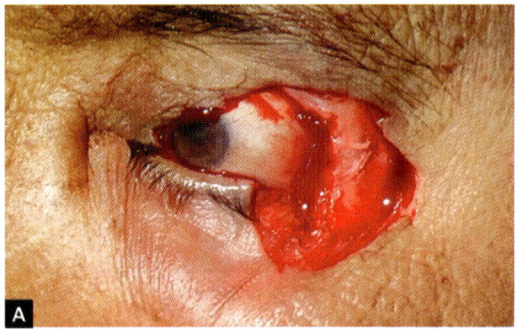

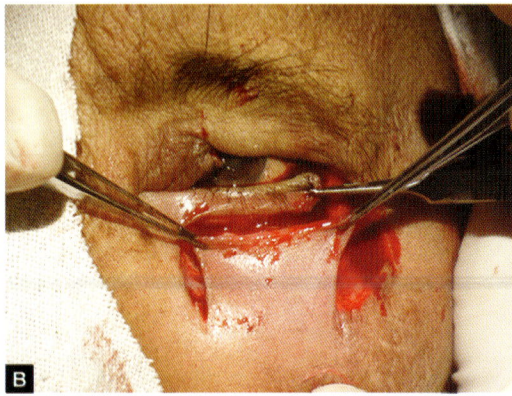

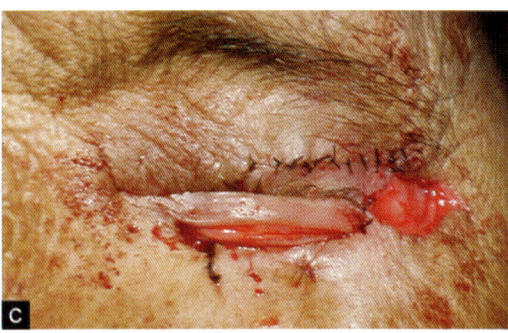

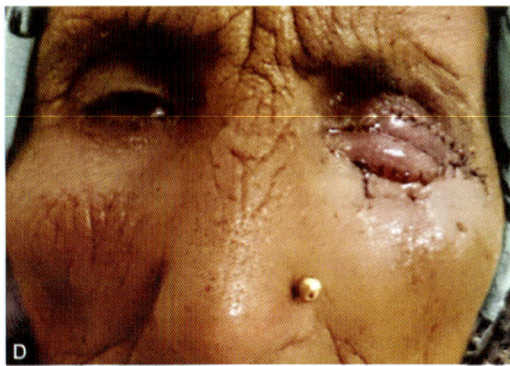

Fig. 11.16 *Extended Cutler-Beard approach: (A) Defect involving upper lid, lateral canthus and lower eyelid; (B) Fashioning of bridge flap; (C) Suturing of bridge flap; (D) Final look after suturing*

Hughes tarsoconjunctival flap technique

It is partial thickness posterior lamellar flap harvested from upper lid to cover lid defects. After everting upper lid, incision is made through tarsus 4 mm above lid margin and flap is mobilized. Flap is sutured with lower lid tarsus to create posterior lamella. Sufficient skin to cover the anterior surface of the flap can be obtained either by harvesting a full-thickness skin graft or by advancing a myocutaneous flap from surrounding skin (Fig. 11.17).

Mustarde cheek rotation flap

It is reserved for the construction of very extensive lower eyelid defects usually involving more than 75% of the eyelid. A large myocutaneous cheek flap is dissected and used in conjunction with an adequate mucosal lining

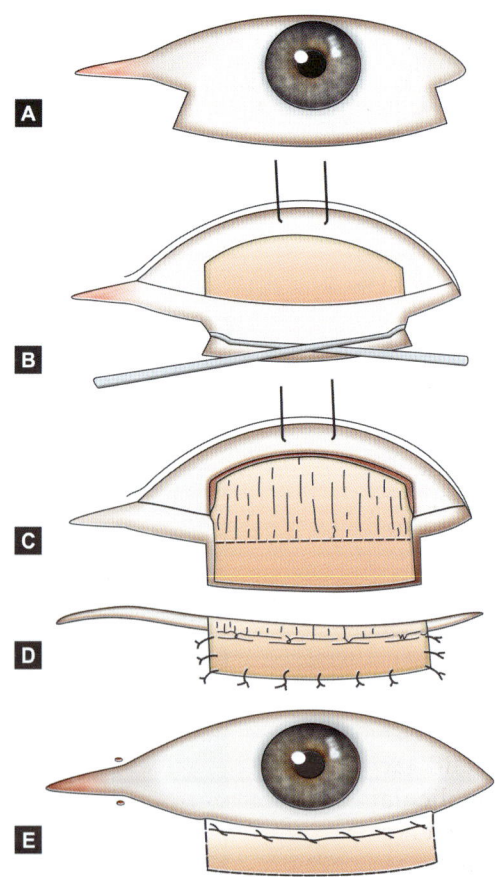

Fig. 11.17 *Eyelid defect repair with Hughes tarsoconjunctival flap*

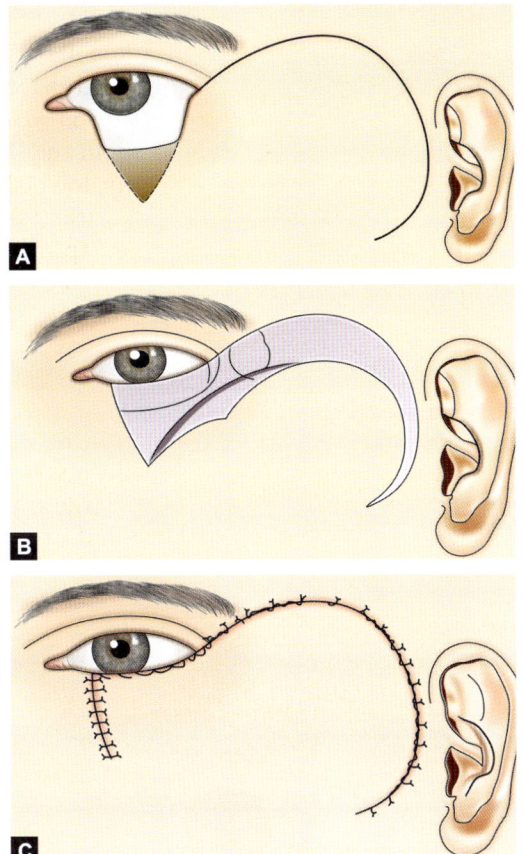

A

B

C

Fig. 11.18 *Eyelid repair using Mustarde cheek rotation flap*

posteriorly. A deep inverted triangle must be excised below the defect to allow adequate rotation of the flap. The side of the triangle nearest the nose should be practically vertical. The advantage of this procedure is that it is a one-stage, complete lower lid reconstruction (Fig. 11.18).

DOG BITES

Profile of injuries

Tearing and crushing injuries occur secondary to dog or human bites, partial or full thickness eyelid lacerations, canthal avulsions and canalicular lacerations are not infrequent. Sometimes serious facial and intracranial injury may be associated and should be looked for. Victims are frequently children and young adults.

Management

At the outset, these wounds need to be liberally irrigated with normal saline. A copious, high-pressure jet flow can be obtained with a large syringe (20 cc or 50 cc) and 18-gauge to 20-gauge needle or plastic catheter number 7, 10. Each wound should be irrigated with a minimum of 100 cc of saline. Such irrigation reduces bacterial inoculums and debrides the wound. Care should be taken not to inflict additional trauma or to inject fluid into the tissues.

Debridement. Dead skin and scabs in and around the wound can be removed and the tissue irrigated for the second time. Excessive debridement in the facial area is not advised since the defect may be enlarged resulting in difficulty in wound closure and a poor cosmetic outcome. The debridement of puncture wounds is unnecessary.

Antirabies vaccine along with antirabies immunoglobulin (40 IU/kg, half dose at the site of wound and half dose intramuscularly after test dose) should be administered.

Tetanus toxoid should be injected, if the wound is found to be contaminated and/or the latest booster has been taken more than 5 years back.

Surgical repair of animal bites which do not result in wound infection is well recognised.
- *Puncture wounds* are cleaned and not sutured.
- *Lacerations* are repaired by standard wound closure techniques for that injured area.
- *Canalicular lacerations* are repaired in a multi-layered fashion with silicone tubing intubation and tubing removal in five or six months.

Infected wounds and those seen after the first 24 hours should be left open. However, cosmetic results are said to be better if facial and eyelid wounds are sutured.

Factors enhancing the cosmetic result in wounds of the face may include the excellent blood supply in the area, copious irrigation, the use of prophylactic antibiotics and the rarity of oedema since the head is rarely a dependent part of the body.

POST-TRAUMATIC EYELID ANOMALIES

TRAUMATIC PTOSIS

Mechanism: Injury to the levator muscle usually includes its transection or complete disinsertion or due to damage to its nerve supply. Sometimes severe lid oedema or inadequate repair may mask levator injury and result in delayed recognition of the traumatic ptosis. As regards to timing of surgery, it is preferably done 10–12 weeks after trauma by which the spontaneous recovery may occur or else surgery can be planned for residual ptosis.

Management: Traumatic ptosis, with its varied etiology, presents a challenging problem. The choice of surgery varies with the etiology, severity of ptosis and levator action.

- *Fasanella-Servat procedure* is the choice in very few cases which present with mild ptosis.
- *Levator aponeurosis surgery*—either reattachment of a dehisced aponeurosis or resection is required in most cases. Resection requires a careful dissection of the levator muscle and making it free from all the fibrotic bands, to get a good correction and avoid excessive lagophthalmos.
- *Sling procedure* is carried out when the levator action is very poor.

Note. The presence of associated abnormalities due to trauma, such as traumatic lid notches, symblepharon, entropion and ocular motility restrictions are often complicating factors and need to be taken into account when planning the surgical approach and may necessitate a multi-staged procedure.

CICATRICIAL ECTROPION

Mechanism: Cicatricial ectropion (Fig. 11.19) of the upper or lower eyelid occurs following loss of skin secondary to thermal or chemical burns consequent to mechanical trauma or as a complication of surgical procedure.

Management: Treatment of the underlying cause, along with conservative medical protection of the cornea, is essential as primary management.

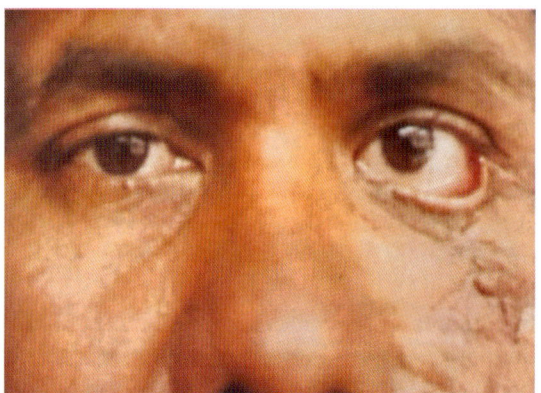

Fig. 11.19 *Photograph of a patient with cicatricial ectropion of lower eyelid*

Cicatricial ectropion of the lower eyelid is usually treated in a three-step procedure (Fig. 11.20):
- *Cicatricial tissue is* surgically excised (Fig. 11.20A).
- *Eyelid is horizontally tightened* with a lateral tarsal strip operation or horizontal lid resection (Fig. 11.20B).

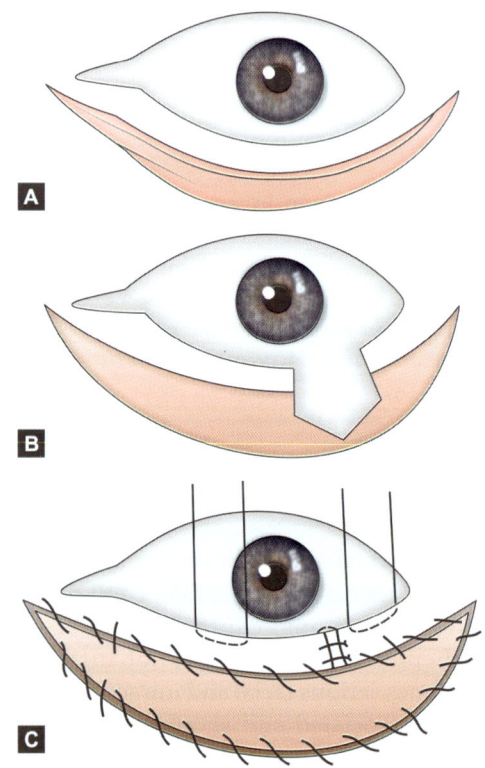

Fig. 11.20 *Surgical technique of repair of cicatricial ectropion*

- *Anterior lamella is vertically lengthened* via a full-thickness skin graft (Fig. 11.20C).

Treatment of cicatricial ectropion or retraction of the upper eyelid usually requires only release of traction and augmentation of the vertically shortened anterior lamella with a full-thickness skin graft. Although skin from the opposite upper eyelid is the best colour and texture match for skin grafting, this source is usually inadequate except in patients with significant dermatochalasis. The postauricular, preauricular, supraclavicular, and medial upper arm areas are other donor-site options for eyelid reconstruction.

CICATRICIAL ENTROPION

Mechanism

It is caused by vertical tarsoconjunctival contracture and internal rotation of the eyelid margin, with resulting irritation of the globe from inturned cilia or the keratinized eyelid margin seen especially after thermal or chemical burns (Fig. 11.21).

Management

The goal of treatment is to eliminate the chronic ocular irritation by removing the lashes and keratinized tissue from contact with the cornea. Cicatricial entropion usually requires surgery, but lubricating drops and ointments, barriers to symblepharon formation, and lash ablation with lash cautery or cryotherapy are sometimes useful adjuncts.

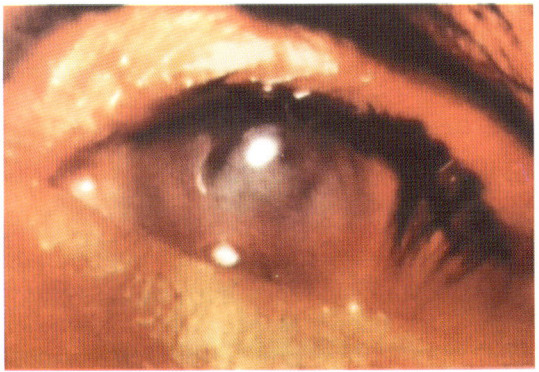

Fig. 11.21 *Photograph of a patient with cicatricial entropion*

When there is only slight inversion of the eyelid margin (with or without trichiasis) and little distortion of other eyelid structures, *resection of anterior lamellar tissue with or without mucous membrane grafting* may be curative.

Anterior lamellar repositioning slides the offending tissues away from the eye. In this procedure, (Fig. 11.22) anterior and posterior lamellae are separated by giving incisions at grey line and 4 mm from lid margin. Blunt dissection is then carried out over the tarsus to join the two incisions. The septum is then opened to expose the levator aponeurosis. The levator and muller are dissected free from conjunctiva and the levator is recessed. Z-myotomies of the levator can be carried out to lengthen it. Both of these procedures help in advancement of posterior lamella to protect the cornea. Double-armed 5–0 vicryl sutures are placed partial thickness through the tarsal plate and emerge through the anterior lamella close to the upper eyelid margin. The bare eyelid margin is allowed to epithelialize. The skin crease is maintained by passing 6–0 vicryl sutures through levator which helps in maintaining upward vector of traction to anterior lamella thus preventing post-surgery ptosis.

Terminal tarsal rotation. Medial and lateral vertical eyelid margin incisions are made (Fig. 11.23A). The two vertical incisions are joined on the tarsal surface superior to any posterior lamella keratinization after everting the eyelid (Fig. 11.23B). The skin crease is incised. This incision should not be deep and also should not extend to other incisions else there is a risk of complete detachment or avascular necrosis of the terminal eyelid (Fig. 11.23C). After recessing the levator (Fig.11.23D), the anterior and posterior lamellae are divided, by exposing the anterior tarsal surface. The tarsal height is now measured. If it is found to be less than 4 mm, rigid mucosal graft is required. Hard palate graft or free tarsal graft from other eyelid can be used for this purpose. Terminal tarsal dissection and outward rotation is then

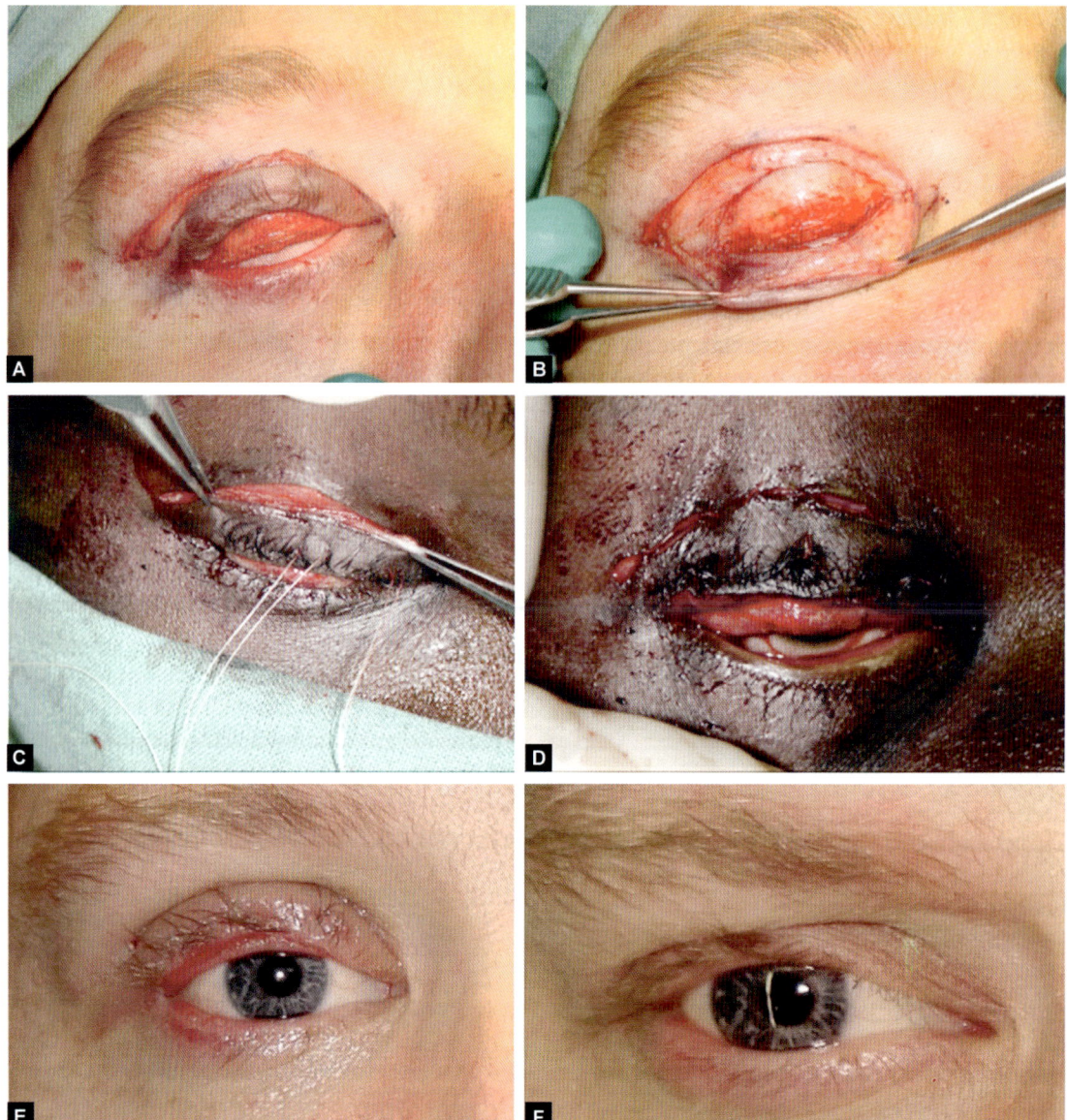

Fig. 11.22 *Steps of the anterior lamellar repositioning technique of repair of cicatricial entropion. (A) Grey line incision and low skin crease incision 4 mm from upper eyelid margin. (B) Exposure of the anterior surface of the tarsal plate. The anterior lamella (skin and orbicularis) has been reflected. (C) Double-armed 5–0 vicryl sutures placed through tarsal plate, emerging through anterior lamella close to eyelid margin. (D and E) Bare eyelid margins are allowed to epithelialize. (F) Postoperative appearance at 3 months*

carried out in order to make the keratinized conjunctiva a part of anterior lamella. Three double-armed 6–0 vicryl sutures are passed partial thickness through the advanced tarsus and the everted terminal tarsus (Fig. 11.23E).

Both bare tarsal edges are left to granulate (Fig. 11.23F). Finally the skin crease is formed in the same manner as that of anterior lamellar repositioning and preventing post-surgical ptosis.

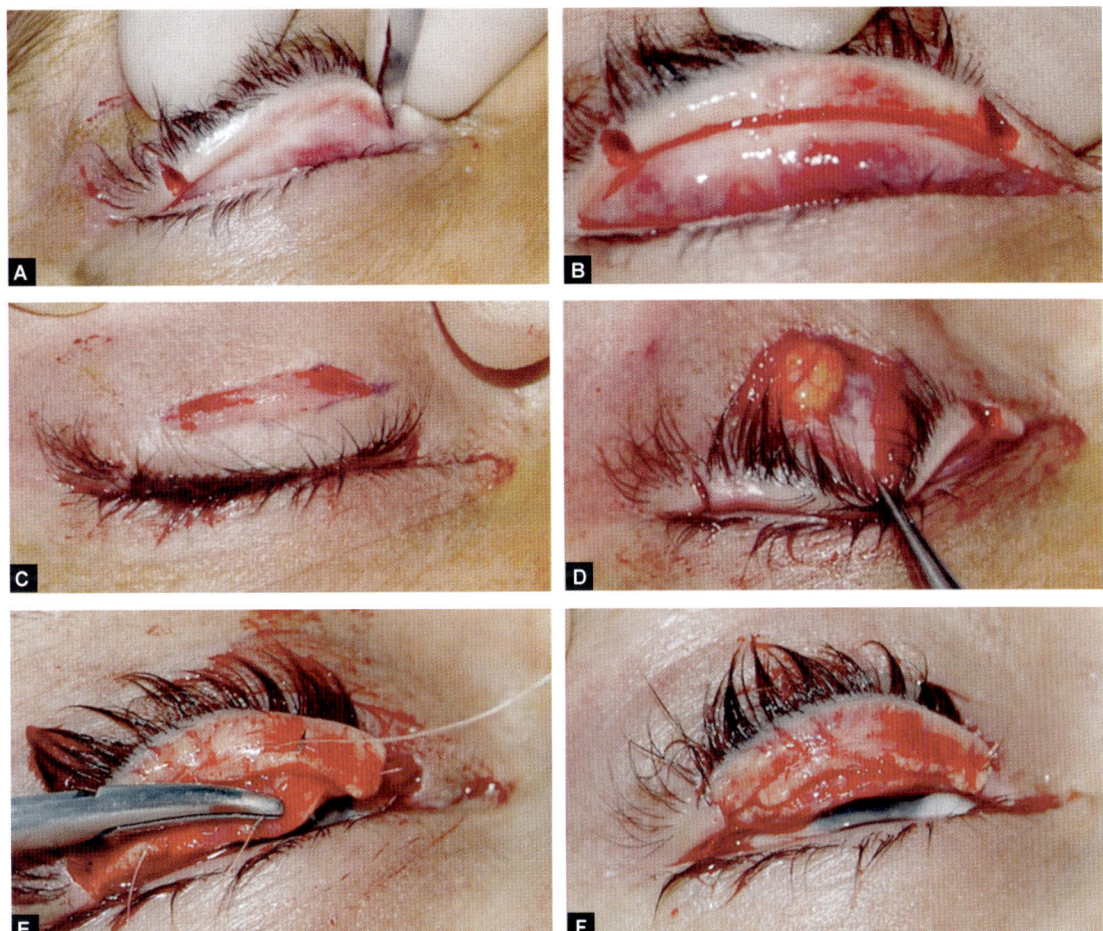

Fig. 11.23 *Steps of correction of cicatricial entropion with the terminal tarsal rotation. (A) Medial and lateral vertical eyelid margin incisions. (B) Two vertical incisions are joined on tarsal surface of everted eyelid. (C) Skin crease incision. (D) Exposure and release of levator. (E) Three double-armed 6–0 vicryl sutures passed through the advanced tarsus and everted terminal tarsus. (F) Bare tarsal edges are left to granulate*

LACRIMAL SYSTEM TRAUMA

Lid lacerations can involve the medial canthus thereby involving the lacrimal system, i.e. the canalicular and lacrimal sac injuries. Canalicular injury is the one which needs to be repaired with the primary repair of the lid laceration since the results when done as a second stage procedure are highly dismal.

CANALICULAR TRAUMA

Pathophysiology

Canaliculus lies in the weakest part of the eyelid and is the first structure to yield being unsupported by tarsal plate. Canalicular injuries

occur by direct laceration or by stab wound or dog bite or by traction leading to sudden lateral discplacement of the lid leading to sudden tear of the medial canthus and associated caniculare tear (Fig. 11.24). So whenever there is full thickness injury involving medial part of the lid, proper evaluation of the canalicular system along with diagnostic probing (if possible) should be undertaken.

Clinical presentation

It has been observed that if primary repair of the injured canaliculus is not undertaken, 40% of the patients develop symptomatic epiphora with ocular irritation.

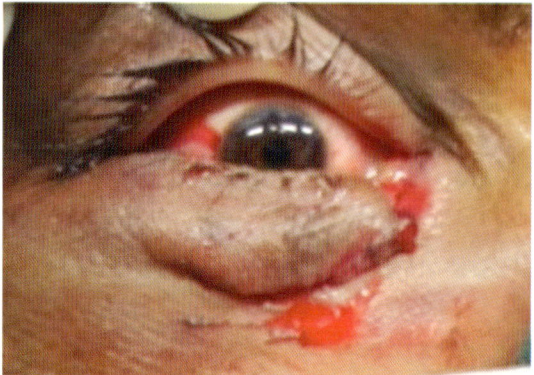

Fig. 11.24 *Lower lid full thickness laceration involving lid margin and thus injuring lower canaliculus*

Management

- *Repair should be done within 48 hrs* preferably and under microscope. As mentioned already, the success rate of primary repair is much higher than secondary repair.

- *Canalicular repair demands peseverence*, patience, expertise and exact knowledge of the anatomy of the structure.
- *Anaesthesia.* In children, it should be done under general anaesthesia, however, in adults it can be done under local anaesthesia.
- *First step is to find out the severed ends of canaliculus* (Figs 11.25A and B). For lacerations away from medial canthus, the distal end of the laceration is located near the eyelid margin but for lacerations close to lacrimal sac, the canaliculus is found to lie deep to the anterior limb of medial canthal tendon. The intact adjacent canaliculus may be irrigated by substances, like air, viscoelastic substance or fluorescein dye and thus the medial end can be identified. Irrigation by pigtail probe can be done but it requires expertise. The probe is passed through upper punctum, intact upper canaliculus, common canaliculus and finally passed through medial cut end.

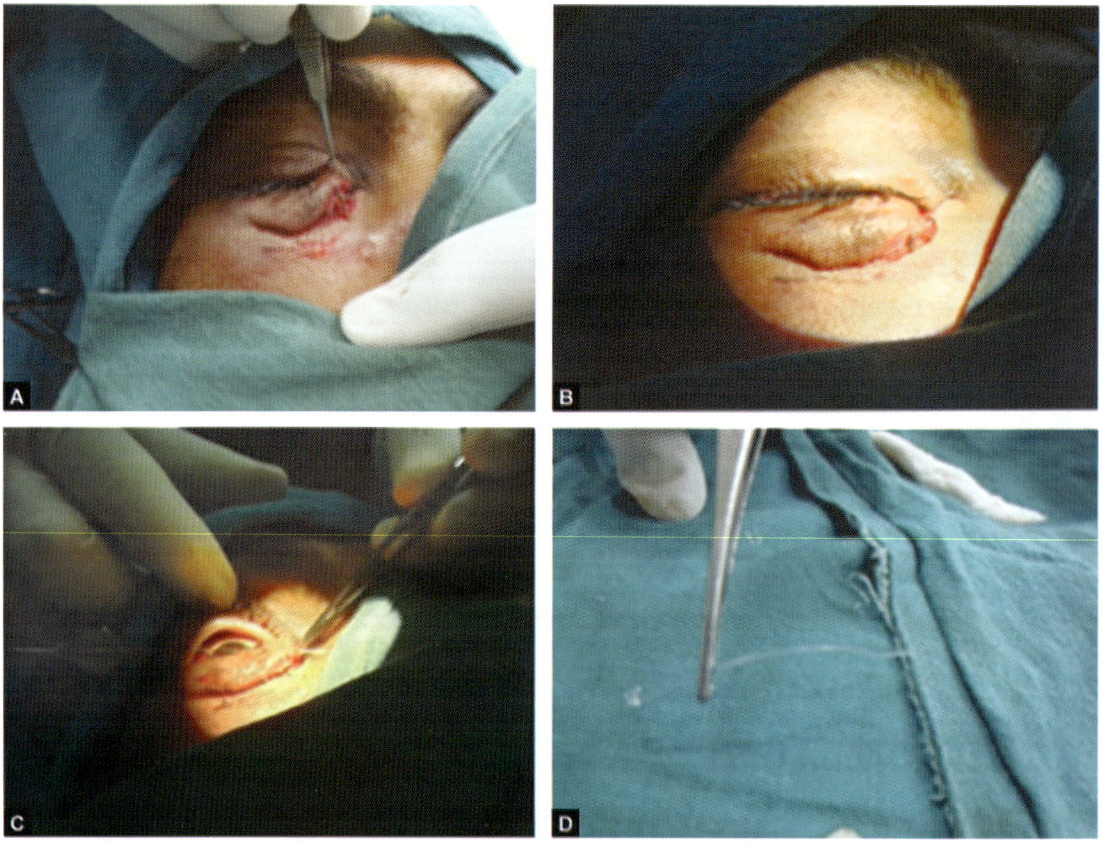

Fig. 11.25 *Steps of canalicular injury: (A and B) Finding out medial end of canaliculus; (C and D) Stenting with mono-canalicular minimonoka implant*

- *The injured canaliculus must be stented* (Fig. 11.25C) to avoid postoperative stricture. The silicon stents (Fig. 11.25D) are most commonly used nowadays and by putting it on traction the severed canailcular ends as well as the soft tissues are apposed together in the normal anatomical relations and placement of sutures are not required. This stenting also facilitates the reconstruction of medial canthal tendon and the repair of eyelid laceration in a standard and layred manner which should follow subsequently.
- *Stents can be monocanalicular or bicanalicular.* The distal end of the monocanalicular stent is attached to metal guiding probe and is passed intranasally (Fig. 11.26). These monocanalicular stents are getting popular day by day because of reduced chances of punctual injury,

easy retrieval, cheese wiring and these mono-canalicular stents can be used in soft tissue approximation easily. Also newer ones have self-retaining property. They are generally retained in place for 3 months. Any evidence of infection, irritation, pyogenic granuloma formation necessitates their early removal. Bicanalicular stents are removed by cutting their medial end and retrieving it intranasally, however, monocanalicular stents are removed by simply pulling through the punctum.

- *Major problem of the repair of the canalicular system is failure to identify the cut end.* A gentle irrigation of fluid into uncut canalicular system may help in the identification. However, if it is not possible, the eyelid should be closed and subsequently the case is taken up for conjunctivodacryocystorhinostomy in case patient presents with epiphora.

LACRIMAL SAC AND GLAND INJURY

Lacrimal sac trauma can occur in direct laceration or stab wounds or fracture of bone surrounding it. In such cases, direct repair of the laceration after doing meticulous dissection and intubation of the lacrimal sac and nasolacrimal duct is carried out. Late treatment may include DCR.

Lacrimal gland trauma. Injuries involving lateral part of eyelids may result in ptosis or prolapse of the lacrimal gland. The lacrimal gland is returned to lacrimal fossa beneath superolateral orbital rim by placing horizontal 5–0 vicryl mattress sutures through the periosteum in this region and through the capsule surrounding the lacrimal gland. On tightening the sutures, the lacrimal gland suspends back in normal anatomic position.

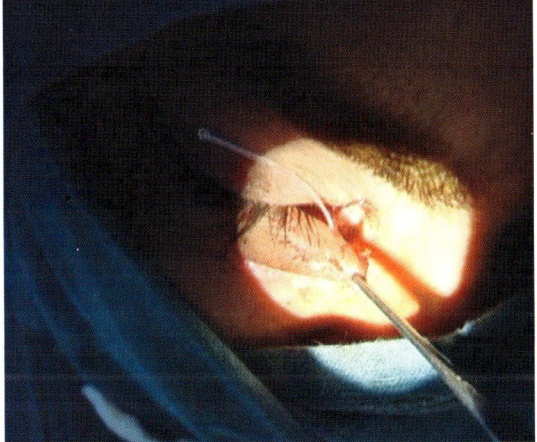

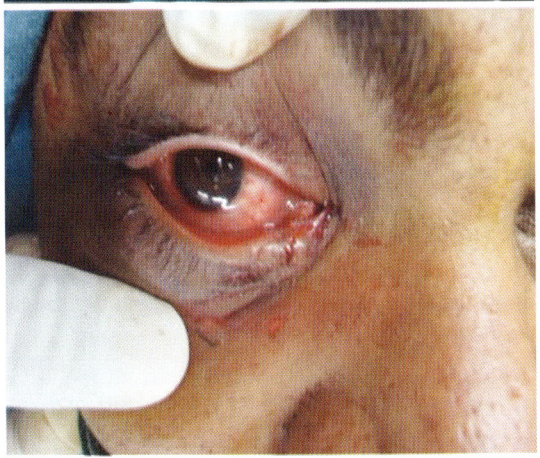

Fig. 11.26 *Insertion of minimonaka implant followed by primary repair of the lid laceration*

BIBLIOGRAPHY

1. Cho SH, Hyun DW, Kang HJ, Ha MS. A simple new method for identifying the proximal cut end in lower canalicular laceration. Korean J Ophthalmol Jun 2008;22(2):73–76.
2. Ing E, Ing T, Emara B. Ocular adnexal injuries from industrial blunt hook trauma. Can J Ophthalmol. Apr 2002;37:177–178.
3. Ross AH, Cannon PS, Selva D, Malhotra R. Management of upper eyelid cicatricial entropion. Clinical and Experimental Ophthalmology 2011;39:526–539.

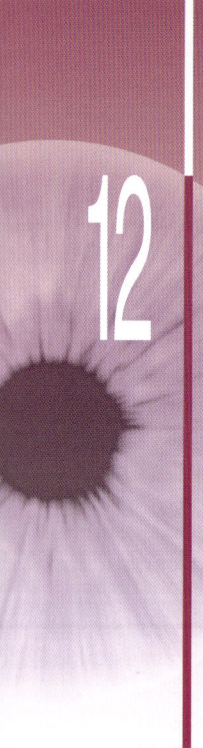

12

ORBITAL TRAUMA

GENERAL CONSIDERATIONS

INTRODUCTION

The bony perimeter of the orbit offers greatest defense against blunt trauma. Concussive forces in a blunt trauma are not only absorbed by bony orbit but also by eyelids, extraocular muscles, and orbital fat pad. Anatomy of bony orbit is such that it provides adequate protection to orbital soft tissue superiorly and nasally, but the protection is inadequate temporally and inferiorly. This defence, however, may be bypassed by relatively small masses, such as fist, table corner, cricket ball, etc. In such circumstances, the traumatic forces are absorbed by orbital soft tissue, extraocular muscles as well as eyelids.

Orbital trauma poses a great challenge to the ophthalmologist not only because of the associated ocular and adnexal injuries but also in management. The bony perimeter of the orbit may be bypassed by strong concussive forces which ultimately lead to soft tissue trauma. Immediate assessment and treatment of such soft tissue injury especially of retro-orbital haemorrhage or caroticocavernous fistula is trivial to preserve the vision. Orbital bony injuries require timely repair to restore the integrity as well as function of associated injured soft tissue, e.g. entrapped muscle. Intraorbital foreign bodies, especially metallic, require special attention and immediate removal.

EPIDEMIOLOGY

The rate of orbital involvement among all serious injuries is 15%; fracture being seen in 78% of cases, haemorrhage in 1% and foreign body in 24 % of these cases. Variety of lesions of the orbital soft tissue and bony injury discussed as under are seen mostly in blunt orbital trauma.

APPLIED ANATOMY

Before discussing the orbital injuries, it is important to briefly review the relevant clinical anatomy (Fig. 12.1).

Roof of orbit: It is triangular in shape. It is formed by orbital plate of frontal bone, lesser wing of sphenoid. Lateral part shows lacrimal gland fossa while at the junction of roof and medial wall, there is a trochlea, 4 mm from the

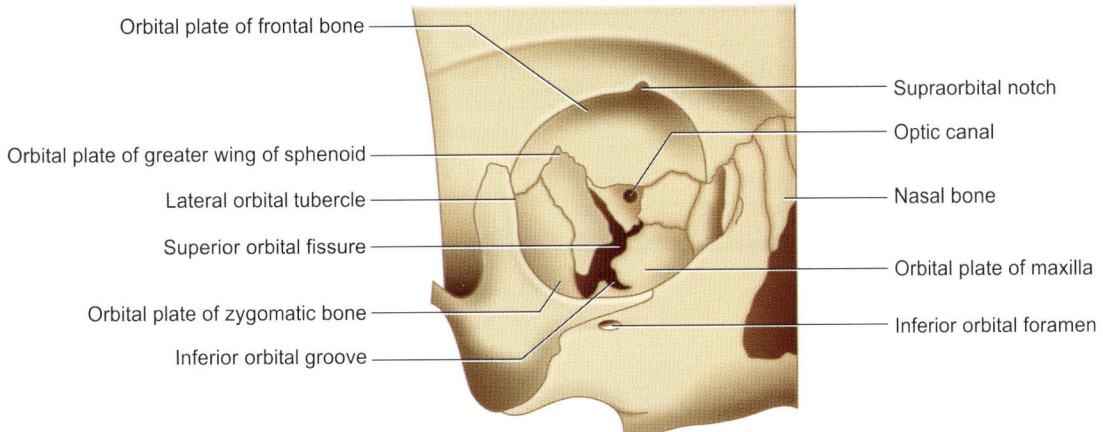

Orbital plate of frontal bone

Orbital plate of greater wing of sphenoid

Lateral orbital tubercle

Superior orbital fissure

Orbital plate of zygomatic bone

Inferior orbital groove

Supraorbital notch

Optic canal

Nasal bone

Orbital plate of maxilla

Inferior orbital foramen

Fig. 12.1 *Gross anatomy of the orbit*

orbital margin, located superonasally for superior oblique tendon.

Medial wall: It is the thinnest orbital wall (0.2–0.4 mm) and quadrilateral in shape. It is formed by frontal process of maxilla, lacrimal bone, orbital plate of ethmoid and body of sphenoid. It also bears a lacrimal fossa: bounded by anterior and posterior lacrimal crests into which rests the lacrimal sac. At the junction of the medial wall and orbital roof are the anterior and posterior ethmoidal foramina. Through these foramina, the anterior and posterior ethmoidal arteries and nerves course between the orbit and the anterior cranial fossa. These structures can be injured directly at the time of trauma, and the surgeon must be aware of their location during repair in order to avoid intra-operative bleeding. Also of anatomic importance is the medial rectus muscle, which is intimately related to the medial wall. One of the most obvious signs of medial wall fracture is a motility disturbance, usually deficient adduction or abduction, caused by damage to or entrapment of the medial rectus. Other significant, medially located structures that must be accounted for in medial wall trauma include the medial canthal tendon, trochlea and lacrimal drainage system.

Floor of orbit: It is triangular in shape. It is formed by orbital plate of maxilla anteromedially, orbital surface of zygomatic anterolaterally, and orbital part of palatine bone posteriorly. The orbital floor lies in close proximity to the inferior

rectus muscle, which can have pathologic involvement in an adjacent fracture. At the junction of floor with lateral wall posteriorly, there is an inferior orbital fissure which transmits infraorbital nerve, infraorbital artery and infraorbital vein. Infraorbital nerve dys-function is common after orbital floor fracture.

Lateral wall: It is triangular and thickest wall of the orbit. It is formed by orbital surface of zygomatic anteriorly and orbital surface of greater wing of sphenoid posteriorly. The anterior half of globe is not covered by bone on lateral side and hence easily susceptible to trauma. Whitnall's tubercle, which serves a critical role in the maintenance of eyelid contour, has the attachment site for the lateral canthal tendon and is located on the zygomatic bone, 2 mm behind the lateral orbital rim.

Apex of orbit: It is the posterior end of orbit which contains two orifices: Optic canal and superior orbital fissure. The optic canal transmits optic nerve surrounded by meninges and ophthalmic artery. The length of the canal is 6–11 mm and is circular in cross-section in the middle while oval in shape at either end. Superior orbital fissure is a comma-shaped aperture bounded by lesser and greater wings of sphenoid. Structures passing through its upper and lateral parts are lacrimal, frontal and trochlear nerves along with superior ophthalmic vein and recurrent branch of ophthalmic artery. The middle part of fissure within tendinous ring transmits superior and inferior divisions of oculomotor nerve, nasociliary branch of ophthalmic nerve and abducent nerve. However, the lower and medial parts transmitt inferior ophthalmic vein.

PROFILE OF ORBITAL TRAUMA

BLUNT TRAUMA TO ORBIT

SKIN INJURIES

Abrasions and lacerations over the skin of orbit may give rise to periorbital cellulitis and therefore, copious irrigation and early prophylactic topical antibiotic therapy of these skin breaks along with skin apposition should be considered. Tetanus prophylaxis is indicated, especially if the wound is deep or much devitalized tissue is present.

Concussive trauma may result in crushing of subcutaneous muscle and connective tissue with secondary haemorrhage and oedema. Cold compresses can diminish this. However, infected, large, tense haematomas may require drainage.

OEDEMA

Eyelid oedema: Because of the absence of fat in the lid skin and its loose adherence to the underlying structures, there is easy spread of leaked intravascular fluid into surrounding soft tissues. However, its lateral spread is limited by adherent fascia beneath eyebrows and by malar and nasojugal folds. Oedema can turn bilateral, if the fluid seeps subcutaneously across the nasal bridge.

Chemosis: The loose adherence of conjunctiva to underlying structures leads to conjunctival oedema; chemosis. This can at times lead to conjunctival prolapse which can be medial, inferior or lateral. Topical antibiotic ointment must be applied to prevent desiccation of chronically exposed conjunctiva.

Orbital oedema: If orbital oedema is present without haemorrhage, it is usually self-limiting. Extraocular movement restriction that develops after orbital oedema is also self-limiting and should not be taken for muscle entrapment. Orbital oedema if associated with pain, diplopia,

chemosis, proptosis, conjunctival and episcleral vascular congestion (corkscrew vessels) along with raised intraocular pressure, a possibility of caroticocavernous fistula must be kept in mind. Patient can have ocular/cranial bruit, choroidal thickening, retinal venous congestion, ptosis and tinnitus.

ORBITAL TISSUE TRAUMA

Orbital tissue trauma can be classified as under for convenience of description:

Intraconal/conal-lesions involving injury to soft tissue contents of the orbit within the muscle cone:
- *Orbital haemorrhage*
- *Optic nerve injury*
  – Optic nerve sheath haemorrhage
  – Optic nerve avulsion
  – Fracture optic nerve canal
- Caroticocavernous fistula

Extraconal-lesions involving the bony socket of orbit:
- Orbital fractures
- Intraorbital foreign bodies

INTRACONAL ORBITAL TRAUMA

ORBITAL HAEMORRHAGE

Clinical profile

Patients with orbital haemorrhage can have dramatic onset of symptoms and rapid progression threatening the vision and may have complete visual loss. Hence appropriate localization of the haemorrhage (preseptal/post-septal) along with timely intervention is must.

Clinical anatomy: Orbital septum is a fibrous sheath that arises from periosteum of orbital rims. It descends and superiorly fuses with levator aponeurosis while inferiorly it fuses with capsulopalpebral fascia creating two compartments—preseptal and post-septal.

Preseptal haemorrhage: An acute haemorrhage in preseptal space, while dramatic in appearance, may not be as vision-threatening as post-septal haemorrhage (Fig. 12.2). Normal pupillary reflexes and normal intraocular pressure along with painless and free extraocular movements

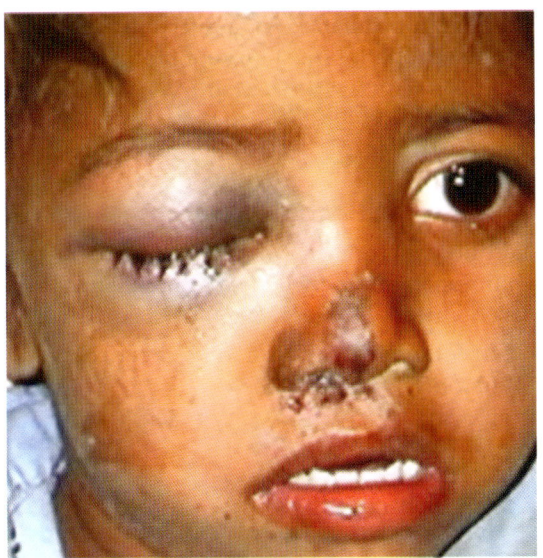

Fig. 12.2 *Preseptal orbital haemorrhage in a 3-year-old child following blunt trauma*

essentially rule out post-septal haemorrhage. Such a haemorrhage must be observed clinically and rapid expansion or any deterioration as regards the above mentioned parameters must be looked for. Any such deterioration, if occurs or if there is no resolution of the haemorrhage, drainage of the haematoma can be carried out through small incision.

Post-septal haemorrhage: Bounded anteriorly by orbital septum a post-septal haemorrhage produces a compartment syndrome—can compromise the enclosed structures namely: the optic nerve and blood supply to the eye. Hence it is the most precarious situation to the patient. In the presence of afferent pupillary defect (APD), decreased vision, raised intraocular pressure (IOP), impaired extraocular movements, proptosis one should treat it on urgent basis by doing canthotomy or cantholysis.

Investigations and tests

Non-contrast CT scan of the orbit must be done in such cases to rule out fractures. Patients with a predisposition to bleeding or having orbital haemorrhage following trivial trauma may undergo laboratory tests including complete blood count, coagulation profile, factor Xa assay and anticoagulant levels. Proper history of such

medications as NSAIDs, like aspirin, herbal agents and other platelet interfering agents must be taken.

Management

Prior to surgical measures, conservative measures, like IOP lowering drops and intravenous 350 cc 20% mannitol, can be administered. Empirically patient can be put on systemic steroids as well which hasten the resolution of orbital oedema due to inflammation. Surgical decompression is kept reserved for patient losing vision following orbital haemorrhage.

Canthotomy: Following local anaesthesia, a haemostat is advanced inferiorly and laterally at the lateral canthus with open blades up to base of fornix and then closed. The haemostat leaves a crush mark which is divided by a scissors up to the lateral canthal tendon (Fig. 12.3).

Cantholysis: To perform this, a surgeon should angle a blunt-tipped scissors downwards away from globe, parallel to the direction of intact superior crus of lateral canthal tendon between the skin and conjunctiva. Using haemostats, clamp the soft tissue between the lateral canthus and the lateral rim of the orbit (approx 1 cm) for 30–60 seconds to further improve haemostasis and mark the site of incision. With blunt-tipped scissors, make an incision laterally from the canthus to the rim of the orbit. Using a haemostat or pickups, retract the inferior portion of the lid in order to visualize the inferior lateral canthal tendon. In one motion, cut down to the lateral orbital rim and sever the inferior crus of the

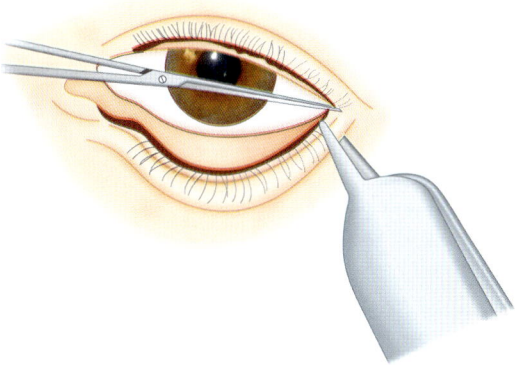

Fig. 12.3 *Incision given at lateral canthus and dissection is done up to canthal tendon*

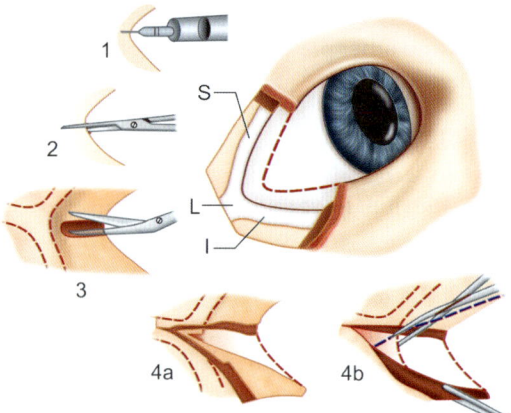

Fig. 12.4 *(1) Local infiltration of anaesthetic solution given. (2) Skin incision given from lateral canthus after applying haemostats for 30–60 sec. (3) With a blunt-tipped scissors, an incision is made laterally from the canthus to rim of orbit. (4a) and (4b) Inferior crus of lateral canthus identified and severed*

lateral canthal tendon (Fig. 12.4). Strum the inferior crus of the lateral canthal tendon to determine whether there are any remaining attachments between eyelid and orbital rim. Such attachments if any should be cut and gentle pressure may be given on globe for easy egress of blood trapped inside.

Follow-up: Observe closely for the pupillary reaction to light and improvement of vision. If the patient's signs and symptoms do not resolve, consider one more cantholysis superiorly in the similar manner. If there is no improvement even after this, orbital evacuation must be considered

in operation theatre. An associated traumatic optic neuropathy must be kept in mind.

OPTIC NERVE INJURY

See Chapter 10.1.

CAROTICOCAVERNOUS FISTULA

Caroticocavernous fistula (CCF) is an abnormal communication between cavernous sinus and carotid arterial system. It can be classified as:

- Direct *v/s* dural (indirect) according to anatomy.
- High flow *v/s* low flow; according to blood flow.

Direct CCFs represent 70–90% of all CCFs.

Applied anatomy

Cavernous sinus: It is the large venous sinus situated in middle cranial fossa one on each side of body of sphenoid bone (Fig. 12.5). Anterior extension of the sinus is up to the superior orbital fissure while the posterior extension is up to apex of petrous temporal bone. It is about 2 cm long and 1 cm wide. It is related superiorly to optic tract, internal carotid artery and anterior perforated substance while inferiorly it is related to foramen lacerum and junction of body and greater wing of sphenoid bone. The pituitary gland and sphenoid sinus are situated medial to cavernous sinus whereas laterally temporal bone and uncus are present. As shown in Fig. 12.5, the structures in the lateral wall of sinus

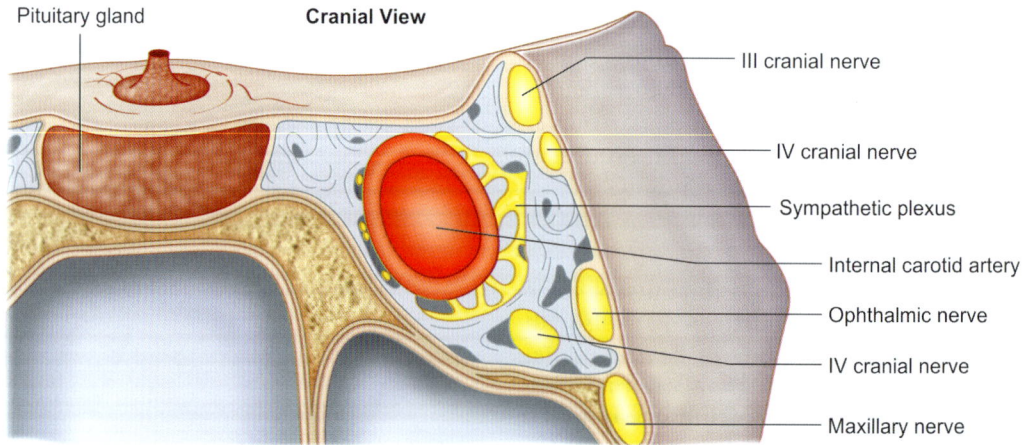

Fig. 12.5 *Anatomy of cavernous sinus, coronal view*

from above downwards are oculomotor nerve (IIIrd cranial nerve), trochlear nerve (IVth cranial nerve), ophthalmic and maxillary divisions of trigeminal nerve. Structures passing through the centre of the sinus are internal carotid artery and abducent nerve.

Internal carotid artery: It enters the middle cranial fossa by passing through the carotid canal and then traversing the foramen lacerum. It runs in the cavernous sinus and emerges in the anterior part of its roof. It lies lateral to optic chiasma and terminates by dividing into anterior cerebral and middle cerebral arteries. Bouthillier et al described a seven segment internal carotid artery (ICA) classification system starting from its origin to its termination during its course (Fig. 12.6):

- C1: cervical segment
- C2: petrous segment
- C3: lacerum segment
- C4: cavernous segment
- C5: clinoid segment
- C6: ophthalmic (supraclinoid) segment
- C7: communicating (terminal) segment

    CCFs are most common in C4 segment of ICA.

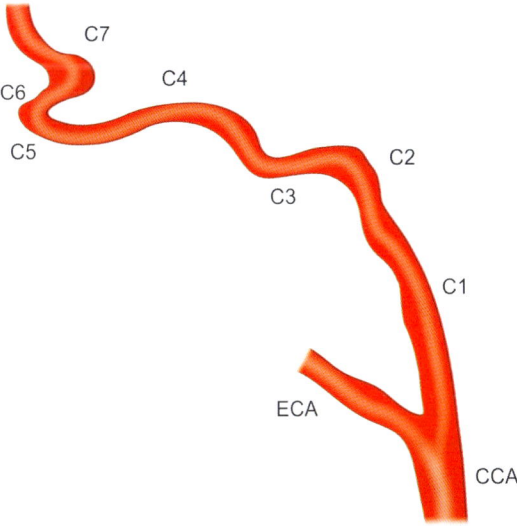

Fig. 12.6 *Seven segments of internal carotid artery from origin to termination according to Bouthillier's classification (ICA—Internal carotid artery; ECA—External carotid artery; CCA—Common carotid artery)*

Pathophysiology

Single tear in the wall of internal carotid artery because of trauma produces a direct connection between carotid artery and one or more venous channels within cavernous sinus. Most of the fistulas arise in the cavernous portion of internal carotid artery. The carotid artery may tear or be perforated by a bone fragment during impact from a sudden deformation or fracture through the carotid canal. CCF has been mostly found to occur secondary to trauma because of road side accident, falls or assaults. In case of assault by an object (knife/pencil/pen) producing stab wound, the object pierces through the superior orbital fissure and lacerates the internal carotid artery within the cavernous sinus. In rare cases, direct CCF results from persistent trigeminal artery originating from internal carotid artery within cavernous sinus.

Clinical features

Non-ocular manifestations

Epistaxis, intracerebral haemorrhage, subarachnoid haemorrhage.

The cavernous sinus drains posteriorly into superior and inferior petrosal sinuses while anteriorly into orbital vein. Hence posteriorly draining CCF may present with isolated ocular motor cranial nerve palsies. However, anteriorly draining fistulas have more severe manifestations as they redirect arterial blood through normal orbital venous channels. This causes diminished arterial blood flow to cranial nerves within the cavernous sinus, stasis of both venous and arterial circulation within eye and orbit and an increase in episcleral and orbital venous pressure.

Ocular manifestations

These can be unilateral (Fig. 12.7), bilateral or even contralateral depending upon the drainage of cavernous and intercavernous connections. Ocular manifestations of CCF include:
- *Proptosis*: Most common sign, mostly on the side of CCF; but can be bilateral or even contralateral
- *Eyelid oedema*
- *Conjunctival chemosis*
- *Arterialization of conjunctival* and episceral veins: corkscrew vessels—hallmark of CCF

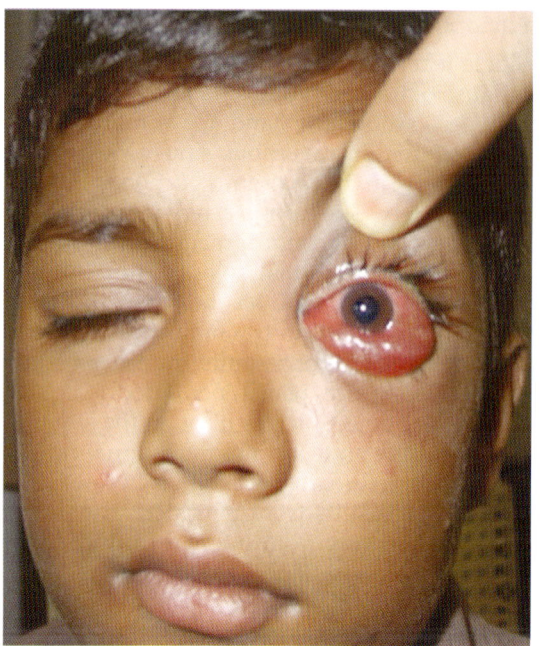

Fig. 12.7 *A case of caroticocavernous fistula in a 10-year-old male child following a blunt trauma to his left eye with an iron rod. Patient presented with proptosis, chemosis and vision loss*

- *Increased ocular pulsations*
- *Pulsating exophthalmos*
- *Exposure keratopathy*: With or without proptosis (because of associated trigeminal neuropathy)
- *Diplopia*: Most commonly because of ocular motor nerve palsies; abducens nerve being commonly affected; may be restrictive because of orbital oedema
- *Vision loss*: Can be immediate because of associated optic nerve damage or delayed because of exposure keratopathy, associated retinal/vitreous haemorrhage
- *Glaucoma*: Can be due to raised episcleral pressure/neovascular glaucoma
- *Ophthalmoscopy findings*: Retinal vein occlusion, stasis retinopathy leading to optic disc swelling, superficial and deep retinal haemorrhages.

Investigations

CT/MR angiography: Enlargement of affected cavernous sinus, abnormal intracranial vessels, dilation of superior ophthalmic vein, enlarged extraocular muscles (Fig. 12.8). However, catheter angiography is most diagnostic.

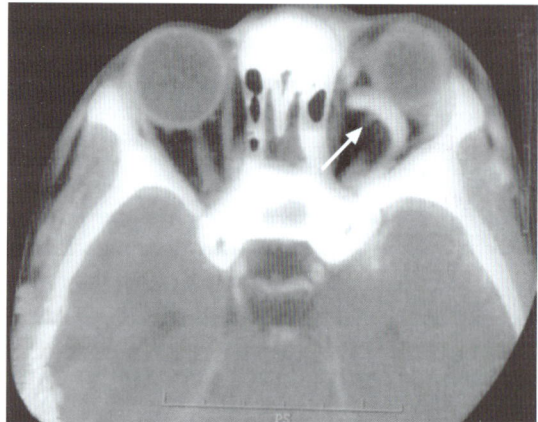

Fig. 12.8 *CT scan of the same patient showing prominent cavernous sinuses (L>>R), dilated left superior ophthalmic vein (arrow), evidence of soft tissues swelling present in the left retro-orbital tissues causing proptosis of left globe. Left optic nerve and extraocular muscles are normal*

Treatment

Aim: Closure of arteriovenous malformation while maintaining internal carotid artery patency.

Procedure used is *endovascular closure of direct CCF with embolization* using platinum coils or detachable balloons. Immediately after doing such embolization, angiography must be performed to confirm the proper placement of the coil/balloon. Most of the ocular signs and symptoms resolve after placement of the balloon/coil (Fig. 12.9). Significant improvement in vision is

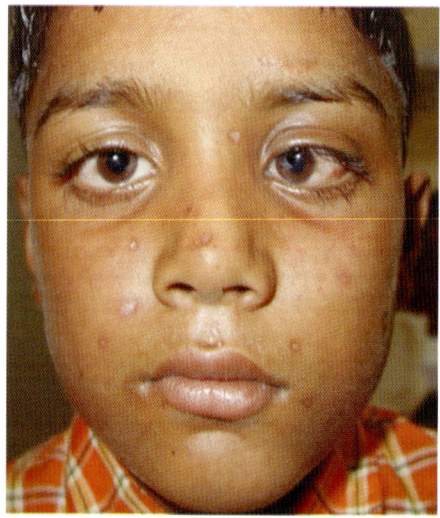

Fig. 12.9 *Postoperative picture of the same patient as in Fig. 12.5 after balloon embolization of CCF*

seen in patients with associated choroidal detachment, effusion, optic neuropathy and retinopathy with timely surgical intervention.

EXTRACONAL ORBITAL TRAUMA

I. ORBITAL FRACTURES

Orbital trauma can lead to fracture of the facial bones as well as injuries to orbital contents, intracranial structures and paranasal sinuses. They can be associated with intraorbital foreign bodies, orbital haemorrhage. In addition associated ocular damage can also include hyphema, angle recession, corneoscleral laceration, retinal tear/detachment/dialysis or vitreous haemorrhage, eyelid malpositions including ptosis. Hence a thorough evaluation of such trauma is a must.

Demographics: Orbital fractures are more commonly found in males than females and mostly in 3rd and 4th decades of life. A high impact trauma (with a stick or cricket ball) is most commonly associated with orbital fractures. Around 60% of the head injury cases involve orbital fractures at single or multiple sites. All four walls are involved in 5%, three walls in 17% and two in 30% of the maxillofacial trauma cases.

A. BLOWOUT FRACTURE ORBIT

Blowout fracture of orbit is defined as fracture of one or more of its internal walls. This injury is typically caused by blunt trauma to orbit. In pure terms, this definition does not involve the orbital rim. If fracture of orbital rim is associated with fractures of one or more of its internal walls, then the term complex blowout fracture is used. Even though there is nothing complex about it, this term is used to stress the importance of non-involvement of orbital rim in blowout fracture. Blowout fracture is actually a protective mechanism which ensures that sudden build up of intraocular pressure which could be detrimental to integrity of eyeball and thereby to vision does not occur following frontal injury to orbit.

Classification of blowout fracture

1. Orbital floor blowout fracture—commonest.
2. Medial wall blowout fracture—this is uncommon even though it is lined by the paper thin lamina papyracea, because of the support it receives from the bony ethmoidal labyrinth.
3. Superior wall blowout fracture—rare.
4. Lateral wall fracture—involves zygoma.

Pathophysiology

There are various theories as under which explain the mechanism of blowout fracture (Fig. 12.10):

A. *Hydraulic theory*: This theory was proposed by Pfeiffer in 1943 which believes that for blowout fracture to occur the blow should be received

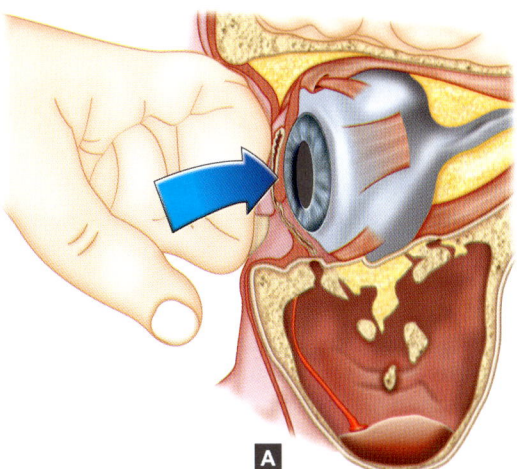 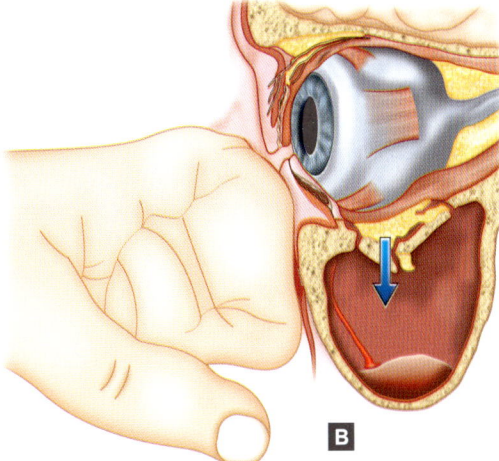

Fig. 12.10 *(A) Hydraulic theory: A blow received by eyeball and the force is transmitted to inferior wall of orbit via hydraulic effect. (B) Buckling theory: Force received at inferior orbital rim getting transmitted to floor of orbit*

by the eyeball and the force should be transmitted to the walls of the orbit via hydraulic effect. So according to this theory for blow out fracture to occur, the eyeball should sustain direct blow pushing it into the orbit. A history of the eye being struck by an object larger than the diameter of the orbital rim is commonly associated in such cases.

B. *Buckling theory*: This theory proposed that if a force strikes at any part of the orbital rim, this force gets transferred to the paper thin weak walls of the orbit (i.e. floor and medial wall) via rippling effect causing them to distort and eventually to fracture. This mechanism was first described by Le Fort.

Blowout fracture of floor of orbit

Clinical features

The primary step in assessing a patient after a trauma, especially for those patients involved in multisystem trauma, requires evaluation of airway, breathing, and circulatory status.

Patients with periorbital trauma frequently present with traumatic pathology of the globe that can threaten visual outcome, especially if not identified in a prudent manner. Patients can present with traumatic iritis, corneal abrasion, hyphema, acute glaucoma, lens trauma, vitreous haemorrhage, commotio retinae, retinal tears and detachment and traumatic optic neuropathy. Decreased visual acuity, colour vision, and, most importantly, an afferent papillary defect can alert the physician to the presence of traumatic optic neuropathy. Careful evaluation for possible globe rupture must be performed. The majority of pathologies can be present even in visually asymptomatic patients. Treatment of any vision-threatening conditions should almost always preclude repair of the fracture until stable.

Signs seen on ocular examination are:
- *Eyelid*: Oedema and ecchymosis, other external signs of injury can be absent (white-eyed blowout).
- *Enophthalmos and globe ptosis*: Seen when in large fractures orbital soft tissue prolapses into maxillary sinus. Along with this if the soft tissue prolapses into medial wall, the degree

of enophthalmos increases. Enophthalmos may be masked by orbital oedema immediately following injury, it becomes more apparent as the orbital oedema subsides. Globe ptosis indicates a sizeable fracture.
- *Hyposthesia* in the distribution of infraorbital nerve.
- *Emphysema* of orbit and lids.
- *Diplopia with limitation of upgaze, downgaze or both*: Inferior rectus entrapment gives rise to vertical movement restriction, vertical diplopia and pain. Limitation of movement can also occur due to haemorrhage or oedema which generally improves as they subside by 1–2 weeks. Forced duction test shows restriction of passive movement in case of entrapment. However, in case of haemorrhage/oedema, it is negative. While doing this test on inferior rectus, the intraocular pressure in primary position and in upgaze usually shows a significant increase in upgaze, if the muscle is entrapped.
- However, in children, a small intensity trauma leads to what is called as trapdoor fracture. Trapdoor fractures result from an acute transient increase in orbital pressure. A linear orbital wall fracture is created. A flap of bone is then outwardly displaced, which immediately returns to its original position. This mechanism is dependent on ample bone elasticity, characteristic of children' bones. Soft tissue may or may not be incarcerated in such fracture. In case of trapdoor fracture with entrapped muscle as seen in children most commonly, the muscle is unable to fully contract, leading to reduced duction in the direction of the fracture (infraduction in most cases). Often more striking is restriction with attempted duction opposite the fracture (supraduction in most cases) (Fig. 12.11).

Indications for surgical repair

1. *Persistent diplopia* in the primary position of gaze along with limitation of upgaze and/ or downgaze within 30° of primary position, i.e. symptomatic disturbance of ocular mobility, if persisting for more than 2 weeks is considered to be an absolute indication by many. This two-week window is considered

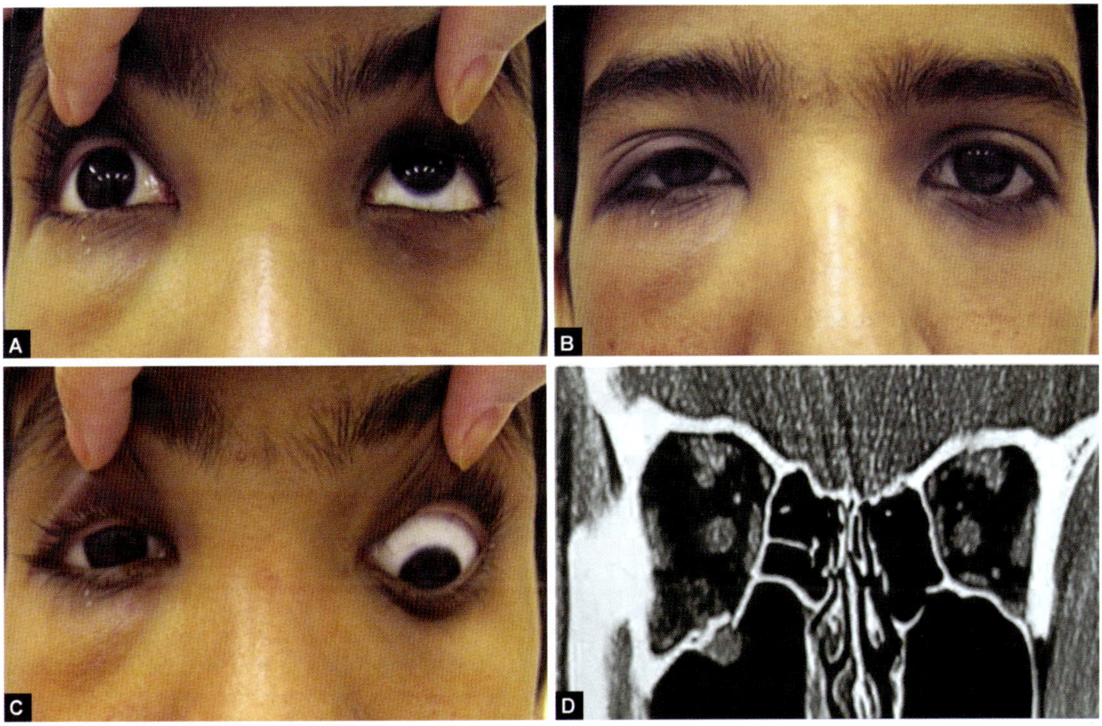

Fig. 12.11 *Trapdoor fracture of the right orbital floor in a teenage male. Note that there is mild swelling and ecchymosis. There is marked limitation of supraduction (A) he is orthophoric in primary gaze;(B) and there is moderate limitation of infraduction; (C) Marked abnormal external findings with the exception of abnormal motility is the hallmark of paediatric trapdoor fractures. Computed tomography demonstrates a non-displaced fracture of the right orbital floor; (D) Note that the inferior rectus muscle is located inferior to the orbital floor*

because it is the time taken by oedema/ haematoma of orbit to resolve. Two weeks after the injury, fibrosis and adhesions begin to develop. Any surgery performed before development of adhesions/fibrosis has best results.

2. *Radiological evidence* of extraocular muscle entrapment.

3. *Enophthalmos* of more than 2 mm; which is cosmetically unacceptable to the patient.

4. *Large fractures* involving the floor of the orbit (more than 50% of the floor is involved).

5. *Infraorbital nerve hypoaesthesia*/anaesthesia.

Imaging

X-ray paranasal sinuses: May show the classical "teardrop sign" of prolapsed orbital contents (Fig. 12.12). The fractured fragment may also be visible. The corresponding maxillary sinus may appear hazy due to the presence of hemosinus.

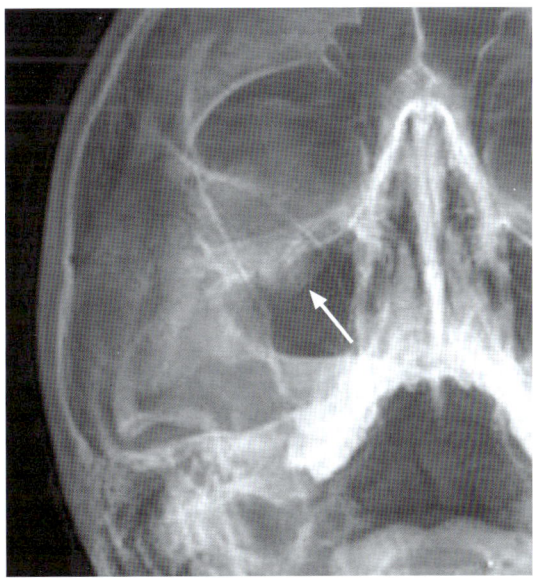

Fig. 12.12 *Teardrop sing as seen on X-ray PNS (Water's view) with prolapsed orbital contents in the maxillary sinus (arrow) following fracture of floor of orbit*

CT scan: The coronal and sagittal views are helpful and they guide the treatment. They help in evaluating the fracture size and extraocular muscle relationships thus helping to predict enophthalmos and possible muscle entrapment (Figs 12.13 and 12.14).

Blowout fracture medial wall of orbit

Fractures involving medial wall of orbit may occur alone or as part of more complex orbital fractures. Pure medial wall fractures are really rare. Fractures involving medial orbital wall may be missed in plain radiographs, hence CT scan is diagnostic.

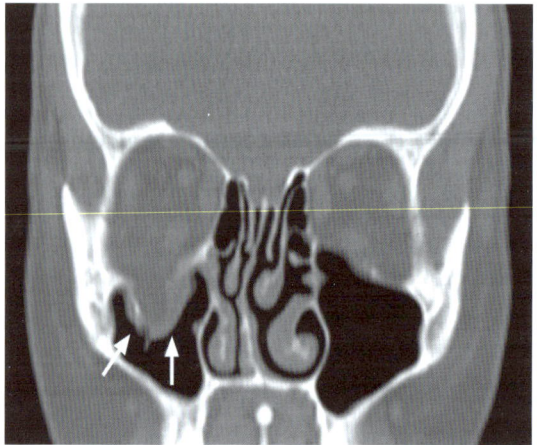

Fig. 12.13 *Non-contrast CT scan orbit coronal cut showing fracture floor of orbit with prolapsed of orbital contents in maxillary sinus: "teardrop sign" (arrows)*

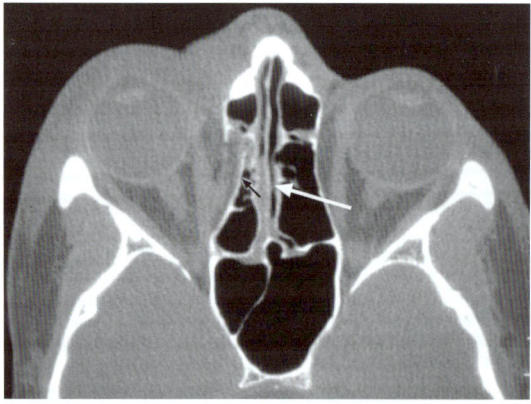

Fig. 12.14 *Non-contrast CT scan right orbit axial cut showing fracture medial wall of right orbit (black arrow)*

Clinical features

1. Periorbital oedema
2. Ecchymosis
3. Subcutaneous emphysema due to escape of air from ethmoid sinus in the periorbital space
4. Epistaxis
5. Enophthalmos—according to Pearl, enophthalmos is worse in medial blowout fractures than fractures involving other walls of orbit (Fig. 12.14).

Management

Repair is preferable within 2 weeks of the trauma. Formation of scar tissue and contracture of the prolapsed tissue make later correction of entrapment and diplopia difficult.

Surgical approaches to orbital floor have been classified into:

1. *Transorbital*—transcutaneous, subciliary approaches and transconjunctival. The subciliary approach can be combined with or without lateral cantholysis
2. *Transantral*—includes endoscopic approach
3. *Combined* approach

1. Transorbital approaches

Transorbital approaches include:

i. *Transcutaneous* orbital rim incision is usually given just below the lower eyelid. This approach is very simple one and easy to perform. The incision area is marked and infiltrated with xylocaine mixed with 1 in 100,000 units adrenaline. Ideally the incision should hug the infraorbital rim. Orbicularis oculi muscle should be slit along its long axis. Orbital contents are retracted to expose the floor of orbit. This approach gives rise to postoperative oedema. This incision also causes visible scar just below the lower eyelid.

ii. *A subciliary incision* is made 2 mm below and parallel to the eyelash line. This incision is usually performed using a 15 blade. Medially this incision should fall short of the punctum, while laterally it can be extended even up to 15 mm beyond the lateral canthus. The lateral extension of this incision is preferred and should be extended horizontally and not inferiorly in order to promote formation of aesthetically acceptable scar. Dissection proceeds in the subcutaneous plane superficial to orbicularis oculi muscle. At the level of lower end of tarsal plate, orbicularis oculi muscle is divided parallel to the direction of muscle fibres. Orbicularis oculi muscle over the tarsal plate should be protected to maintain lower lid structure and support. The dissection now follows the preseptal plane down to the level of orbital rim. The periosteum is incised over the anterior portion of infraorbital rim. This elevation of the periosteum proceeds up to the level of orbital floor.

Advantages of this approach:
• Easy to perform
• Gives broad access to the floor of orbit

Disadvantages include:
• Lower lid malposition
• Scarring of lower eyelid

iii. *Transconjunctival* approach is the most preferred approach for orbital surgeries because of low complication rates and excellent cosmesis. In this method, the lower eye lid is pulled forward. To increase the laxity, a lateral cantho-tomy should be performed. However, this approach is fraught with complications which include eyelid avulsion, button holing of eyelid, canthal dehiscence, haematoma, prolonged chemosis and lacrimal sac laceration. Further, cicatricial entropion, ectropion and lower lild retraction can also occur as late complications.

Associated proptosis, orbital swelling, severe chemosis, severe swelling of lower eyelid, laceration of conjunctiva can pose problem in transconjunctival approach. In addition, it is not suitable for medial wall fracture of orbit.

2. Transantral–endoscopic reduction/repair of blowout fracture

Indications are more or less identical to that of traditional repair procedures. These are as under:
• Isolated fractures involving the floor of the orbit with extraocular muscle entrapment.
• Preoperative enophthalmos.
• More than 50% disruption of orbital floor.

Trapdoor fractures of floor of orbit respond the best to endoscopic repair. In large blow-out fractures of orbital floor, endoscopic repair will jeopardize the infraorbital nerve as extensive dissection is necessary in that area. Hence it is contraindicated in such cases.

In trapdoor fracture of orbital floor, there is mild to moderate degree of orbital fat herniation. Strangulation of herniated orbital contents are common in these patients. This area appears endoscopically as enlarged and tense. These fractures can be managed by reduction and repositioning of the fractured and displaced fragments. No prosthesis is necessary.

Medial blowout fractures pose real challenges during endoscopic reduction. These fractures are usually comminuted and unstable; hence require more dissection and an implant for reconstruction of orbital floor. In fact in majority of these fractures having large void require orbital implant to fill up the gap.

Miniplating and microplating systems and their various metallic orbital implants has significantly improved the management of large, unstable orbital floor fractures.

Orbital implants can be:
• *Alloplastic*: Porous polyethylene, supramid, gore-tex, teflon, silicone sheet, titanium mesh
• *Autogenous*: Iliac bone crests, septal cartilage, split cranial bone, fascia

Delayed treatment of blowout fractures to correct diplopia/strabismus/enophthalmos may include exploration of the orbital floor in an attempt to free the scarred tissues entrapped or prolapsed through the fracture and to replace them in orbit.

B. MEDIAL ORBITAL FRACTURES

These fractures result from direct trauma (face striking to solid surfaces). These involve frontal process of maxilla, lacrimal bone, ethmoid bone along the medial wall of orbit. They are categorized as type I–III, with type I being a central fragment of bone attached to canthal tendon, type II having comminuted fracture of central fragment and type III having commi-nuted tendon attachment or avulsed tendon. Patients generally present with depressed nose bridge with traumatic telecanthus. Complica-tions include cerebral and ocular damage, severe epistaxis due to avulsion of anterior ethmoidal artery, orbital haematoma, CSF rhinorrhoea, damage to lacrimal drainage system, lateral displacement of medial canthus and associated fractures of medial orbital wall and floor. Treatment includes repair of nasal fracture and miniplate stabilization which is usually carried out in collaboration with ENT surgeons.

Indirect (blowout) fractures are frequently extensions of blowout fractures of orbital floor. Surgical intervention is generally not necessary. Isolated blowout fractures of the medial wall are rare but they may result in cosmetically noticeable enophthalmos and its risk further increases when both floor and medial wall are fractured.

C. ZYGOMATIC FRACTURES

These are mainly caused by involovement of zygomaticomaxillary complex (ZMC) and are also called as tripod fractures. Here the zygoma is fractured at four of its articulations with the adjacent bones (lateral orbital rim, inferior orbital rim, zygomatic arch, and lateral wall of the maxillary sinus). These fractures can cause globe displacement, cosmetic deformity, diplopia and trismus. Open reduction of such fractures and fixation with miniature metal plates that are attached with bone screws achieve best results.

D. ORBITAL APEX FRACTURES

These fractures involve optic canal, superior orbital fissure and structures that pass through them. Hence it can damage the optic nerves causing decreased visual acuity, cerebrospinal fluid (CSF) leaks and carotid cavernous sinus fistulas. Canalicular portion of the optic nerve can receive indirect trauma because of stretching, twisting or tearing of this fixed part of nerve as the cranial skeleton receives sudden deceleration.

E. ORBITAL ROOF FRACTURES

These are mainly caused by blunt trauma or missile injuries. Frontal traumatic forces are absorbed by frontal sinus and prevent their extension along orbital roof. Frontal sinus is, however, not pneumatized in young children. Hence, they are common in young age group.

Complications include intracranial injuries, CSF rhinorrhoea, pneumocephalus, subperiosteal haematoma, ptosis and extraocular muscle imbalance. Muscle entrapment is, however, rare. In severely comminuted fractures, pulsating exophthalmos may occur as a delayed complication. Most roof fractures do not require repair, indications are generally neurosurgical.

II. *INTRAORBITAL FOREIGN BODIES*

Intraorbital foreign bodies usually occur after a high-velocity injury, such as a gunshot or industrial accident but may occur after relatively trivial trauma to the extent that the history may be unclear. A high index of suspicion is required in the setting of projectile injuries or in the setting of orbital inflammation after a history of periocular trauma, no matter how trivial it seems, because a retained foreign body may give rise to severe orbital complications. Inorganic foreign bodies usually cause visual loss or orbital complications from direct trauma, whereas organic foreign bodies also have a higher incidence of developing severe orbital infections thereby producing severe inflammatory reactions. Hence, a history of trauma in patients with orbital infections or inflammation must be taken because they may harbor a foreign body. Children, or patients under the influence of various substances, may not give such a history, so clinicians must maintain a high index of suspicion.

Diagnosis

Appropriate imaging studies should be performed. A CT scan is the standard diagnostic test, because it demonstrates most of the foreign bodies, and it is safe in the presence of metallic foreign bodies (Figs 12.15 and 12.16).

Wooden foreign bodies may be missed on CT scanning or may be misdiagnosed as intraorbital air. MRI scans are better at demonstrating wooden foreign bodies and should be performed after a negative CT scan, if there is a possibility of a wooden foreign body.

Management

Whether to remove the foreign body or not depends on the size, type and location of foreign

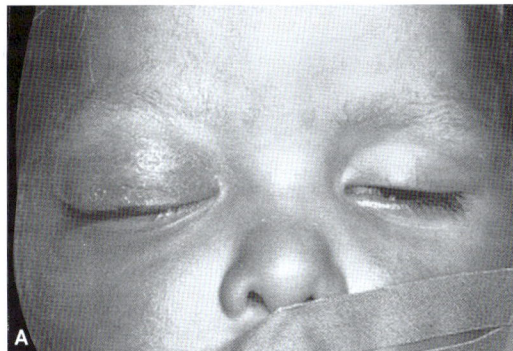

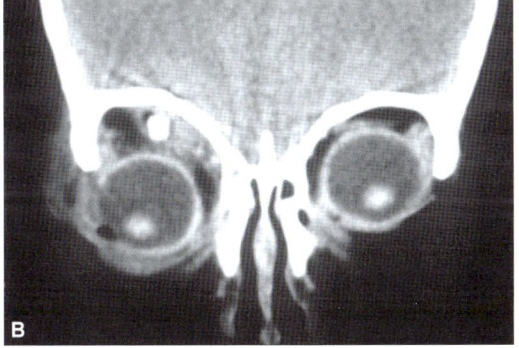

Fig. 12.15 *(A) A 1-year-old boy was seen with right periorbital swelling and inflammation 1 week after falling on to a pencil. (B) A computed tomography scan revealed a pencil fragment and orbital abscess in his right superior orbit*

body. Figure 12.17 depicts the protocol for management of intraorbital foreign bodies. Posteriorly located foreign bodies have an increased risk of motility disturbances or optic neuropathy after surgical removal, whereas anteriorly placed foreign bodies are more easily removed. The removal of anteriorly located metallic foreign bodies also allows patients to undergo future MRI investigations without concerns regarding dislodgment of the foreign body with potential complications.

Organic foreign bodies have a much higher incidence of potentially sight-threatening complications than inert, nonorganic foreign bodies.

Three types of non-organic foreign bodies are not inert and require specific mention.
- *Copper-containing compounds* may incite a marked inflammatory response necessitating removal.
- *Lead shot or pellets* may cause systemic toxicity; however, in the orbit this seems unlikely.
- *The exact risk of iron foreign bodies* causing siderosis with loss of vision is difficult to predict, but retinal photoreceptor function could be assessed with electroretinography to monitor for this.

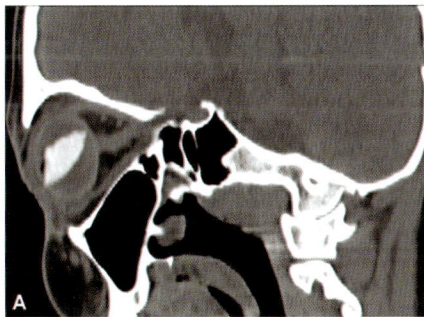

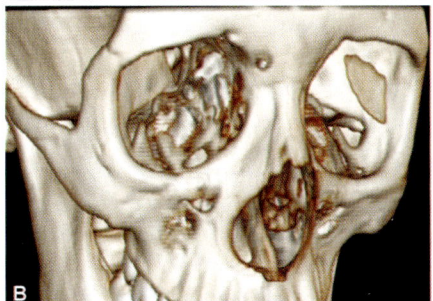

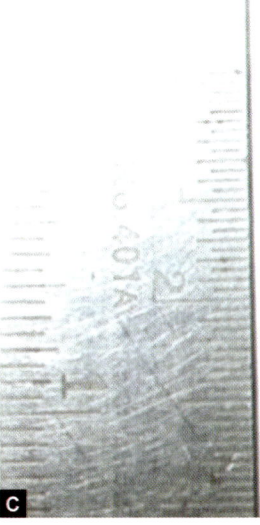

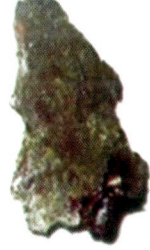

Fig. 12.16 *A. Non-contrast CT scan sagittal view of the left orbit showing a metallic foreign body in the superotemporal region of the orbit, B. 3-D reconstructed view of the CT scan as in A, C. The foreign body following removal*

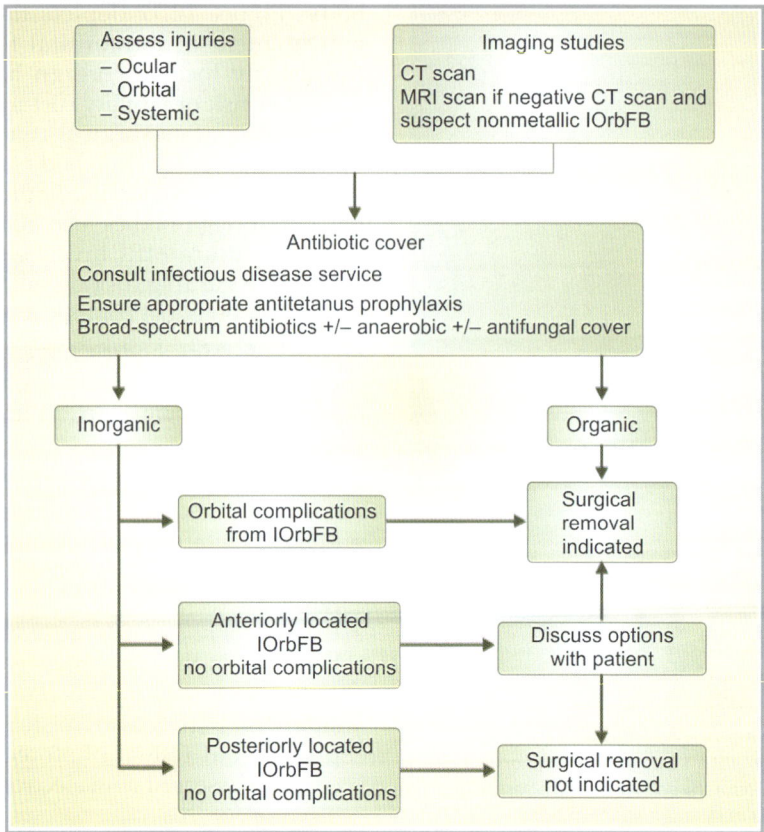

Fig. 12.17 *Protocol for management of intraorbital foreign bodies*

BIBLIOGRAPHY

1. Al-Mujaini A, Al-Senawi R, Ganesh A, Al-Zuhaibi S, Al-Dhuhli H. Intraorbital Foreign Body: Clinical Presentation, Radiological Appearance and Management. Sultan Qaboos University Medical Journal, 2008;8(1),69–74.

2. Boffano P, Roccia F, Gallesio C, et al. Diplopia and orbital wall fractures. J Craniofac Surg Mar 2014;25(2):e183–185.

3. Bord SP, Linden J. Trauma to the globe and orbit. Emerg Med Clin North Am Feb 2008; 26(1):97–123, vi–vii.

4. de Keizer R. Carotid-cavernous and orbital arterio-venous fistulas: ocular features, diagnostic and hemodynamic considerations in relation to visual impairment and morbidity. Orbit Jun 2003;22(2):121–142.

5. Jordan DR, Allen LH, White J, Harvey J, Pashby R, Esmaeli B. Intervention within days for some orbital floor fractures: the white-eyed blowout. Ophthal Plast Reconstr Surg Nov 1998;14(6): 379–390.

6. Lake D, Mearza A, Thompson GM. Intraorbital foreign bodies. Ophthalmology. 2003 Jun;110(6): 1269.

7. Yu JS, Lei T, Chen JC, He Y, Chen J, Li L. Diagnosis and endovascular treatment of spontaneous direct carotid-cavernous fistula. Chin Med J (Engl) Aug 20 2008;121(16):1558–1562.

Section

III

Non-Mechanical Injuries

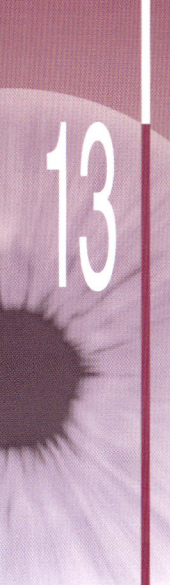

CHEMICAL INJURIES

INTRODUCTION AND EPIDEMIOLOGY

INTRODUCTION

Chemical (alkali and acid) injuries of the eye represent one of the true ocular emergencies as they can cause extensive damage leading to visual impairment in a short time span. More than 25000 chemical products—oxidizers, reducing agents, corrosive, dyes, etc.—can cause chemical burns and all such injuries should receive prompt intervention. Besides causing ocular surface damage, chemicals, such as alkalis, readily penetrate the cornea, entering the anterior chamber and injure the corneal stroma and endothelium. Other anterior segment structures, such as iris, lens and ciliary body, are also damaged resulting in blinding complications, especially in cases of bilateral chemical exposure. Alkali injuries are more common and more deleterious. Usually, there occurs no permanent visual impairment but the outcome is highly dependent on the agent responsible for the injury as well as the treatment received.

EPIDEMIOLOGY

Chemical injuries of the eye form a small but significant fraction of ocular trauma. Three major studies put the incidence at 7, 8.7, and 9.9% of all ocular trauma, respectively.[1-3] Ocular chemical injuries can occur under diverse circumstances and in varied locations as the home, the workplace, and school. These injuries are common in industrial chemical laboratories, in machine factories, in agriculture, and among labourers and construction workers. They also are frequently reported from fabric mills, automotive repair facilities, and cleaning and sanitizing crews. Most of these injuries are accidental (89.4%) and the rest occur as a result of chemical assault. Chemical burns of the eyes are seen mostly among young patients between 16 and 45 years of age, with men being more affected than females (58.4% versus 41.6%). The mean age among all categories is 33.6 years.

CAUSATIVE CHEMICALS

LIST OF ALKALIS AND ACIDS

Common acids and alkalis causing chemical injuries are depicted in Table 13.1.

ALKALI VERSUS ACID INJURIES

Alkali injuries occur twice more frequently than acid injuries and are more damaging due to more effective ocular penetration. The hydroxyl ion (OH) of the alkali saponifies the fatty acid components of cell membranes, resulting in cell disruption and death, whereas the cation of the alkali is responsible for penetration of a specific alkali. The cations react with carboxyl groups (COOH) present in the stromal collagen and glycosaminoglycans (GAGs), with their subsequent hydration. Hydration of the GAGs results in a loss of stromal clarity and hydration

Table 13.1 *List of alkalis and acids causing chemical injuries*

Alkalis

Agent	Source	Comments
NH_3	Fertilizers, refrigerators, cleaning agents, charging of NH_3 applicators	*Most serious alkali injury* Rapid penetration of the alkali (reaches the AC within 5 sec)
Lime — $Ca(OH)_2$	Plaster, cement, whitewash, mortar	*Most common* chemical at workplace Poor ocular penetration Toxicity more due to retained particulate matters
Lye — NaOH (Caustic soda)	Drain cleaner	Reaches the AC within 1 minute
Potassium hydroxide — KOH	Caustic potash	Reaches the AC within 1 minute
$Mg(OH)_2$	Sparklers, fireworks	Both thermal and chemical injury

Acids

Agent	Source	Comments
Sulphuric acid (H_2SO_4) [Oil of Vitriol]	Industrial cleaners, battery acid	*Commonest agent* With water produces corneal thermal burns If injury at the time of explosion may be associated with mechanical component and RIOFB
Sulfurous acid (H_2SO_3)	Bleach, refrigerants, preservatives for fruits and vegetables	Penetrates into the AC easily when compared to other acids
Hydrofluoric acid (HF)	Glass polishing, glass frosting, mineral refining, semiconductor industry	*Most serious acid injury*
Hydrochloric acid (HCl)	31–38% solution	Severe injury if high concentration of acid and prolonged exposure
Acetic acid (CH_3COOH)	Vinegar, glacial acetic acid, essence of vinegar	Mild to severe injury depending upon the concentration of the acid
Chromic acid (Cr_2O_3)	Chrome plating industry	Chronic conjunctivitis with brownish discolouration
Methyl isocyanate gas	Bhopal gas	Severe burning, chronic dry eye, corneal opacity

of collagen fibrils results in their thickening and shortening. This distorts the architecture of the trabecular meshwork as well and there occurs a release of prostaglandins. Both these factors cause a rise in intraocular pressure which is seen immediately following alkali injuries.

Depending on degree of penetration by the alkali, there occurs damage to the corneal and conjunctival epithelium, basement membrane, stromal keratocytes, stromal nerve endings, endothelium, lens epithelium, vascular endo-thelium of conjunctiva, episclera, iris and ciliary body. Penetration into the anterior chamber is seen immediately after ammonia injury and within 3–5 minutes after sodium hydroxide injury. This causes damage to the ciliary body epithelium resulting in decreased secretion of ascorbate, thereby compromising subsequent corneal keratocyte collagen synthesis and stromal repair. Changes also occur in the chemical milleu of the anterior chamber aqueous and prolonged aqueous pH levels of 11.5 or more leads to irreversible intraocular damage with hypotony and later on, phthisis bulbi.

Acid injuries. Acids penetrate much less readily into corneal stroma. The hydrogen (H^+) ion of the acid causes damage due to pH alteration, whereas the anion produces protein precipita-tion and denaturation in corneal epithelium and superficial stroma. Coagulation of proteins produces characteristic "ground glass" appea-rance of epithelium, and it also functions as a barrier to further penetration by the acid, limiting further intraocular injury.

Therefore, tissue alterations, which occur if the chemical agent penetrates into the stroma, are as follows:

- Precipitation of extracellular glycosamino-glycans and corneal opacification
- Hydration and shortening of collagen fibrils
- Transient elevation in IOP due to trabecular meshwork distortion
- Anterior chamber pH alterations
- Anterior segment damage
- Lowered aqueous ascorbate levels

PATHOPHYSIOLOGY OF CHEMICAL INJURY

The severity of chemical injury depends upon the following factors:

- Surface area of contact
- Time of contact
- Depth of penetration
- Time of interference
- Concentration of the chemical
- Degree of limbal stem cell injury

EPITHELIAL INJURY, REPAIR AND DIFFERENTIATION

Corneal epithelium

The cornea consists of a 5–6 cell-layered stratified squamous epithelium overlying basal epithelial cells, which are affixed to their underlying basement membrane (Bowman's layer) through hemidesmosomes. The presence of an intact extracellular matrix, with fibronectin, laminin, GAGs and collagen is essential for secure binding of the epithelial cells. The corneal epithelium is non-keratinized and contains no goblet cells. It plays a very important optical role by maintaining smoothness of the optical surface and the transparency necessary to transmit images with minimal distortion. It also helps prevent entry of microorganisms into the corneal stroma, maintains deturgence of the stroma and regulates the metabolic activity of stromal keratocytes.

Limbal stem cells

At the limbus, the stratified squamous epi-thelium thickens to approximately 10 cell layers. Thoft and Friend proposed the X,Y,Z hypothesis according to which epithelial cells arising from multipotent stem cells at the corneoscleral limbus migrate continuously in a centripetal pattern towards the corneal center and replace the epithelial cells that have moved toward the surface during their normal maturation and have then desquamated from the cornea. The basal epithelial cells of the limbal zone maintain the ocular surface epithelium, in normal health and also following injury. In the uninjured cornea, complete replacement of epithelial cells occurs every 5 to 7 days. The rate at which migrating cells move over the corneal surface increases after trauma.

Conjunctival epithelium

The conjunctival epithelium consists of 2 or more layers of stratified columnar epithelium with numerous goblet cells. These goblet cells help in the production of mucin which forms an important component of the tear film and ensures complete wetting of the ocular surface. Along with the corneal epithelium, the conjunctival epithelium forms a relative barrier to the passage of microorganisms and noxious chemical agents and also participates in local immune reactions. It is also capable of re-populating corneal epithelial surface following traumatic injury.

LIMBAL STEM CELL/OCULAR SURFACE INJURY

Following corneal epithelial injury, recovery depends upon the centripetal movement of most proximal, viable epithelium. Complete corneal epithelial defect requires epithelium from limbus. When there is extensive corneal and limbal injury, the surrounding conjunctival epithelium provides the only source for epithelial regeneration. Rate of re-epithelialization and the ultimate functional competence of ocular surface depends upon the source of regenerating epithelium.

Transdifferentiation

When conjunctival epithelium resurfaces cornea, it undergoes progression from a histologically undifferentiated initial phase (showing neither goblet cells nor corneal epithelial basal cells) to the appearance of numerous goblet cells throughout corneal epithelium, multicentric nests of corneal cells in midst of evanescent conjunctival cells and finally, histologically normal corneal epithelium. The pseudo-stratified, columnar conjunctival epithelium becomes pseudostratified, squamous, and there is an attrition of goblet cells. After several weeks, the biochemical functions of the healing cells begin to resemble more closely those of corneal epithelium. Transdifferentiation of conjunctival epithelium is rarely complete following severe chemical injuries.

Rate of migration of surrounding epithelial cells towards the corneal surface is slowed down by persistent inflammation, epithelial basement membrane damage and degradation of basement membrane fibronectin by plasminogen activator, released during the inflammatory process. Therefore, resurfacing of the cornea with conjunctival epithelium after a severe chemical injury is associated with:

- Delayed re-epithelialization
- Superficial and deep stromal neovascularization
- Persistence of goblet cells within corneal epithelium
- Recurrent epithelial erosions due to abnormal basement membrane epithelial adhesion

If limbal stem cell loss is complete, severe superficial pannus invariably occurs (often in association with stromal vascularization) resulting in complete conjunctival phenotypic characteristics or "conjunctivalization" of the new ocular surface. Because of poor trans-differentiation and "conjunctivalization" of ocular surface following complete limbal stem cell loss, Kenyon and Tseng proposed that limbal stem cells are the most qualified cells to restore functional competence after extensive ocular surface and limbal stem cell injury.

CORNEAL STROMAL MATRIX INJURY, REPAIR AND ULCERATION

Nearly 80% of the corneal stroma is collagen, predominantly type I collagen. It is produced by the stromal keratocytes and provides major tensile strength to the corneal tissue. Sufficient synthesis by keratocytes is essential for successful repair and prevention of corneal ulceration and perforation. The stromal keratocytes besides synthesizing collagen also produce GAGs, which regulate the water content in the stroma and help in maintaining corneal transparency. Matrix metalloproteinases (MMPs), responsible for initial rate-limiting cleavage of collagen molecules and regulate wound healing are also secreted by keratocytes. The important corneal MMPs are type I collagenase, stromelysin and gelatinase. MMPs are regulated in vivo by tissue inhibitors of metalloproteinases (TIMPs) and other inhibitors.

After a chemical burn, there occurs an increase in the number of keratocytes and they migrate into the region of damage. Migration of keratocytes occurs only under an intact epithelium. EGF (Epidermal Growth Factor) and fibroblast growth factors both help to regulate the influx of new keratocytes. The energized keratocytes produce new collagen and proteoglycans. Although the new collagen is type I, its structure is irregular, decreasing transmission of light through the resulting scar. Meanwhile, the new proteoglycans bind water more avidly, resulting in excess hydration of the scar, which further insures irregular spacing (with lack of transparency) of the new collagen. In addition, stromal keratocytes develop intracytoplasmic contractile elements that cause contraction of the scar and irregular astigmatism.

INFLAMMATORY PROCESS

Following any insult to the ocular surface, infiltration of inflammatory cells into injured tissue occurs. Within 12–24 hours after chemical injury, polymorphonuclear neutrophils (PMN) and mononuclear leucocytes infiltrate the peripheral cornea. A second wave of inflammatory cell infiltration begins at 7 days and peaks between 14 and 21 days, when corneal repair and degradation are maximal. Stromal inflammation persists as long as epithelial defect remains, or till necrotic conjunctival tissue provides a focus of inflammatory infiltration. Persistent inflammation, enzymatic products of degranulating PMN leucocytes, stimulation of keratocyte collagenase by mononuclear leucocyte cytokines cause sterile enzymatic digestion of corneal stroma during second and third post-injury weeks and retard epithelial recovery. Therapeutic strategies used for chemical burns aim to exclude PMN and mononuclear leucocytes from corneal stroma, thereby preventing and arresting stromal ulceration. Prompt debridement of necrotic bulbar and tarsal conjunctival tissue helps to eliminate a source of continuous leucocyte infiltration and release of proteolytic enzymes. Treatment of first-wave infiltration with citrate is effective in preventing second wave and reducing the incidence of corneal ulceration in experimental alkali injuries.

CLINICAL PROFILE

CLINICAL FEATURES

A detailed history regarding the mechanism of injury, whether it was simply a splash of chemical into the eye or if it was a high velocity blast, should be taken. High velocity blasts have associated component of mechanical injury besides the injury caused by the chemical itself. Patients usually give history of a liquid or a gas being splashed or sprayed into the eyes or a history of fall of particles of a certain chemical falling into the eye.

Symptoms. The most common complaints are pain in the eye (often extreme), foreign body sensation, blurring of vision, excessive tearing, photophobia and redness in the eye.

Signs depend upon the grade of chemical burn and the pathophysiologic and clinical phase of the chemical injury (given by McCulley).

CLASSIFICATION OF CHEMICAL INJURIES

Hughes classification (modified by Ballen and Roper-Hall)

Hughes classification modified by Ballen and Roper-Hall is summarized in Table 13.2 and depicted in Figs 13.1 to 13.4.

Table 13.2 *Hughes classification of chemical injuries (modified by Ballen and Roper-Hall)*

Grade	Prognosis	Cornea	Conjunctiva or limbus
1.	Excellent	Corneal epithelial damage	No limbal ischaemia
2.	Good	Corneal haze, iris details visible	<1/3 limbal ischaemia
3.	Guarded	Total epithelial loss, stromal haze, iris details obscured	1/3–1/2 limbal ischaemia
4.	Dismal	Cornea opaque, iris and pupil obscured	>1/2 limbal ischaemia

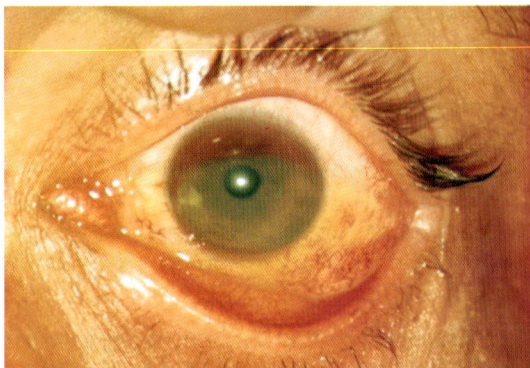

Fig. 13.1 *Grade I chemical injury showing corneal epithelial defect on fluorescein staining*

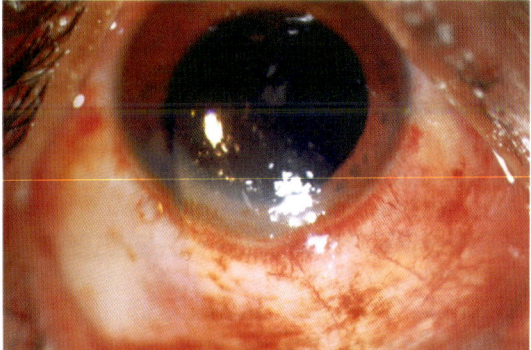

Fig. 13.2 *Grade II chemical injury showing corneal stomal haze with less than one-third limbal ischaemia*

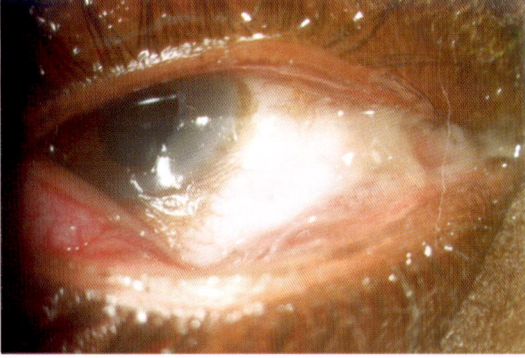

Fig. 13.3 *Grade III chemical injury showing epithelial loss with stromal haze and limbal ischaemia more than one-third*

Roperhall classification correlates the loss of stromal clarity and degree of limbal ischaemia with the ultimate prognosis in various grades of injury as below:

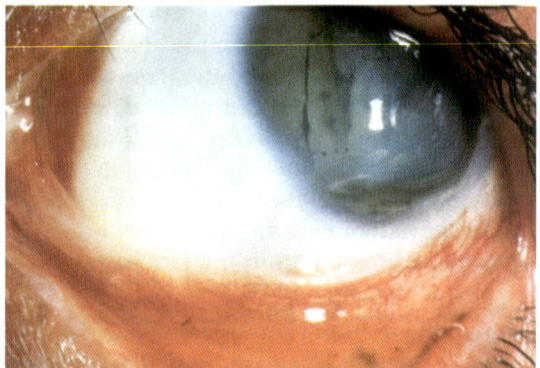

Fig. 13.4 *Grade IV chemical injury showing opaque cornea with limbal ischaemia more than half*

- *Grade I* (Fig. 13.1). There is no corneal opacity or limbal ischaemia and the prognosis is excellent.
- *Grade II* (Fig. 13.2). Prognosis is good
- *Grade III* (Fig. 13.3). Prognosis is guarded
- *Grade IV* (Fig. 13.4). Prognosis is dismal

Modified Hughes classification scheme evaluated the extent of injury by degree of limbal ischaemia without realizing that this is an excellent indirect means of assessment of limbal stem cell injury. Using a limbal-stem-cell-injury based model:

- *Grade I injury* involves little or no loss of stem cells,
- *Grade II injury* involves subtotal stem cell loss,
- *Grade III injury* has complete stem cell loss with retention of some proximal conjunctival epithelium and vascularity, and
- *Grade IV injury* has complete stem cell loss and loss of proximal conjunctival epithelium. Grade IV injuries may also be associated with necrosis of bulbar and conjunctival epithelial and subepithelial tissue, significant conjunctival and limbal ischaemia, and extensive damage to the entire anterior segment.

Drawbacks in the above classification:
- In Grade IV, i.e. 50–100% limbal ischaemia, the prognosis is poor. Nowadays, however, with 50–75% limbal ischaemia, prognosis is good.
- No conjunctival involvement is considered. If conjunctiva is normal, prognosis is better.

Dua's classification

A new classification system was given by Harminder S Dua. In this classification, chemical burns are graded according to the percentage of conjunctival and limbal involvement. Limbal involvement is assessed according to the number of clock hours involved and is a better term to be used than limbal ischaemia (Table 13.3).

Note. The Roper-Hall classification is more practical and easier to use in the emergency setting and is thus the most common system used for grading chemical injuries.

CLINICAL COURSE AND EVALUATION

There are four distinct pathophysiologic and clinical phases of chemical injury (McCulley):

1. *Immediate phase.* The clinical findings immediately following a chemical injury are related to:
- The area of involvement (extent of positive staining with fluorescein)
- The area of penetration by the chemical—corneal penetration is characterized by a loss of stromal clarity while conjunctival penetration is determined by observation of vascular ischaemia and/or necrosis of limbal and bulbar conjunctiva.

2. *Acute phase.* This phase lasts from day 0 to day 7
- *Grade I* injuries usually heal
- *Grade II* injuries show early re-epithelialization and slow recovery of stromal clarity
- *Grade III* and *Grade IV* injuries show a little or no re-epithelialization, with early keratocyte proliferation, first wave of inflammatory cell infiltrates and no corneal vascularization.

3. *Early repair phase.* During the early repair phase (day 7–21), epithelial migration continues in less severe injury (Grade II) but becomes alarmingly delayed in more severe grades of injury (Grades III and IV).

- *Grade II injury*: Normal epithelial recovery occurs in the quadrants with intact limbal stem cells but there may be delayed re-epithelialization from the quadrant(s) of limbal stem cell loss. In areas of stem cell loss, either transient amplifying cells from limbal stem cells may migrate circumferentially into the area of limbal stem cell loss and then migrate centripetally or epithelialization may occur from conjunctival epithelium with transient neovascularization.

- *Grade III/IV*: Because complete limbal stem cell loss has occurred, epithelial recovery is rate-limited by the total reliance on the slow migration of conjunctival epithelium on to the cornea. In Grade IV injuries, there is a little change in clinical appearance. Additional inflammation, loss of limbal blood supply and lack of vascularly derived collagenase inhibitors lead to anterior segment necrosis and sterile ulceration.

4. *Late repair phase (after 21 days).* Based on the epithelial healing which has occurred by this stage, it is possible to classify the injury into a confirmed healing pattern. This classification can accurately predict the functional outcome in the absence of aggressive intervention and form the basis of recommendations for surgical intervention.

- Type I—normal epithelial recovery
- Type II—delayed differentiation
- Type III—fibrovascular pannus
- Type IV—sterile corneal ulceration

Table 13.3 Dua's classification of chemical injuries

Grade	Prognosis	Limbal involvement	Conjunctival involvement	Analogue scale
1.	Very good	0 clock hours	0%	0/0%
2.	Good	≤3 clock hours	≤30%	0.1–3/1–29.9%
3.	Good	>3 – 6 clock hours	>30% – 50%	3.1–6/31–50%
4.	Good to guarded	>6 – 9 clock hours	>50% – 75%	6.1–9/51–75%
5.	Guarded to poor	>9 – <12 clock hours	>75% – < 100%	9.1–11.9/75.1–99.9%
6.	Very poor	Total limbus (12 clock hours)	Total conjunctiva (100%)	12/100%

The analogue scale records accurately the limbal involvement in clock hours of affected limbs/percentage of conjunctival involvement. While calculating the percentage of conjunctival involvement, only the bulbar conjunctiva up to the including fornices is considered.

Eyes entering into this phase can be broadly divided into the following two groups:

Group I includes:
- Re-epithelialization complete/ nearly complete
- Persistent goblet cell and mucin abnormalities
- Slow migration of new basement membrane and epithelial adhesions
- Persistent epitheliopathy, prolonged suboptimal vision
- Severe cases—fibrovascular pannus

Group II includes:
- Corneal epithelialization poor or not at all
- Conjunctival re-epithelialization required for all resurfacing
- Lack of epithelial migration at this stage—high chances of sterile stromal ulceration
- Severe corneal vascularization (Fig. 13.5)
- Conjunctival and corneal scarring
- Goblet cell and mucin deficiency
- Recurrent or persistent epithelial erosions
- Progressive symblepharon formation—lid abnormalities (cicatricial entropion) and trichiasis (Fig. 13.6)

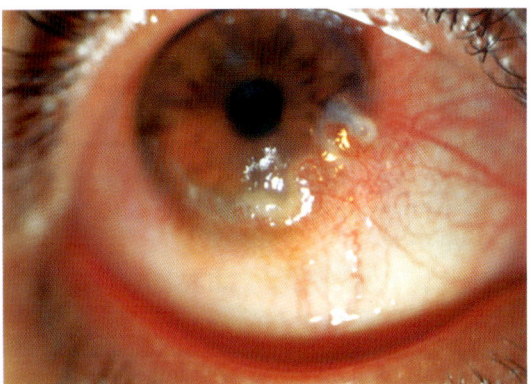

Fig. 13.5 *Post-chemical injury severe corneal vascularization*

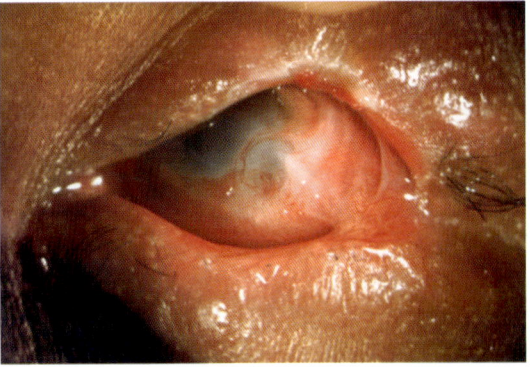

Fig. 13.6 *Post-chemical injury symblepharon formation*

- Permanent corneal anaesthesia—neurotrophic keratitis.

MANAGEMENT

Management of chemical injuries can be discussed under the following heads:
- Treatment in the immediate (acute) period
- Treatment in the intermediate (subacute) period
- Treatment in the late (chronic) period

A. IMMEDIATE MANAGEMENT

1. Irrigation

The initial treatment of every chemical injury should be immediate flushing with water; this may be the most important determinant in the ultimate prognosis of the injury. Copious irrigation should be done prior to any ophthalmic examination as this helps to remove the inflammatory substances and the rapidity of neutralization determines the subsequent clinical course. Irrigation should not be interrupted during transport to a professional eye-care unit and the eye should be rinsed for at least 30 minutes to 2–4 hours with 500–1000 ml of fluid via an intravenous infusion set. To overcome blepharosopasm, lids are passively held open or topical anaesthetic drops are used. A polymethylmethacrylate scleral lens with an attached perfusion tube (Medi-flow or Morgan Therapeutic Lens) has been designed for ocular irrigation with an intravenous delivery apparatus (Fig. 13.7). There is also a perforated silicone tube (Oklahoma Eye Irrigating Tube) shaped to fit the conjunctival fornices and adaptable to an intravenous delivery system. Another method of irrigation, perhaps better suited for prolonged continuous perfusion, is a thin (PE 20) polyethylene tube inserted percutaneously into the conjunctival fornix and attached to either an intravenous drip apparatus or a mobile ocular perfusion pump.

Water is the most commonly used irrigation fluid but fluids with higher osmolarities are preferred. Copious amounts of water have a

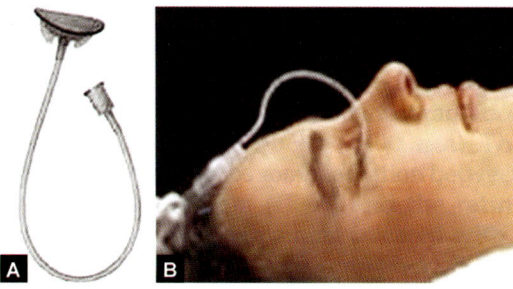

Fig. 13.7 *Medi-flow or Morgan therapeutic lens*

dilutive effect but being hypotonic, there occurs an increased uptake of additional water into the corneal stroma drawing the corrosive agent along with. The most suitable fluids to be used are sterile ringer lactate (RL) and balanced salt solution (BSS). A new amphoteric solution, Diphoterine (0.4%), is also available but a delay to obtain irrigants other than water is not warranted. Every moment that passes without treatment allows longer contact time with undiluted chemical and increases the risk of more serious injury. The effectiveness of rinsing can be checked by a universal indicator paper to determine the external pH of the eye. Ectropinization and intensive cleaning of cul-de-sac are mandatory and EDTA 1% soaked cotton-tipped applicator used to facilitate cleaning of cul-de-sac from calcium hydroxide.

2. Debridement

Once irrigation has been initiated, the lids should be doubly inverted over a Desmarre's lid retractor and fornices should be extensively searched to locate any sequestered particles of caustic material. If allowed to remain, these particles dissolve slowly, allowing additional toxic substances to leach into surrounding tissues. Therefore, deep swabbing of the conjunctival recesses using moistened cotton-tipped applicators should be done. Careful attention must be directed to those regions where extreme chemosis is likely to hide particulate matter in crypts and folds. Debridement of necrotic corneal epithelium is necessary to allow proper re-epithelialization and in severe injuries, it helps remove the nidus of continued inflammation from retained caustic materials, and sustained release of detrimental proteolytic enzymes.

3. Proper examination

After emergency treatment with irrigation and debridement, a critical evaluation of the severity of injury dictates the nature of further therapy. The following points should be looked after:

- Visual acuity, repeated on subsequent visits
- Examine eyelids for laceration
- Palpate orbital rim to look for fractures or crepitus (traumatic chemical explosion)
- Intraocular pressure
- Presence of particulate matter in fornices
- Extent of corneal and conjunctival epithelial cell loss
- Presence and extent of conjunctival ischaemic necrosis
- Slit-lamp examination—use fluorescein stain and cobalt blue light to determine presence and extent of any corneal epithelial defect or abrasion
- Corneal clarity
- Degree of limbal ischaemia
- Anterior chamber inflammation
- Lenticular clarity

The management of chemical injuries aims to:
- Promote ocular surface epithelial recovery with proper corneal phenotypic trans-differentiation,
- Augment corneal repair by supporting keratocyte collagen production and minimize ulceration related to collagenase activity,
- Control inflammation

4. Antibiotics

Topical antibiotics are essential in the period immediately after chemical injury to decrease the risk of secondary infection in an inflamed eye with surface defects and necrotic, avascular conjunctiva. Adequate coverage usually can be achieved using a fluoroquinolone agent, such as moxifloxacin or ciprofloxacin, four times a day. An aminoglycoside, such as gentamicin or tobramycin, four times a day may also suffice, but may be more irritating to the damaged ocular surface because of higher concentration of preservative.

5. Cycloplegics

Cycloplegics are essential for all but the most insignificant chemical injuries. Within the first few hours of any chemical burn resulting in corneal epithelial loss or tissue necrosis, there occurs an element of iridocyclitis. Posterior synechiae may form later, impeding transfer of aqueous between the posterior and anterior chambers and leading to a rise in intraocular pressure. A cycloplegic, such as atropine1% solution or homatropine 2%, three times a day should be included in the initial regimen.

6. Corticosteroids

Judicious use of topical corticosteroids under close observation during the first six days is probably safe, and may be beneficial in its reduction of inflammation. Topical cortico-steroids reduce inflammatory cell infiltration and stabilize PMN leucocyte cytoplasmic and lysosomal membranes. But on the downslide, corticosteroids also inhibit healing and the reformation of new collagen. The enhancement of collagenase by corticosteroids is greatest during the second and third weeks after an alkali burn but insignificant during the first six days or in the fourth or fifth week. Therefore, beyond the initial 1 week, it is inadvisable to continue these agents unless the patient is hospitalized or can be examined daily as an outpatient.

7. Ocular hypotensive agents

Trabecular outflow obstruction, caused by inflammatory debris and distortion of the trabe-cular beams, results in an increase in intraocular pressure. Oral carbonic anhydrase inhibitors, such as acetazolamide and methazolamide, decrease aqueous production. Topical agents, such as dorzolamide, another carbonic anhydrase inhibitor, and the beta-adrenergic blockers, such as timolol and betaxolol, also reduce intraocular pressure by decreasing aqueous production. Sometimes, ocular hypotony can also occur because of intense iridocyclitis causing ciliary body shutdown.

8. Ascorbate and citrate

Ascorbate is an essential water-soluble vitamin and its supplements help in restoring depleted aqueous ascorbate levels and decrease the incidence of corneal thinning and ulceration following chemical injuries. Topical application (sodium ascorbate 10% solution hourly) has been found to be superior to systemic adminis-tration (500 to 1000 mg oral ascorbic acid four times a day). However, ascorbate supplements do not halt the progression of established ulceration and therefore, they should be started early in the course of management. Sodium citrate 10% solution, which inhibits movement of PMNs into the injured area and their release of proteases, also can be applied hourly.

9. Tetracyclines

In moderate to severe burns, the use of oral tetra-cycline (250 mg four times a day), doxycycline (100 mg twice a day), or minocycline (100 mg twice a day) helps in reducing collagenase activity and corneal ulceration. They also inhibit PMN leucocyte activity and scavenge the PMN-generated reactive oxygen compound.

10. Hydrophilic and collagen binding lenses

Hydrophilic lenses promote epithelial migra-tion, Bowman's membrane regeneration and epithelial-stromal adhesion by protecting the ocular surface from the "windshield-wiper" effect of lids. But they are not very well tolerated by the acutely injured eye. Antibiotic coverage and close observation are necessary, especially if the patient is also receiving topical cortico-steroids. Although a collagen bandage lens may be useful in delivering topical medications such as antibiotics, it does not seem to facilitate the rate of healing of epithelial defects.

Summary of management strategies during the immediate (acute) period is depicted in Fig. 13.8.

B. INTERMEDIATE (SUBACUTE) PERIOD

1. Topical antibiotics, cycloplegics and corticosteroids

After the first week of treatment, continued assessment of the risk of infection is essential. Persistent epithelial defects, necrotic corneal stroma, and corneal melting all facilitate infec-tion and, therefore, necessitate the continued use

Irrigation is critical. Use water or ringer lactate for at least 1 to 2 hours. Check pH of fornices with litmus paper	Debridement is essential to remove residual caustic particles	Antibiotics are essential. Use singly or in combination
Cycloplegics are necessary, if there is an anterior chamber inflammatory reaction	Corticosteroids (such as dexamethasone 0.1% solution four times a day) are helpful in reducing inflammation during the first week	Ocular hypotensives, such as timolol 0.5% solution, twice a day with or without 250 mg oral acetazolamide thrice a day, to reduce elevated intraocular pressure
Sodium ascorbate 10% solution every hour and 500 to 1000 mg ascorbic acid four times a day	Sodium citrate 10% solution applied hourly inhibits PMN facilitation of ulceration in moderate to severe burns	250 mg tetracycline four times daily or 100 mg doxycycline every 12 hours in moderate to severe burns
	A therapeutic soft contact lens may facilitate corneal re-epithelialization in burns of minimal grade	

Fig. 13.8 *Summary of management strategies during the acute period*

of topical antibiotics. Long-term use of topical antibiotics, however, can lead to development of bacterial resistance or corneal toxicity from preservatives.

The continued use of a cycloplegic is based on therapeutic need and they should be continued in cases where anterior segment inflammation still persists. If the cornea is opaque or necrotic, and if there is still considerable external ocular inflammation, there is very little risk in maintaining cycloplegic therapy.

The case against continued use of topical corticosteroids after the first week is a strong one, especially if damaged stroma remains unprotected by epithelium. After the initial 1 week, milder steroids, such as fluorometholone 1% or loteprednol 0.5% suspension, can be substituted for topical corticosteroids. These agents minimally interfere with corneal stromal repair and collagen synthesis. Anti-inflammatory activity can also be maintained by using a topical nonsteroidal antiinflammatory agent, such as diclofenac or ketorolac. These do not seem to favour corneal ulceration.

2. Ocular hypotensive agents

Persistent anterior segment inflammation and distortion of the trabecular meshwork compromise aqueous outflow pathways, necessitating continued use of ocular hypotensives.

3. Ascorbate, citrate and tetracycline

These agents tend to reduce corneal ulceration after a chemical injury; they should be continued in cases where re-epithelialization is incomplete.

4. Collagenase inhibitors

Examples include cysteine, acetylcysteine (available commercially as mucomyst 10% and 20%), sodium EDTA, calcium EDTA and penicillamine. N-acetylcysteine (mucomyst) 10% solution can be applied as often as every hour without significant toxicity, aside from an occasional transient superficial stromal haze. Although these early collagenase inhibitors have largely fallen into disfavour, recent discovery of the potent inhibition of collagenase by tetracycline derivatives and promising new synthetic inhibitors have reopened this area of therapy. Recombinant tissue inhibitors of metalloproteinases (TIMP) also have anti-collegenolytic properties but clinical trials of its use in chemical injuries are still undergoing. Disodium EDTA (endrate) and calcium disodium EDTA (calcium disodium versenate) inhibit collagenase through chelation.

5. Homologous or autologous serum

The α2-macroglobulin of serum is a powerful inhibitor of collagenase and the other MMPs. α1-antitrypsin is considerably less effective against collagenase, but it too has been documented to prevent corneal ulceration after ocular chemical injuries. Blood drawn into dry, sterile containers containing no anticoagulants it subsequently clots and yields serum that can be separated and refrigerated until needed. If autologous blood is available, its therapeutic use need not be delayed by testing for human immunodeficiency virus or hepatitis. Gentamicin sulphate sufficient to achieve a concentration of 0.003% can be added to the serum before its administration by drops or by continuous perfusion.

6. Continuous perfusion

Continuous delivery of therapeutic fluids to the ocular surface has been achieved by a direct drip from an intravenous delivery system, from a variety of perfusing devices inserted into the conjunctival recesses, and through percutaneous tubes exiting in the conjunctival fornices. One portable method involves a small electrolytic pump carried in a bag suspended around the neck that delivers fluid through a percutaneous (PE 20) polyethylene tube terminating in a flared end in the lower conjunctival fornix.

7. Maintenance of the conjunctival fornices and ocular motility

Transudation of intravascular fluid from an ocular chemical injury results in bridges of fibrin that threaten to obliterate the conjunctival fornices leading to formation of true symble-phara and ankyloblephara. Dividing these adhesions at the earliest stage can be beneficial because otherwise their inexorable progression may lead to an immobile eye with non-functional lids in the late cicatricial stages. A glass rod greased with an antibiotic ointment can be used to sweep the fornices daily to lyse early adhesions. A flush-fitting scleral shell or acrylic ring can be employed for preventing symble-pharon progression.

8. Limbal stem cell transplantation

If no significant epithelialization has taken place over a denuded cornea by the third to sixth week after a severe chemical injury, eventual conjunctivalization with vascularization will probably occur unless the eye also has suffered profound loss of conjunctiva. Because of its instability and its tendency to vascularize after minor trauma, this new epithelial covering derived from conjunctiva is less desirable than true corneal epithelium.

To re-establish corneal epithelium over the exposed stroma after a severe chemical injury, it may be necessary to consider a limbal stem cell autograft or homograft (Fig. 13.9). In cases of monocular chemical burn, an autograft can be used, but homologous tissue must be used in cases of binocular damage. Limbal stem cell transplantation is the best method of re-establishing tissue protection over denuded stroma, providing a clear, adherent and stable epithelial layer (Fig. 13.10).

9. Lamellar keratoplasty

Progression of stromal ulceration to the descemetocele stage may threaten to perforate the cornea. The presence of anterior chamber inflammation, precludes penetrating kerato-plasty, but lamellar keratoplasty may be the procedure of choice to re-establish the architectural integrity of the eye. Restoration of vision by penetrating keratoplasty can be attempted at a later date. Collagenase inhibitors should be continued after a lamellar graft for descemeto-

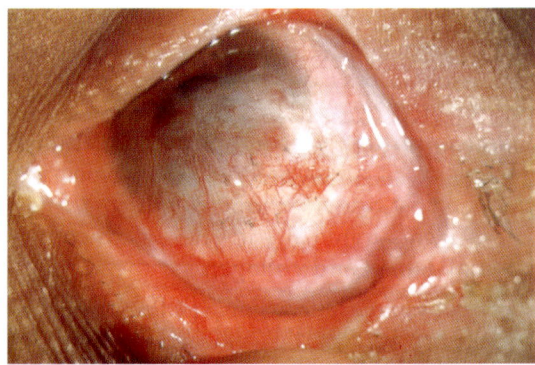

Fig. 13.9 *Limbal stem cell transplantation*

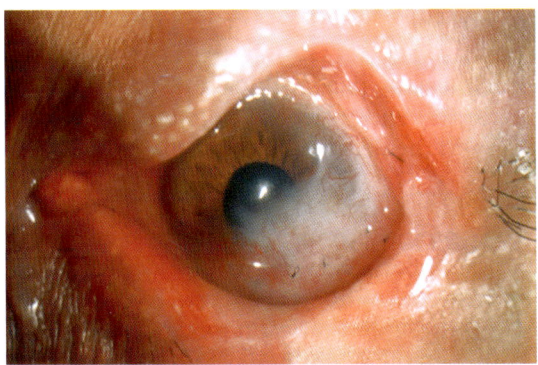

Fig. 13.10 *Corneal clarity improved two months after limbal stem cell transplantation*

cele, but topical corticosteroids are withheld whenever possible. Protection of the grafted cornea with a therapeutic soft lens helps in healing.

10. Tissue adhesive

They are used in the management of impending or actual perforation (<1 mm) as they provide immediate tectonic support and also arrest further ulceration by excluding PMN leucocytes from the site of inflammation and by inducing fibrovascular scarring.

11. Blowout patch and penetrating keratoplasty

Once frank perforation has occurred, a lamellar transplant is difficult to perform and is less likely to seal the perforation. A full-thickness blowout

patch can be cut freehand from corneal donor material, or a standard trephine can be used to excise a circular button for penetrating kerato-plasty. In either case, a metal scleral expander should be sutured to the eye before further manipulation, and a viscoelastic substance may be helpful in reforming a flat anterior chamber before placing the graft.

With both the blowout patch and the penetrating keratoplasty, the primary goal is to restore the anterior chamber and preserve the eye. The need for a repeat penetrating keratoplasty for optical reasons can be reassessed months or years later. *Summary of management strategies during the intermediate (subacute) period* is shown in Fig. 13.11.

C. LATE (CHRONIC) PERIOD

1. General considerations

The goal of treatment in the late or chronic period is to restore the ocular function and appearance, but the obstacles that lie in the way may be nearly insurmountable. After control of inflammation, many long-term sequelae may complicate the outcome of chemical injuries. Some of these are:

• Fornix foreshortening
• Symblepharon formation
• Cicatricial entropion
• Trichiasis

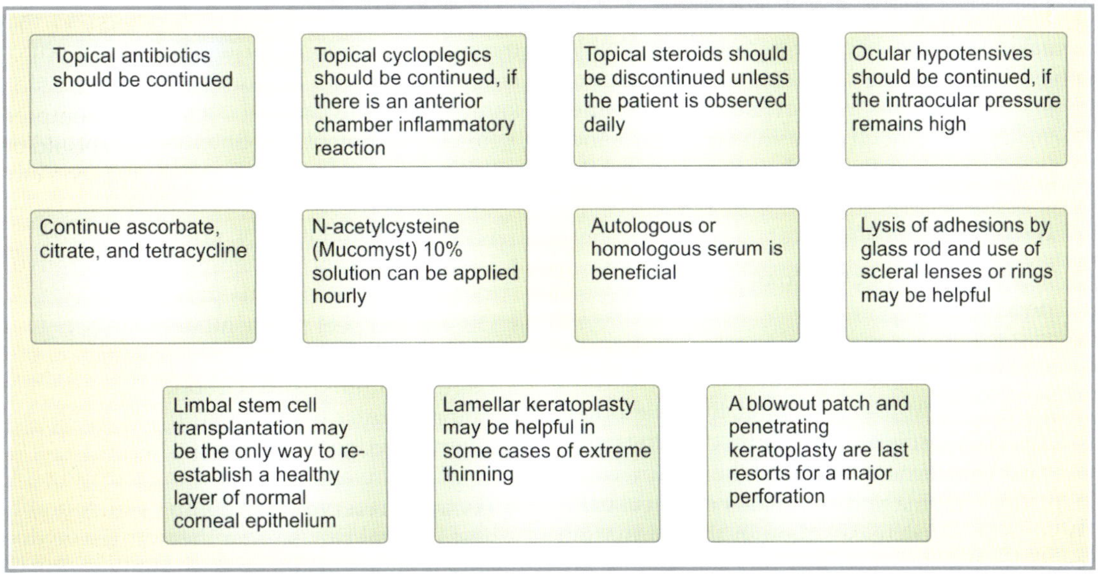

Topical antibiotics should be continued	Topical cycloplegics should be continued, if there is an anterior chamber inflammatory reaction	Topical steroids should be discontinued unless the patient is observed daily	Ocular hypotensives should be continued, if the intraocular pressure remains high
Continue ascorbate, citrate, and tetracycline	N-acetylcysteine (Mucomyst) 10% solution can be applied hourly	Autologous or homologous serum is beneficial	Lysis of adhesions by glass rod and use of scleral lenses or rings may be helpful
	Limbal stem cell transplantation may be the only way to re-establish a healthy layer of normal corneal epithelium	Lamellar keratoplasty may be helpful in some cases of extreme thinning	A blowout patch and penetrating keratoplasty are last resorts for a major perforation

Fig. 13.11 *Summary of management strategies during intermediate (subacute) period*

- Distichiasis
- Ocular surface keratinization
- Vascularization
- Secondary cataract
- Secondary glaucoma

Major goals of therapy in the chronic phase include re-establishment of lid motility with lid-corneal congruity, supplementation of a deficient tear film, and restoration of a clear visual axis.

2. Lysis and control of symblepharon and ankyloblepharon

Progressive cicatrization in the late phase of a severe ocular chemical injury fuses the lids to each other or to the globe, impairing blinking and preventing adequate surfacing of the tear film. Restoration of the conjunctival fornices and establishment of functional lid motility are essential before performing keratoplasty. Unfortunately, lysis of symblephara provides only transient relief because the fibrous bands almost always form again, especially if the raw edges of apposing mucosal surfaces are allowed to contact each other before healing is complete.

Division of symblephara may be followed by a mucosal graft from the upper conjunctival fornix of an unaffected fellow eye or from buccal mucosa. An interim prosthesis, such as an acrylic shell or ring, must be used to separate the lids from the globe, or symblephara rapidly recurs. Preservation of the deepened fornices remains a major challenge because regrowth of symblephara is almost the rule. Retention of a scleral shell or silicone rubber sheets becomes increasingly difficult once the cicatrical bands reform. Beta-irradiation has been used after excision of the scar tissue to inhibit reformation of lysed symblephara.

3. Management of cicatricial entropion and trichiasis

Cicatricial entropion and trichiasis hinder uniform tear film surfacing and may result in corneal scarring. In cicatricial entropion, the lid shortens and its margin rotates inward, directing the lashes toward the corneal surface, where they cause repetitive trauma and stimulate neovascularization. In pure trichiasis, though the lid margin is in its proper position but the lashes are misdirected backward against the cornea.

Surgical management of entropion and trichiasis includes procedures using either full-thickness or partial-thickness transverse lid incisions, with placement of sutures designed to evert the lid margins to normal position.

4. Amniotic membrane transplantation

AMT promotes normal conjunctival epithelialization while preventing excessive subconjunctival fibrosis formation. The Type IV collagen in amniotic membrane acts as a substrate for conjunctival re-epithelialization and growth factors from the amniotic membrane modulate proliferation and differentiation of stromal fibroblasts. There is no risk of rejection due to lack of human leucocytic antigen. It has antimicrobial actions as well. Its anti-adhesion effects prevents symblepharon formation in chemical injuries.

5. Penetrating keratoplasty

The success of penetrating keratoplasty in the late or chronic period after an ocular chemical injury depends on the skill of the surgeon, the quality of the donor material, and also on the extent of inflammatory response from surgical manipulation. Eyes with chemical burns which have remained quiet for months can develop a sudden surge of neovascularization, a non-healing epithelial or stromal defect, anterior uveitis, or a retrocorneal membrane. Keratoplasties done two or more years after the initial injury appear to have a better prognosis than the procedures done earlier. Following important steps improve the outcomes of penetrating keratoplasties in cases of chemical burns:

- Re-establishment of obliterated fornices and lid motility before keratoplasty is essential.
- Correction of cicatricial entropion avoids repetitive trauma to the graft.
- Use of intravenous mannitol preoperatively to decrease the vitreous pressure.
- Dissect and peel off the inflammatory pannus from the underlying corneal stroma.
- Use of vacuum-assisted trephination provides a more regular wound margin in the host and a vertical edge on the donor tissue, assuring more secure apposition during suturing.
- Try and preserve 1.5 to 2 mm of surrounding host corneal rim, so that the new tissue does not impinge directly on the heavily vascularized limbus.

- Hydrophilic soft lenses are usually necessary for extended periods to prevent persistent postoperative epithelial defects.
- Topical corticosteroids (such as dexamethasone 0.1% solution every 2 to 4 hours) are essential to curb postoperative inflammation and graft vascularization but their dose should be decreased promptly at the first sign of wound melting or in cases of persistence of an epithelial defect.
- Collagenase inhibitors should be started if postoperative melting is observed.
- A topical antibiotic (such as a fluoroquinolone with a low concentration of preservative) should be used postoperatively.
- A topical beta-blocker with/without an oral carbonic anhydrase inhibitor may be used to keep the intraocular pressure under control.

6. Keratoprosthesis

They are useful for bilateral severe chemical injuries where prognosis is not good for penetrating keratoplasty due to irreparable damage to the ocular surface or repeated immunological rejection. But use of keratoprosthesis for corneal reconstruction after chemical injury has been largely unsatisfactory. The greatest limiting factor has been collagenolytic erosion of the interfaces at which corneal tissue adjoins prosthetic material.

Summary of management strategies during the late (chronic) period is depicted in Fig. 13.12.

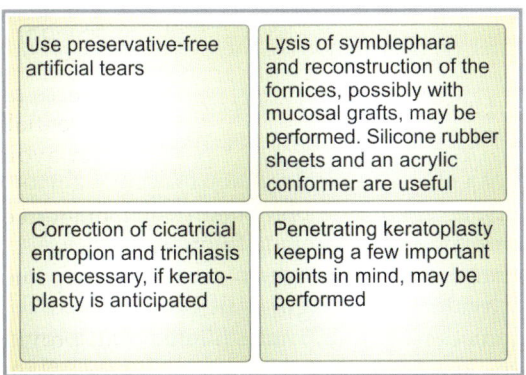

Use preservative-free artificial tears	Lysis of symblephara and reconstruction of the fornices, possibly with mucosal grafts, may be performed. Silicone rubber sheets and an acrylic conformer are useful
Correction of cicatricial entropion and trichiasis is necessary, if kerato-plasty is anticipated	Penetrating keratoplasty keeping a few important points in mind, may be performed

Fig. 13.12 *Summary of management strategies during late (chronic) period*

COMPLICATIONS AND SUMMARY

COMPLICATIONS OF CHEMICAL BURNS

- Necrosis of bulbar conjunctiva
- Persistent inflammation due to retention of contaminated particles
- Ischaemic necrosis of conjunctiva leads to limbal ischaemia
- Corneal ulceration and perforation
- Retrocorneal membranes
- Hypotony
- Phthisis bulbi

SUMMARY

Chemical injuries of the eye are potentially devastating ocular surface injuries that may result in permanent visual disability and blindness. The alkalis are more damaging than the acids since they permeate deeper into the corneal tissue. However, aggressive therapy in the early stages and appropriate treatment at the subsequent stages may help in restoring the damaged ocular surface partially. The advent of ocular surface transplantation techniques by which the depleted limbal stem cell population can be restored, has added a new dimension in the ocular surface reconstruction therapy, thereby vastly improving the prognosis of the severely chemically injured eyes.

REFERENCES

1. Jones NP, Hayward JM, Khaw PT, Claoue CMP, Elkington AR. Function of an ophthalmic 'accident and emergency' department:results of a six month survey. Br MedJ 1986;292:188–190.

2. Vernon SA. Analysis of all new cases seen in a busy regional centre ophthalmic casualty department during a 24 week period. J R Soc Med 1983;76:279–282.

3. Pfister RR. Chemical injuries of the eye. Ophthalmology 1983;90:1246–1253.

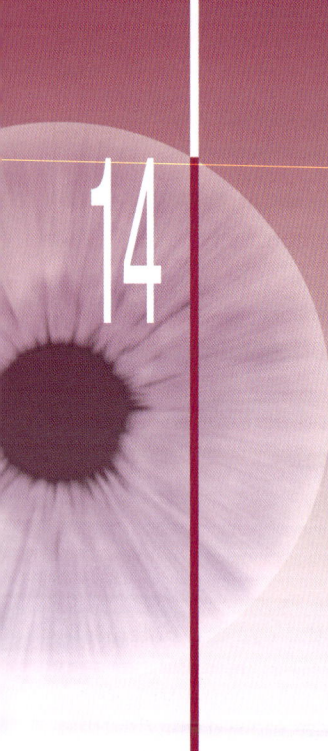

RADIATIONAL INJURIES

14

GENERAL CONSIDERATIONS

The eyes of human beings are able to capture and perceive a small part of the electromagnetic spectrum, the visible light. Energy in this spectrum travels in the form of an electromagnetic wave and has the propensity to cause damage to the ocular tissues. The electromagnetic spectrum comprises the following:

- Gamma rays ($\lambda < 10^{-2}$ nm)
- X-rays ($\lambda - 10^{-2}$ nm – 10 nm)
- Ultraviolet rays ($\lambda - 100$ nm – 400 nm)
  - UV-A (315–400 nm)
  - UV-B (280–315 nm)
  - UV-C (100–280 nm)
- Visible light ($\lambda - 400$ nm – 750 nm)
- Infrared rays ($\lambda - 760$ nm – 1 mm)
- Microwaves ($\lambda - 1$ mm – 10 cm)
- Radio waves ($\lambda > 10$ cm)

Microwaves and radio waves have not been reported to cause any significant ocular trauma and hence the discussion in this chapter will be limited to ionising radiations (gamma rays and X-rays), ultraviolet rays, visible light and infrared rays. The shorter the wavelength of light, the greater the energy, and therefore greater potential for biological damage. However, though the longer wavelengths are less in energy, they penetrate the eye more deeply.

OCULAR MEDIA—TRANSMISSION AND ABSORPTION OF ELECTROMAGNETIC SPECTRUM

For a photochemical reaction to occur, light must be absorbed by a particular ocular tissue. The primate eye has unique filtering characteristics that determine in which area of the eye each wavelength of light will be absorbed. UV radiation below 295 nm is filtered from reaching the lens by the human cornea. This means that the shortest, most energetic wavelengths of light (all UV-C and some UV-B) are filtered out before they reach the lens. The lens has a very efficient defence system against light and radiation damage. It contains antioxidant enzymes, like superoxide dismutase and catalase; and antioxidants, like vitamins E and C, lutein, glutathione that serve to protect it against oxidative and photo-induced damage. Most UV light is absorbed by the lens, but the exact wavelength depends upon age as well as species. Lenses of mammals other than primates transmits UV radiation longer than 295 nm to the retina but the adult human lens absorbs part of UV-B (which is not absorbed by cornea) and all of UV-A (295–400 nm), therefore, only allowing visible light to reach the retina. However, the lens in young children transmits a small window of UV-B (320 nm), while the elderly lens filters out much of the short blue visible light (400–500 nm). Besides the lens and cornea which protect the eye from ultraviolet radiations, the aqueous humour also contains high concentrations of various antioxidants and the retina has protective pigments which absorb radiation and dissipate its energy without causing damage. But after middle age, there is a decrease in the production of ocular antioxidants and the protective pigments are chemically modified, and now, these modified ocular pigments permit damage to the lens and retina on exposure to ambient radiation.

MECHANISM OF RADIATION INJURY TO EYE

There are two major mechanisms for light damage to the eye: An inflammatory response and photo-oxidation. Intense light can induce direct DNA damage, but with less intense light, the eye is damaged through a photo-oxidation reaction.

Inflammatory response

The human eye is unique in the sense that it is immune privileged, that is, under ordinary stress its immune response is suppressed. However, in the presence of very intense UV and visible light (for instance, emitted from lasers), this suppression is overwhelmed. There occurs release of interleukin-1 and invasion of macrophages at the site of irritation with subsequent release of superoxides, peroxides and other reactive oxygen species, which eventually damage the ocular tissues.

Photo-oxidation

Chronic exposure to less intense radiation damages the eye through a photo-oxidation reaction. In photo-oxidation reactions, a pigment in the eye absorbs light, produces reactive oxygen species such as singlet oxygen and superoxide, and these damage ocular tissues. The pigment may be endogenous (natural) or exogenous (drug, herbal medication, or nanoparticle that has accumulated in the eye).

INJURIES DUE TO IONIZING RADIATION (GAMMA RAYS AND X-RAYS)

Medical professionals, like interventional cardiologists, interventional radiologists and other doctors using fluoroscopy in operating theatres and paramedical personnel who remain close to the patient during the procedure, are at risk for damage due to ionizing radiation. These individuals are within a high-scatter X-ray radiation field for several hours a day during procedures and the risk for eye injuries is particularly high for professions involving high workload unless suitable protective tools and proper operational measures are used. Use of lasers in eye surgery and for treatment purposes, without proper filters may cause ocular damage to personnel present in the working area. X -rays, beta rays, UV rays and other radiation sources in adequate doses can cause ocular injury.

MECHANISM OF INJURY

Radiation damage starts at the cellular level. Radiation which is absorbed in a cell has the potential to impact a variety of critical targets in the cell, the most important of which is the DNA. Evidence indicates that damage to the DNA is what causes cell death, mutation, and carcinogenesis. The mechanism by which the damage occurs can happen via one of two scenarios.

1. *Direct action.* In the first scenario, radiation may impact the DNA directly, causing ionization of the atoms in the DNA molecule.

2. *Indirect action.* In the second scenario, the radiation interacts with non-critical target atoms or molecules, usually water. This results in the production of free radicals, which can then attack critical targets, such as the DNA. Damage from indirect action is much more common than damage from direct action, especially for

radiation that has a low specific ionization. Radiation injuries may range from trivial to severe injuries. Various structures are affected because of various type of radiation.

OCULAR LESIONS BY IONIZING RADIATIONS

1. *Lids lesions.* The eyelid is particularly vulnerable to X-ray damage because of its thin skin. Loss of lashes and scarring can lead to inversion or eversion (entropion or ectropion) of the lid margins and prevent adequate closure.

2. *Conjunctival lesions.* Scarring of the conjunctiva impairs the production of mucus and function of the ducts of lacrimal gland, thereby causing dry eyes.

3. *Lens lesions.* X-ray radiation in a dose of 500–800 rads directed towards the lens surface can cause cataract, sometimes with a delay of several months to a year before the opacities appear. A number of studies in the last decade indicate that there is risk of lens opacities at doses below 1 Gy and the threshold may range from none to 0.8 Gy. However, the International Commission on Radiological Protection (ICRP) has recently accepted the threshold of 0.5 Gy. In a recent statement, ICRP now recommends an equivalent dose limit for the lens of the eye of 20 mSv in a year, averaged over a defined period of 5 years, with no single year exceeding 50 mSv. The time required for cataract to form can range from 6 months to 35 years, and appears to be inversely related to the dose. The lens is highly radio sensitive and ionizing radiation can cause coagulation of lens proteins producing lenticular opacities. Human evidence for radiation cataractogenesis is derived mainly from a relatively small number of workers inadvertently exposed to large doses of radiation to the eye, including several nuclear physicists working with cyclotrons, patients exposed to therapeutic radiation (sometimes from radium plaques applied to the eye) and Japanese atomic bomb survivors who were heavily irradiated.

Ionizing radiation is generally (but not exclusively) associated with posterior subcapsular (PSC) and sometimes cortical opacities. Historically, PSC opacification was thought to be a characteristic of radiation damage to the

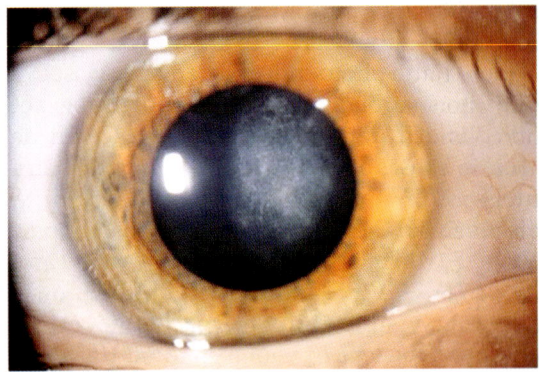

Fig. 14.1 *Post radiation subcapsular cataract*

lens, although more recent data suggest that radiation induced opacities can be found in the lens cortex as well (Fig. 14.1).

PROTECTION OF THE EYE

The use of radiation-protection tools must be promoted to decrease the risk of ocular pathologies. Best practice includes the use of ceiling suspended screens, wearing leaded glass eyewear, positioning of the X-ray tube below the table as far away from the patient as possible and positioning oneself as far away as clinically possible from the X-ray tube and patient. Maintaining X-ray equipment in optimum operating condition, using pulsed fluoroscopy, minimizing fluoroscopy time, limiting radiographic images, collimation and reduced use of magnification will help reduce X-ray exposure to staff as well as to patients. Anything that increases the amount of radiation exposure, e.g. longer fluoroscopy times, more radiograph images generated, proximity to the radiation source, positioning the X-ray source above the patient, and a person's closeness to the patient will increase the radiation dose and potential risk from ionizing radiation.

Currently available protective measures and devices (lead glass screens and eyewear) are quite effective and practical for day-to-day use. Proper and regular use of these radiation protection tools is among the most efficient ways to prevent lens injuries.

Use of leaded glasses alone reduced the lens dose rate by a factor of 5 to 10; scatter-shielding screens alone reduced the dose rate by a factor of 5 to 25. Use of both simultaneously is even more efficient than either used alone, reducing the dose rate by a factor of 25 or more. Available estimation on effectiveness of protective devices indicates that their appropriate use can lead to situations where radiation cataract risk in interventional medical procedures may be effectively controlled.

The ocular protection of the patients undergoing radiotherapy by ionizing radiations for various head and neck malignant tumors is equally important. The eyes of the patients undergoing radiotherapy can be protected by eyeshields which are of two types. *External eyeshields* are used in megavoltage radiation of head and neck and maxillary cancers, e.g. pencil lead eyeshields for blocking the eye completely. *Internal eyeshields* are used with electron beam and orthovoltage radiation for the treatment of superficial cancers of the eyelid and basal cell carcinoma of the skin around the eye region. These eyeshields are generally made of tungsten, steel alloy and even gold plated lead. They are generally placed underneath the eyelids to protect the cornea and the lens.

INJURIES DUE TO ULTRAVIOLET RADIATION

The sun is a natural source of ultraviolet (UV) energy. Apart from skin, the organ which is most susceptible to sunlight-induced damage is the eye. Though the consequences of skin exposure to UV rays are well understood by the general population, the same does not exist, when it comes to the eye. Ultraviolet light is the most common cause of radiation injury to the eye.

UV radiation does not form part of the visible light spectrum, but comprises wavelengths between 100 and 400 nm of the electromagnetic spectrum of light. Although it comprises only 5% of the sun's energy, it is the most harmful. It is further categorized as;

- UV-A 315–400 nm
- UV-B 280–315 nm
- UV-C 100–280 nm

Solar UV rays that reach the earth's surface contain 95% UV-A and 5% UV-B. UV-A mainly causes skin tanning and photosensitivity reactions, while UV-B is the one which is responsible for the more harmful effects. The shorter and arguably more toxic wavelengths of UV-C are blocked by the ozone layer of the stratosphere and it also decreases the proportion of UV-B reaching the surface of earth. With the thinning of the ozone layer, UV protection has become critically important for our population. Also, it is important to note that as the atmosphere is thinner at higher altitudes, it absorbs less UV radiation, increasing exposure. The equatorial regions of the earth also receive high UV radiation levels and with global climate change, humans are receiving excessive UV exposure on a chronic or acute basis making themselves susceptible to adverse consequences.

MECHANISM OF INJURY

The mode of action of UV rays depends upon its wavelength. As energy is inversely proportional to wavelength, the short wavelength UV radiation has the highest potential for damage. For example, UV-B at 300 nm is roughly 600 times more biologically active at damaging ocular tissues than UV-A at 325 nm. Conversely, longer wavelengths have more penetration into the living tissues. The extent of damage from UV radiation is determined by the wavelength, duration and intensity of exposure.

UV-B causes direct DNA damage and changes the shape of the molecule via disruption of hydrogen bonds, formation of protein-DNA aggregates and strand breaks. This results in formation of distorted proteins. UV-A does not damage DNA directly but generates highly reactive chemical intermediates, such as hydroxyl and oxygen radicals, which in turn can damage DNA. Other mechanisms of damage by UV radiations include enzyme dysfunction, ion pump inhibition, p53 mutation and cell membrane damage.

A large number of ocular conditions can be caused by UV exposure. The cornea and lens are the most important ocular tissues which absorb UV radiation. Below 300 nm (UV-B), it is the cornea that absorbs most radiation, whereas the lens primarily absorbs UV-A radiation of less than 370 nm. Conjunctiva and retinal pathologies can also be caused by UV exposure and some of these are discussed further.

OCULAR LESIONS BY UV RAYS

1. Eyelid lesions

The eyelid skin is continually exposed to UV-A and UV-B rays from direct and reflected solar radiation and is, therefore, at risk for UV related damage. Acute and chronic exposure of skin to UV rays can produce erythema, and histopathological changes. Melanin pigmentation is protective against UV ray-related damage. People with a poor ability to tan, who burn easily, and have light eye and hair colour are at a higher risk of developing skin-related malignancies, such as basal cell carcinoma.

2. Conjunctival lesions

The conjunctiva is easily damaged by UV rays, which activates a complex series of oxidative reactions and distinct pathways of cell death. It is a risk factor for squamous cell carcinoma of the conjunctiva. The only other ocular cancer associated with UV radiation is epidermoid carcinoma of the bulbar conjunctiva, which occurs with increased frequency in the tropics and subtropics and has been experimentally replicated in animal models using UV radiation. There is also strong epidemiological evidence to support an association between chronic UV exposure and formation of pterygium, which is particularly more common in population exposed to the sun. A weaker link has also been observed between UV radiation and the occurrence of pingueculae.

3. Corneal lesions

The corneal epithelium and endothelium are prone to damage by UV radiation. UV-B exposure damages the anti-oxidant protective mechanism of the eye resulting in injury. A significant amount of UV-B is absorbed by corneal stroma, so thinning with keratoconus or refractive surgery allows more UV-B to reach the lens, though it is not yet known whether surgical stromal thinning increases the risk of cataract.

UV radiations reaching the cornea can cause acute or chronic damage.

i. Acute damage

Ultraviolet radiation of wavelengths shorter than 300 nm (actinic rays) can damage the corneal epithelium. This is most commonly the result of exposure to the sun at high altitude. Other sources of UV radiation injury include sun-tanning beds, carbon arcs, photographic flood lamps, lightning, electric sparks, and halogen desk lamps.

I. *Snow blindness.* Exposure to the sun on highly reflective snow fields at high elevation can lead to direct corneal epithelial injury known as snow blindness, a type of photokeratitis. This reversible condition is characterised by severe pain, lacrimation, blepharospasm and photophobia. The corneal epithelium and Bowman's layer absorb about twice as much UV-B radiation than the posterior layers of the cornea. It is the superficial epithelium that becomes irritated in photokeratitis. A one hour exposure to UV rays reflected off snow around midday is enough to cause a threshold snow blindness. At levels below this there may still be mild symptoms of ocular discomfort.

II. *Sea blindness.* Exposure to sun rays at sea surface can lead to sea blindness. Compared to snow, which reflects 80 to 94% of UV-B rays, water reflects only 5 to 8% and, therefore, this type of blindness is less common.

III. *Photo-ophthalmitis.* Exposure to radiation generated by a welding arc can cause welding flash burn or arc eye, a form of keratitis labelled as photo-ophthalmitis. Patients with photo-ophthalmitis (UV keratitis) experience the onset of a foreign-body sensation, irritation, pain, photophobia, tearing, blepharospasm, and decreased visual acuity 6–12 hours (latent period) after the exposure. This unexplained pattern of corneal sensory loss and return is thought to indicate a probable photochemical injury rather than thermal injury to the cornea. Examination of the lids and conjunctiva may reveal varying lid edema and conjunctival hyperemia. A diffuse corneal haze may be seen in severe cases. Fluorescein staining reveals superficial punctate epithelial surface irregularities, which usually cover the entire surface of the cornea (Fig. 14.2). If the patient's eyelid was

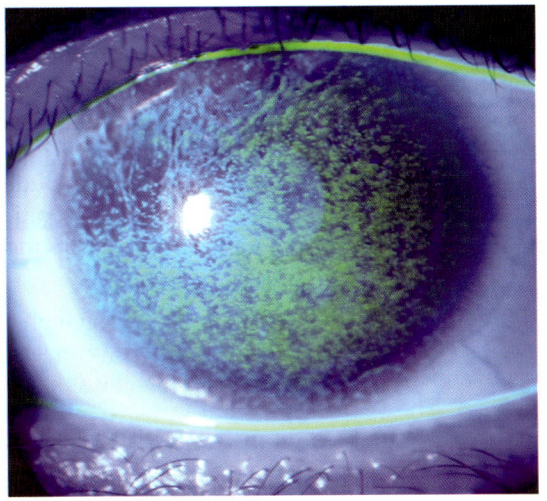

Fig. 14.2 *Photo-ophthalmitis*

partially closed during the exposure, a well-demarcated line separates normal from damaged corneal epithelium. Involvement of the lens is rare and occurs only after intense exposure.

Treatment

Fortunately, arc eye is almost always a temporary condition. If ultraviolet (UV) keratitis is suspected, flush eyes for several minutes with water or saline solution. Nonsteroidal anti-inflammatory drugs (NSAIDs) are a reasonable first-choice analgesic. Use of a lubricating ointment or eyedrops may also help reduce pain. Short-acting cycloplegics also help in relieving pain of reflex ciliary spasm. Oral vitamin C helps in early recovery. The eyes can be patched for 12 to 24 hours for symptomatic improvement. The damage is transient and recovery occurs in 24–48 hours.

ii. Chronic damage

Prolonged exposures to UV radiation can lead to chronic solar toxicity, which is associated with several ocular surface disorders (e.g. pinguecula, pterygium, climatic droplet keratopathy, squamous metaplasia and carcinoma).

Herpes simplex keratitis following ultraviolet-induced immunosuppression

Ultraviolet radiation is known to cause a reduction of cell-mediated immunity. Clinically, there is a risk for reactivation of latent herpes simplex virus (HSV) in the cornea when these eyes are exposed to surface UV rays either through sun exposure or excimer laser treatments. Excimer laser treatments have been shown to increase the risk of reactivation of latent HSV. Prophylaxis with acyclovir (or derivatives thereof) has been shown to reduce UV-induced HSV reactivation and is recommended in clinical situations in which corneas with known HSV are subjected to UV radiation.

4. Lens lesions

Ultraviolet radiation is considered one of the major risk factors for cortical cataract. It has been demonstrated in many epidemiologic studies that sunlight increases the risk for cortical cataract. The antioxidant ascorbic acid which is present in high concentration in the aqueous humour, scavenges free radicals and acts as a filter for both UV-A and UV-B, thereby protecting against UV induced lenticular damage. Following UV exposure, there occurs a significant decrease in ascorbic acid, exposing the lens to damage by these radiations. The lens absorbs both UV-A and UV-B. It is exposed to three times more UV-A, but both types of radiation damage the lens via different mechanisms as mentioned previously. Epidemiologic studies suggest that exposure to solar radiation in these wavelengths near the equatorial regions of earth is correlated with a higher incidence of cataracts, with a possible association with cortical and posterior subcapsular cataract. These studies have also shown that workers exposed to bright sunlight in occupations, such as farming, truck driving and construction work, appear to have a higher incidence of cataract than those who work primarily indoors.

5. Retinal lesions

Although the amount of UV radiation reaching the retina in the adult eye is very low, with protection by the filtering power of the crystalline lens (1% UV below 340 nm and 2% between 340 and 360 nm), studies have linked the early development of age-related macular degeneration with greater time spent outdoors, while some studies have found no association. The young retina is at particular risk for damage from UV exposure because the young lens has not yet synthesized the protective yellow pigments which prevent UV transmission to the retina. The effect of UV damage to the retina is cumulative and there is an increased risk of developing eye disorders like ocular melanoma and macular degeneration later in life.

The retinal pigment epithelium and choroid contain melanin, which absorbs UV and protects the retina against UV-induced damage to the eye. With age, the ocular melanin is photo-bleached and this decreases its protective effect against UV damage. Also other pigments like lutein and zeaxanthin, which are present at the macula, protect the retina against both the inflammatory and photo-oxidative damage caused by these radiations. Unfortunately, as these pigments get depleted with age, the retina loses its protection against free radicals and reactive oxygen species. More recently, a significant link between the 10-year incidence of early age-related macular degeneration and extended exposure to summer sun has been reported.

i. Solar maculopathy

Other examples of retinal damage by UV rays are *solar retinopathy or eclipse blindness* and intra-operative photochemical damage inflicted by the operating microscope. Solar retinopathy occurs due to prolonged sun gazing or watching a solar eclipse. During a solar eclipse, the sunlight is dim and a curious gazer can watch the sun continuously when the pupil remains dilated, thereby allowing more of UV rays to enter the eye and get focussed on fovea centralis thus causing a solar burn. The condition is rare (approximately 1/10,000) and mainly reported in at risk groups, namely military personnel, sun bathers, religious sun gazers, solar eclipse viewers and users of psychotropic drugs. Retinal damage results from thermal rather than photochemical injury, and primarily affects the macula. There is intense bleaching and shedding of photoreceptor outer segments and loss of RPE function.

Symptoms: There is usually a history of solar exposure or viewing an eclipse. Typically, symptoms first occur several hours after exposure. There may be complaints of blurred vision, central or paracentral scotomata, metamorphopsia, chromatopsia or headache.

Signs: Vision loss is typically reversible, lasting for as short as one month to over a year. Vision may be decreased to 20/40 or even 20/100, often bilaterally. A solar maculopathy is usually less than 0.2 mm in diameter, corresponding to the size of the retinal image of the sun. First signs of phototoxicity occur in the first one to two days, with a small yellowish foveal or parafoveal lesion and mild pigmentary changes and retinal oedema. The yellow spots are intraretinal and are presumed to be xanthophyll pigment. Chronic RPE pigmentation effects are variable, ranging from depigmentation to hyper-pigmentation or RPE hyperplasia. Classically, the chronic lesion is described as a reddish dot with surrounding pigmentation, somewhat like a stage 1A macular hole (Fig. 14.3).

ii. Operating microscope light retinopathy

It was first reported in 1983. Such photic injuries are sustained in cataract and other anterior segment surgeries when carried out under operating microscope. The lesion clinically appears as a solitary, perifoveal, round to oval in shape which corresponds to the shape of the illuminating source used during the surgery. It is usually located inferior to fovea and outside the foveal avascular zone. It is initially greyish yellow in colour and later on becomes pigmented (Fig.14.4) FFA shows a sharply.

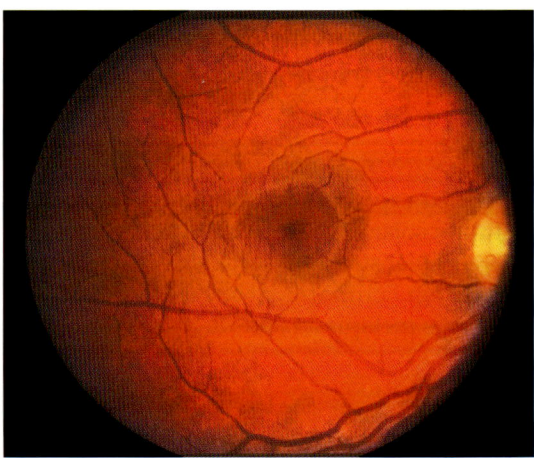

Fig. 14.3 *Solar maculopathy*

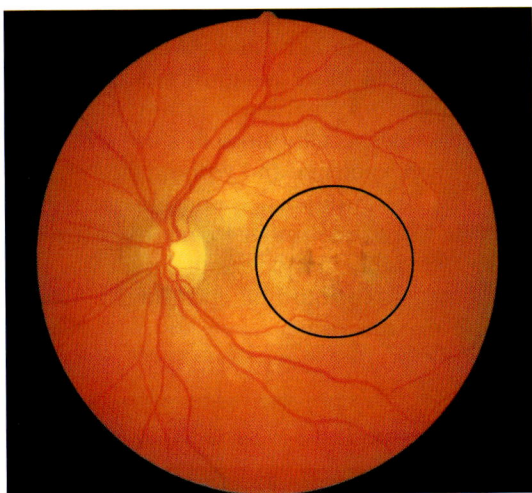

Fig. 14.4 *Pigmentary lesion in operating microscope light retinopathy*

demarcated lesion with mottled hyperfluorescence. The mechanism is said to be a photochemical injury of the exposed macula. The UV and/or IR filters in the modern operating microscopes have reduced but not eliminated the incidence of this photic injury of the macula. The most important risk factor is the duration of the surgery. Therefore, in addition to incorporation of filters in the operating microscope, decreasing the duration of surgery and reducing the intensity of light helps in lowering the incidence of photic maculopathy.

PROTECTION FROM UV RAYS

The eye is exposed to both UVA and UVB; the latter, although present in smaller quantities, is arguably more dangerous due to its higher energy and ability to affect DNA directly. Epidemiological and experimental evidence exists for the role of UV radiation in a number of ocular pathologies such as pterygia, photokeratitis and cataract. The effects of UV radiation are cumulative over our lifetime, and young eyes are particularly vulnerable. Importance should be placed on starting ocular UV protection from a young age. Avoidance of UV light by using appropriate sunglasses, brimmed hats and UV protective contact lenses may dramatically decrease the risk of developing blinding diseases. Maximum exposure to ocular UV occurs at unlikely times, so people should be advised to use combined protection, like appropriate sunglasses, brimmed hats and UV protective contact lenses.

Though the shape of the orbit provides some anatomical protection from direct UV radiation and spontaneous closure of eyes in bright light reduces exposure further, reflected light can still reach the eye. Therefore, one must use brimmed hats, sunglasses and UV protective contact lenses to reduce exposure. The frequent use of sunglasses has been associated with a 40% decrease in the risk of posterior subcapsular cataract. A recent research found that ocular UV exposure is greatest during early morning and late afternoon for all seasons except winter. Similarly, most clouds don't protect from UV; making overcast days, where people are usually reluctant to take protective measures, particularly dangerous. Research is also ongoing into the protective effects of UV-blocking contact lenses which have shown promise in protecting the cornea, aqueous humour and the crystalline lens from UV-induced pathological processes.

INJURIES DUE TO VISIBLE LIGHT RAYS

Visible light has a spectrum of 400–750 nm. Light is the essential component of the output of illuminating lamps, visual displays and a wide variety of illuminators. Some light sources, besides being important sources of illumination, pose unwanted physiological reactions, such as disability and discomfort glare, flicker and other forms of eye stress due to poor ergonomic design of workplace tasks. The emission of intense light is also a potential hazard of some industrial activities, such as arc welding. If the wavelengths of visible spectrum penetrate fully into the eye, they can cause thermal, mechanical, or photic injuries.

1. Thermal injuries

These are produced by light, intense enough to increase the temperature of the retina by 10–20°C. Lasers used for treatment purposes can cause this type of injury. The light is absorbed by the retinal pigment epithelium, where its energy is converted to heat, and the heat causes photocoagulation of retinal tissue. The local burning of the retina results in a blind spot (scotoma).

2. Mechanical injuries

These can be produced by exposure to laser energy from a Q-switched or mode-locked laser, which produces sonic shock waves that disrupt the retinal tissue.

3. Photic injuries

These are caused by prolonged exposure to intense light, which produces varying degrees of cellular damage in the retina (especially the macula) without a significant increase in the temperature of the tissue. "Blue light" photo-retinitis, a hazard principally associated with blue light of wavelengths from 400 to 550 nm is a type of photochemical injury to the retina.

Sun gazing is a very common cause of this type of injury. Exposure to sunlight has long been suggested as a cause of age-related macular degeneration especially in the elderly population. Although capable of handling the normal photo-oxidative stress in youth, with age the defence mechanisms of the eye are no longer able to protect the retina against previously non-damaging exposures and irreversible changes start to accumulate.

The intensity of light, length of exposure, and age are all important factors. The retina is much more sensitive to damage from blue light than it is from longer wavelengths of visible light. Elderly people are more sensitive, and also pseudophakes and aphakes because filtration of blue light by the lens is lost.

Protection

Whatever the mechanisms for the various types of ocular damage, it seems prudent to protect the eyes from unnecessary solar radiation. Since there is an association between ocular exposure to blue or visible light and AMD, the use of sunglasses that block a significant amount of broad-spectrum visible radiation should be encouraged, especially since this use would be relatively inexpensive and without side effects. Similarly, the middle-aged and elderly would do well to reduce unnecessary exposure to intense sunlight, and the use of sunglasses and a brimmed hat should be encouraged during outdoor excursions.

INJURIES DUE TO INFRARED RADIATION

INFRARED RADIATIONS AND SOURCE

Infrared radiation (IR) lies beyond the red end of the visible spectrum, with wavelengths between 780 and 10000 nm. It is divided into three sub-ranges:

- *IR-A, or near infrared* (from 780 to 1400 nm),
- *IR-B or far infrared* (1400 to 3000 nm), and
- *IR-C* (3000 to 10000 nm)—This band does not normally reach the earth's surface because it is absorbed by the atmosphere, but non-natural sources of IR-C can be a significant hazard.

Source of infrared rays and their effects are summarized in Table 14.1.

MECHANISM OF INJURY

The occupations of glass blowing, metal working, chain making and tin plating are those in which infrared levels can be significant. Arc lamps and electric radiant heaters also give off infrared rays, and various lasers are rich sources, for example, the neodymium: YAG laser (IR-A)

Wavelength	Laser sources	Other sources	Symptoms	Tissue affected
Near IR (IR-A) **780–1400 nm**	Neodymium: YAG 1064 nm Helium-neon 1150 nm Iodine 1315 nm	Sun, furnaces, lamps, glass blowing	Dull after image, pain, rapid onset of scotoma	Retina (pigment epithelium) Iris Lens (cataract) choroid
Far IR (IR-B) **1400–3000 nm**	Erbium 1540 nm Holmium 2060 nm (pulsed lasers)	Sunlight, furnaces, lamps	Pain, blepharospasm, visual loss	Cornea (opacity) Lens (cataract)

Table 14.1 *Infrared sources and their effects*

and carbon dioxide laser (IR-C). Some IR is absorbed by each ocular structure. In general, the cornea absorbs almost all wavelengths greater than 3000 nm (IR-C) and most radiation with a wavelength above 1400 nm. The crystalline lens absorbs some radiation between 900 nm and 1400 nm (IR-A) and the retina absorbs most of the remaining infrared with a wavelength less than 1400 nm (IR-A). When human tissues absorb IR radiation, significant changes occur at the cellular level and in the eye, the greatest concern is with the thermal effect on the lens and retina.

OCULAR LESIONS BY INFRARED RAYS

1. Eyelids and periorbital skin lesions

The effect of IR exposure on eyelids ranges from lid edema and mild erythema to third degree skin burns produced by very high levels of IR delivered over a short time or low levels over a long period. The IR radiation emitted by normal welding arcs causes damage only within a comparatively short distance from the arc. There is an immediate burning sensation in the periorbital skin, if it is exposed to arc heat.

2. Corneal lesions

The cornea transmits 96% of the incident IR in the range 700–1400 nm and the radiation effects from these wavelengths involve protein coagulation within different layers of cornea. High dose infrared damage to the cornea causes immediate pain and vascularization. Subsequently, corneal ulcers occur which lead to opacification and loss of transparency.

3. Iris lesions

The iris absorbs between 53 and 98% of incident infrared in the 750–900 nm range, depending upon the amount of iris pigmentation. Overall, the iris is sensitive to IR, and suffers swelling, cell death, hyperaemia and pupillary miosis. Iris gets inflamed on exposure to IR and this causes leakage of proteins from iris vessels into the anterior chamber leading to aqueous flare.

4. Lens lesions

Chronic exposure to IR rays is seen in glass blowers and metal furnace stockers. Cataracts associated with occupational infrared exposure have been known since 1739 and, historically, it is on this problem that the greatest attention has been focused. La *"cataracte des verriers"* *(glassblower's cataract or furnace men's cataract)* is an example of thermal injury caused by infrared radiation that damages the anterior lens capsule among unprotected workers. Denser cataractous changes can occur in unprotected workers who observe glowing masses of glass or iron for many hours a day. Evidence suggests that when IR is incident on the eye, it is absorbed by the cornea and converted to heat which is conducted to the lens and induces cataract. Also compositional and conformational changes in the lens proteins decrease the total soluble proteins leading to increased incidence of cataract.

5. Retina and choroid lesions

Any infrared rays that are transmitted through the ocular media to the retina are absorbed by the pigment epithelium of the retina. The effect of the infrared on the retina and choroid is to cause a rise in temperature, which causes enzymes to denature; in general, temperatures more than 10° above ambient body temperature produce permanent thermal damage. IR exposure produces retinal structural damage and retinal burns.

Welding emits a wide-spectrum of radiation, from IR to UV light and beyond. UV and far-IR radiation are adsorbed by the cornea and the lens, whereas visible light and near-IR radiation penetrate to the retina. Retinal lesions induced by arc welding are known as *"phototoxic maculopathy"/"retinitis photoelectrica"/"photic maculopathy"* or *"macular photo-injury"*. The distance between the worker and the source of radiation is an important factor while considering IR radiation. In the case of arc welding, infrared radiation decreases rapidly as a function of distance, so that farther than 3 feet away from where welding takes place, it does not pose an ocular hazard anymore but, ultraviolet radiation still does. That is why welders wear tinted glasses to protect themselves from IR rays and surrounding workers only have to wear clear ones. Early diagnosis may be difficult, because maculopathy can be masked in the first few days by a phototoxic keratitis. In most cases, retinal injuries heal spontaneously without loss of vision. Several burns on the retina, on the other hand, may lead to permanent complete or partial loss of central vision.

Summary of typical damage to ocular tissues caused by IR exposure is given in Table 14.2.

PROTECTION

Finally, it is worthwhile considering methods for protecting eyes against infrared radiation. Spectacles containing reflective metallic coatings and materials that filter out infrared are the ideal means. Aluminium and inconel (and alloy of iron, nickel and chromium) provide excellent infrared reflectance. The main difficulty with using reflective metallic coatings is that they are susceptible to scratching, abrasions and other faults that cause the breakdown of the coating. Hard protective secondary coating over the metallic coating overcomes this problem, or sandwiching the reflecting metal between two optical layers; the layer adjacent to the eye can then be designed to absorb other unwanted radiation such as ultraviolet. A typical combination protective filter is 'Pfund's glass' developed by American Optical, in which a gold layer reflects 96% of infrared while transmitting 75% of visible light. The metal is sandwiched between clear optical crown glass and Crookes A glass, which absorbs 100% of ultraviolet. The major advantage of reflective coatings is that while protecting the wearer from infrared, they remain cool and so more acceptable. Thus, metallic coatings provide a measure of protection against low level chronic infrared exposure and reduce the total heat load reaching the eye.

Table 14.2 *Summary of typical damage to ocular tissue from IR exposure*

Ocular structure	Typical damage
Cornea	Loss of transparency, corneal haze, exfoliation
Aqueous humour	Rare
Iris	Swelling, miosis, hyperaemia, iridocyclitis
Lens	Anterior opacities
Vitreous humour	Haze
Retina	Oedema, burns, depigmentation

BIBLIOGRAPHY

IONIZING RADIATION

1. Blakely EA, Kleiman NJ, Neriishi K, Chodick G, Chylack LT, Cucinotta FA, et al. Radiation cataractogenesis: epidemiology and biology. Radiat Res 2010;173:709–717.
2. Martin CJ. Personal dosimetry for interventional operators: when and how should monitoring be done? Br J Radiol 2011;84:639–648.
3. Minamoto A, Taniguchi N, Yoshitani S, Mukai S, Yokoyama T, Kumagami T et al. Cataract in atomic bomb survivors. Int J Radiat Biol 2004; 80:339–345.
4. Vano E, Kleiman NJ, Duran A, Rehani MM, Echeverri D, Cabrera M. Radiation cataract risk in interventional cardiology personnel. Radiat Res 2010;174:490–495.

ULTRAVIOLET RADIATION

1. Cejkova J, Stipek S, Crkovska J, Ardan T, Platenik J, Cejka C, Midelfart A. UV rays, the prooxidant/antioxidant imbalance in the cornea and oxidative eye damage. Physiol Res. 2004;53:1–10.
2. Roberts J. Ocular phototoxicity. J Photochem Photobiol B 2001:64:136-143.
3. Walsh K. UV radiation and the Eye. Optician 2009: 237;6204:26–33.
4. Wittenberg S. Solar radiation and the eye: A review of knowledge relevant to eye care. Am J Optom Physiol Opt 1986;63:676–689.
5. Young A. Acute effects of UVR on human eyes and skin. Prog Biophys Mol Biol 2006;92:80–85.
6. Young S, Sands J. Sun and the eye: Prevention and detection of light-induced disease. Clin Dermatol. 1998;16(4):477–485.

INFRARED RADIATION

1. Agrawal LP, Malik SRK. Solar retinitis. Br J Ophthal 1959;53:366–370.
2. Aly EM, Mohamed ES. Effect of infrared radiation on the lens. Indian J Ophthalmol 2011;59:97–101.
3. Goldmann H. Genesis of heat cataract. Arch Ophthal 1933;9:314.
4. Langley RK et al. The experimental production of cataracts by exposure to light and heat. Arch Ophthal 1970;63:473–488.
5. Magnavita N. Photoretinitis: An underestimated occupational injury? Occup Med 2002;52:223–225.
6. Sliney DH, Freasier BC. Evaluation of optical radiation hazards. Applied Optics 1973;12:1–24.

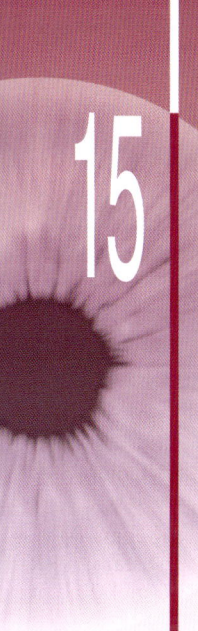

15

ELECTRICAL, THERMAL AND BAROMETRIC INJURIES

ELECTRICAL INJURIES TO THE EYE

INTRODUCTION

Since its inception in 1849, commercial use of electricity has been one of the most potentially dangerous commodities in our society. Electrical injuries are the fourth leading cause of work-related traumatic death and with the advances in technology, they are becoming more common. Electrical burns can be caused by a variety of ways, such as touching or grasping electrically live objects, short-circuiting, inserting fingers into electrical sockets, and falling into electrified water. Lightening strikes are also a cause of electrical burns, but this is a less common event.

EPIDEMIOLOGY

Electric trauma is not uncommon in India where majority of the population lives in the rural setting. Electrical burn injuries account for about 3–4% of burns unit admissions. According to statistical data, 0.8–1% of accidental deaths are caused by an electric injury, with approximately one-quarter caused by natural lightening. Death most often occurs in young males with a Male: Female ratio of 9:1. Electricians and linemen are at highest risk but those working with electrical tools also form a significant proportion of this patient group. Approximately 20% of all electrical injuries occur in children (with a bimodal peak incidence in toddlers and adolescents), usually involving cable extensions or wall outlets and for every death, there are two serious injuries and 36 reported electric shocks. Most of the deaths occur in the spring and summer months.

PATHOPHYSIOLOGY

Electrical current causes damage through:

- *Direct process of physiological changes* by altering cell resting membrane potential.
- *Conversion of electrical energy into thermal energy,* which gets subsequently absorbed by the tissues, thus causing end-organ ischaemia by generalized vascular constriction and coagulative necrosis.
- *Secondary damage* associated with falls and violent muscle contractions.

Factors affecting degree of damage

There are several factors that affect the degree of damage:

1. Current

Type of current. This may be direct or alternating. The latter is significantly more dangerous in a number of respects:

- It may result in tetanic muscular contraction which prevents the patient from letting go of the source, thereby causing severe damage.
- An alternating current of more than 10 milliampere (mA) induces sweating. Skin moisture decreases its resistance which increases conduction.
- Human tissue is most sensitive to frequencies between 40 and 150 hertz (Hz). The frequency best suited for household use is about 50 Hz, making household current particularly dangerous. This is all the more important, as this frequency is capable of producing ventricular fibrillation (VF).

Amount of current. The biological effects differ depending upon the intensity of the current

- 1 mA = Threshold of perception, resulting in a tingling sensation
- >7–9 mA = Leads to muscular tetany preventing release of grip from current source (this is lower for children and women)
- 20–50 mA = Pain and severe breathing difficulties leading to respiratory arrest.
- 50–100 mA = Ventricular fibrillation
- >2 A = Asystole

Current path. The key issue affecting mortality is whether the current passes through the heart. For example, contact of the electrical source with both hands effectively results in a transthoracic pathway which is thought to account for about 60% of mortalities, whereas there is very low mortality related to a pathway passing through one leg and out of the other.

2. Voltage

Generally, the greater the voltage, the greater the damage (the exception being with high-tension voltage: Above this level, greater voltage doesn't necessarily influence the degree of injury).

Low-voltage:
- <50 V: No danger.
- 240 V: UK household supply (±10%). This creates small, deep entrance and exit wounds.

High-voltage:
- ≥1,000 V: There is often extensive tissue damage and limb loss. Contact with >70,000 V is invariably fatal.
- 100 million V: Lightening—this is quite different from a high-voltage electric shock.

3. Resistance

As the current travels through the body, it follows the path of least resistance. Resistance varies in different tissues and will have a great influence on the extent of injuries.

- At a cellular level, the injury resembles a crush injury more than a burn.
- The electrical current will pass through low-resistance tissues in preference, causing necrosis along the way.
- Since the skin resistance can be affected by moisture, electric current can be transmitted to deeper structures before it causes significant skin damage (there may be serious injury deep inside with sparing of overlying skin).
- A current passing along the surface of the body to earth can cause very deep burns over a large surface area.
- There will be a range of clinical manifestations with different effects on different organs.
- There may be potentially dangerous injuries secondary from falling or being thrown to the ground.

OCULAR LESIONS IN ELECTRICAL INJURY

Electric injuries to the eye occur chiefly when current enters the body through the patients head. Both eyes can be equally affected, or one can be affected more than the other. A wide range of voltages, from 220 to 50,000 volts, results in cataract in 5 to 20% of electrical injuries (Figs 15.1 A and B). Lesions of the cornea, fundus, and optic nerve, without alteration of the lens, have also been reported. The optic nerve and retina have a low resistance and are thought to be primarily affected by ischemia resulting from coagulation and necrosis of the vascular tissues that feed them. There has been a recent case report of a 20-year-old boy who suffered an electric injury shock, following which he showed peripapillary retinal opacification and increased

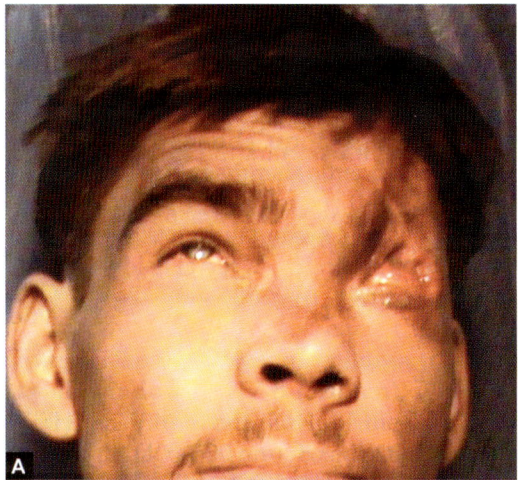

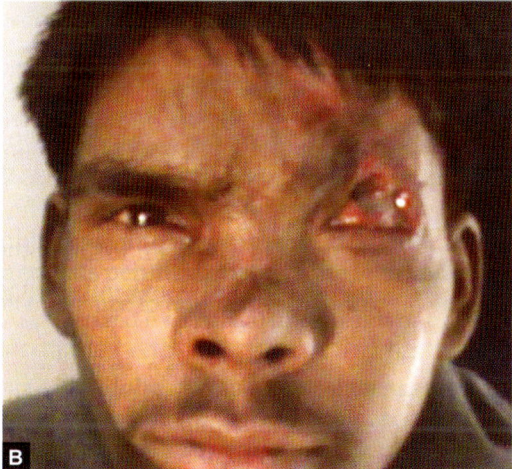

Fig. 15.1 *(A) Loss of the left eye with development of a mature cataract in the right eye following passage of a high-tension electric current. (B) The patient regained 20/20 vision in the right eye following cataract surgery*

retinal thickening that subsequently progressed to retinal atrophy. Common lesions of ocular adnexa and eyeball are described below.

Burns of eyelid and face

- *Burns range from first-degree to third-degree*: There is typically a depressed charred central area with surrounding oedema. There may be several entry and exit wounds (the latter characteristically have an explosive appearance—round or oval grey craters with no inflammatory changes).
- *Arc burns* are produced by the passage of a current of electricity from the source to the

ground and may be associated with extensive skin damage.

- *'Kissing burns'* are produced in flexor creases when muscle tetany causes the joint to flex and the current flows through opposing skin.
- *Flame burns* occur when the current ignites clothing.

Electric Cataract

Electrical cataracts may occur following contact with high-tension conductor, lightening or electric shock therapy. The earliest record of cataract development from lightening shock was made by Saint Yves in 1722. Only a few cases of electric cataract have been reported in the literature probably because a few patients survive the high voltage of current that induces cataract formation. The incidence of cataracts following electrical injury has been reported to be 6 to 20% according to available data.

Cataractogenesis following electrical trauma is usually bilateral; and unilateral involvement as well as exclusive involvement of the lens sparing other ocular structures is rare. Most patients with electric cataract have no subjective complaints early on but become aware of the reducing visual function 1–12 months after the accident. Usually there is no other observable ocular damage. However, the degree of lenticular change seems to bear no definite relation to the strength of the current. In most cases, the electric current has passed through the head in the vicinity of the eye with a contact electrical burn. The nearer the point of contact of the current to the eye, the greater is the potential for cataract formation. A typical electric burn may occur at the point of contact leaving its imprint as a sharply defined necrotic mark without surrounding hyperemia. A similar exit wound may be seen. Young patients with a clear lens are more liable to develop damage following electrical burns than elderly patients with sclerosed lenses (Fig. 15.1 A).

Pathogenesis of electric cataract

The exact pathogenesis of cataract development is unknown. The high water content of the crystalline lens and its surroundings make it a good conductor of electricity. Direct coagulation of lens proteins and the osmotic changes following damage to the subcapsular epithelium are thought to be responsible for the lenticular opacities. The earliest recognizable change in the lens is the appearance of multiple fine vacuoles just beneath the anterior capsule which are replaced later on by fine irregular or mossy *anterior subcapsular opacities*. Sometimes the posterior cortex may also be affected. Though the exact pathogenesis of the effect of electric current on the proteins of the crystalline lens and the process of lenticular opacification is unclear, *five different mechanisms* have been postulated.

1. *Extensive epithelial damage* has been proposed by Hess and Croci as the cause of the lenticular opacities. However, epithelial damage alone does not explain the development of the extensive posterior subcapsular changes, which have been observed to occur almost simultaneously with the anterior changes in several cases.

2. *Direct injury to the lens fibres* by the electric current is the second possible mechanism. This causative mechanism is supported by the observation that the earliest signs of injury are generally confined to the region immediately beneath the capsule.

3. *Uveitis and circulatory changes* have been postulated as cause of cataract by Kiribuchi. Long's experimental report demonstrated the formation of cataract with little associated uveitis, which contradicts this theory.

4. *Mechanical effects,* including capsule rupture, contraction of the ciliary body, local heat production, and ultraviolet and infrared radiations, suggested as the fourth mechanism, have been disproved.

5. *Alteration in the permeability of the lens capsule* or altered osmotic relationships with imbibition of fluid into the lens, demonstrated by the experimental work of Kuwabara, Bellows and Chinn, and Cogan and Donaldson, has also been suggested as a factor in the development of electric cataract.

While the exact cause of electric cataract remains doubtful, a change in the capsular permeability as the direct or indirect result of electric damage seems to be the most important factor.

Clinical course of the cataract

Regression may occasionally occur, they may remain stationary, or maturation may occur slowly over an average period of 6 months. Sometimes with startling rapidity after a long static period, the cataract may mature to complete milkiness resembling *hammered silver or mother of pearl*. The cataract may become intumescent and as a rarity cause acute angle closure glaucoma as it swells, and pushes the iris forwards.

Other lesions

Other lesions affecting the eye are:

• Conjunctival hyperemia,

• Interstitial corneal opacities,

• Uveitis which may be mild or severe, miosis, spasm of accommodation, etc.

• Electric energy can also damage the retina and choroid. Optic nerve coagulation, necrosis of retina, choroid and optic atrophy have all been reported. Retinal oedema, papilloedema and haemorrhages with patches of chorioretinal atrophy in the periphery, rupture of choroid, optic neuritis or even retinal detachment may occur. Macular oedema may lead to development of macular cysts or holes.

• *Paresis of extraocular muscles* has been frequently observed.

PROGNOSIS

When lenticular opacities are the sole manifestations of electrical injury, cataract extraction is expected to produce a functional outcome (Fig. 15.1B). However, with concurrent damage to the optic nerve and retina, complete visual rehabilitation may be limited.

THERMAL INJURIES TO THE EYE

PROFILE OF THERMAL INJURIES

An ocular burn is an ophthalmic emergency, whether it is a chemical or thermal injury, because of the rapid ocular tissue damage that it can cause. Thermal burns represent 16% of ocular burn cases.

Thermal injuries can involve hot liquids, hot gases or molten metals.

Severity of an ocular burn is related to the duration of exposure, and the offending agent.

Burns inflict damage primarily by denaturing and coagulating tissue proteins, and secondarily through ischemic vascular damage.

Thermal eye injury triggers inflammatory processes, including inflammatory cell influx and/or the activation of various inflammatory cells, which result in the rapid accumulation of extravascular fluid in the ocular tissue.

Hot water facial scalding leading to blindness is rare among adults. However, it can result from assault and accidents.

• A hot water burn is a thermal injury, and direct contact with the eye may result in blindness, if not properly managed.

• The thermal burn causes superficial epithe- lium cell death, although thermal necrosis and deeper tissue penetration can occur.

• The ocular effect depends on the temperature of the water, and the final visual outcome depends on many factors, including the promptness of presentation to the hospital, severity of the burn, application of traditional medication, and available expertise (Fig. 15.2).

COMPLICATIONS OF OCULAR THERMAL INJURIES

It is of note that complications sometimes follow ocular burns, including eyelid contractures,

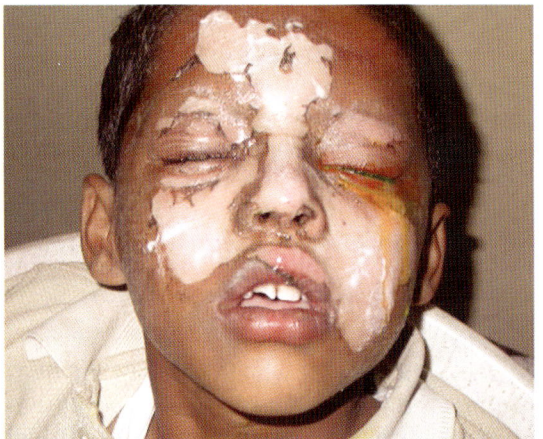

Fig 15.2 *Facial scalds involving the lids of both eyes following spillage of hot water*

conjunctivitis, corneal defects (epithelial defects/ulcer, perforation, scarring), cataracts, raised intraocular pressure/glaucoma, retinal detachment and impaired vision/blindness.

PROGNOSIS

The prognosis of an ocular burn depends on the depth of the injury. In mild to moderate cases, the outcome is good, while severe cases may require serious intervention, including corneal transplant or rehabilitation services. The major concerns with ocular burns are final visual acuity and cosmesis. With prompt treatment and early ophthalmologic intervention, thermal burns generally have good visual outcome.

BAROMETRIC INJURIES

INTRODUCTION

Barotrauma is physical damage to the body tissues caused by a difference in pressure between a gas space inside, or in contact with the body, and the surrounding fluid. It usually occurs when a subject is exposed to a significant change in ambient pressure, such as when a scuba diver, a free diver or an airplane passenger ascends or descends, or during uncontrolled decompression of a pressure vessel, but can also be caused by a shock wave. Middle ear, para- nasal sinuses, lung and sometimes the teeth or bowel, are the most common sites of baro- traumas in scuba diving. Rarely, eyes can also be affected by such injuries. Gases are frequently used as a tamponading agent in vitreo-retinal surgeries and their use is also associated with barotrauma in a variety of settings.

OCULAR AND ORBITAL INJURIES IN DIVERS

Divers who do not wear a face mask and have no air space contiguous to the eye will not experience ocular barotraumas. Use of a face mask creates an air-filled space of which eye and ocular adnexa form one side. Pressure differen- tials created by an inadequately equalized face mask may result in injury to the eye and adnexa. At the surface, both the air in the face mask and the ocular tissues are at one atm but during descent in water, the ambient pressure rises. If air is not added to the gas space in the face mask to equalize the pressure, a relative vacuum may form inside and result in barotrauma such as subconjunctival haemorrhage, lid edema and ecchymosis, hyphema and rarely, orbital haemorrhage.

EXPANSILE GASES IN THE EYE

Intraocular gas injections are used to treat various conditions, including retinal detachment and macular hole surgery with the aim of achieving long term tamponade. Air, sulphur hexafluoride (SF_6) and perfluoropropanes (e.g. $C_3 F_8$) are the most commonly used gases and majority of the vitreoretinal procedures require temporary intraocular gas injection. These gases can provide retinal tamponade for two to six weeks owing to the high surface tension between the gas bubble and retina which is necessary to treat retinal disorders successfully. However, the procedure entails risks and can lead to blindness if patients receive repeated anaesthesia within this time window or travel to high altitudes, as these factors lead to expansion of the intraocular gas bubble.

Many physical laws influence the behaviour of expansile gases in the eye. The volume of intraocular gas bubble increases gradually after injection of pure (100%) SF_6 or C_3F_8, because of diffusion of gases, such as oxygen, nitrogen and carbon dioxide, from the blood into the intraocular space. A bubble consisting of pure SF_6 will expand to twice its injected volume within 24 hours and reabsorbs in 14 days, and a pure C_3F_8 bubble quadruples over three to seven days and total reabsorption takes place in 25 days. Therefore, a mixture of 20% gas in air is commonly used which becomes non-expansile and if at all it expands, expands only to a minimal extent.

Ocular complications of expansile gases

Complications of the expansile gases in the eye are as under.

1. Complications at higher altitude

There have been case reports mentioning sudden visual loss in patients with intraocular gases when travelling to high altitudes and during air travel. At high altitudes, the atmospheric pressure is lower and it falls by 100Pa every 8 metres, starting at sea level. According to Boyle's law (p × v = constant), the gas bubble expands. Since the ascent rate of an aircraft on a scheduled flight is 600 to 900 mt/min, the volume of the gas bubble changes rapidly (~40% increase) leading to raised intraocular pressure. This causes transient retinal ischaemia which subsequently affects vision. Early manifestations include pain and decreased vision, which may be treated by prompt decent to a lower altitude. Scleral expansion and increased drainage of aqueous from the anterior chamber compensate for the rise in IOP (in extreme cases, even globe rupture via surgical wounds can occur). If the volume of the intraocular gas is only 10% of the vitreous volume, and the compensatory mechanisms are functioning properly, the expansion of the gas can be compensated sufficiently. In healthy subjects, no long term sequelae occur if the increase in IOP during the trip last less than 90 minutes. But in glaucoma patients, with disrupted compensatory mechanisms and previously damaged optic nerve, the effects may be long lasting.

2. Diving-related complications

Just like fall of atmospheric pressure above sea level, the atmospheric pressure increases during diving. In accordance with Boyle's law, during the descent in water, the intraocular gas bubble decreases in size leading to hypotony and partial globe collapse. Conversely, as the eye goes from hyperbaric conditions to normal sea level, atmospheric pressure during the ascent to water surface decreases, resulting in expansion of the intraocular gas bubble and can cause a large increase in intraocular volume. Such pressure-induced changes in the volume of the gas bubble can result in vitreous, retinal or choroidal haemorrhage.

3. General anaesthesia-related complications

Nitrous oxide (N_2O) which is one of the most common gases used by anaesthesiologists, has a very high blood gas distribution coefficient compared to nitrogen. This means that during anaesthesia, N_2O diffuses more quickly from the blood into an air filled cavity than nitrogen diffuses from the same cavity into the blood. Therefore, during anaesthesia preoperatively intraocular gas injection must only be given once the application of N_2O has stopped for 15 minutes and it has been flushed out of the body. This is done to avoid a dangerously rapid increase in IOP which might occur after intraocular gas injection. Patients with pre-existing intraocular gas are also at a risk of rapid bubble expansion, if N_2O is used during anaesthesia. This can lead to anterior shift of the lens-iris diaphragm and subsequent angle closure. If the IOP exceeds the perfusion pressure in the central retinal artery, retinal ischaemia can occur. Occlusion of the central retinal artery for more than 90 minutes causes irreversible ischaemic damage to the retina with subsequent optic nerve atrophy. The risk of central retinal artery occlusion after gas injection increases in patients with compromised perfusion pressure such as those with diabetes mellitus or atherosclerosis and elderly individuals.

Patient information

All patients receiving intraocular gas injections must be informed about the associated risks preoperatively. Air travel and travel to high altitudes should be prohibited for a few weeks postoperatively. In case the patient requires anaesthesia for any medical condition, the anaesthesiologist must always be informed about the intraocular gas. An intraocular gas injection that is more than three months old can be assumed to present no contraindication to travel at high altitudes or use of N_2O.

BIBLIOGRAPHY

ELECTRICAL INJURIES

1. Al Rabiah SM, Archer DB, Millar R, Collins AD, Shepherd WF. Electrical injury of the eye. Int Ophthalmol. 1987;11:31–40.
2. Archer DM. Injuries of posterior segment of eye. Tran Ophthal Soc UK 1985;104:597.
3. Boozalis GT, Purdu GF. Ocular changes from electric burn injuries: A literature review and report of cases. J Burn Care Rehab 1991;12: 458–462.
4. Fraunfelder FT, Hanna C. Electrical cataracts. I. Sequential changes, unusual and prognostic findings. Arch Ophthalmol 1972;87:179–183.
5. Kiribuchi K. Experimentelle Untersuchungen über Cataract und sonstige Augenaffektionen durch Blitzschlag. Albrecht von Graefes Arch Ophthalmol 1900;50:1–43.
6. Noel LP, Clark WN. Ocular complications of lightning. J Paediatric Ophthalmol Strabismus 1950;17:245.
7. Rodriguez Valde's R, Garcia Torres V, et al. Electric cataract. Burns 1975;1:317–318.
8. Saffle JR, Crandall A. Cataracts a long-term complication of electrical injury. J Trauma 1985; 25(1):17–21.

THERMAL INJURIES

1. Kuckelkorn R, Schrage N, Keller G, Redbrake C. Emergency treatment of chemical and thermal eye burns. Acta Ophthalmol Scand 2002;80(1): 4–10.
2. Merle H, Gerard M, Schrage N. Ocular burns. J Fr Ophthalmol. 2008;31(7):723–734.
3. Monsudi KF, Ayanniyi AA. A 14-year-old girl who regained normal vision after bilateral visual impairment following hot water injury to the eye. Saudi J Ophthalmology 2011;25(2):2207–2210.
4. Stern JD, Goldfarb IW, Slater H. Ophthalmological complications as a manifestation of burn injury. Burns 1996;22(2):135–136.
5. Xiang H, Stallones L, Chen G, Smith GA. Work-related eye injuries treated in hospital emergency departments in the US. Am J Ind Med 2005; 48(1):57–62.

BAROMETRIC INJURIES

1. Briggs M, Wong D, Groenewald C, McGalliard J, Kelly J, Harper J. The effect of anesthesia on the intraocular volume of the C3F6 gas bubble. Eye 1997;11:47–52.
2. Butler FK. Diving and hyperbaric ophthalmology. Surv Ophthalmol 1995;39:347–366.
3. Lincoff H, Weinberger D, Reppucci V, Lincoff A. Air travel with intraocular gas. I. The mechanisms for compensation. Arch Ophthalmol 1989; 107:902–906.
4. Vote BJ, Hart RH, Worsley DR, Borthwick JH, Laurent S, McGeorge AJ. Visual loss after use of nitrous oxide gas with general anesthetic in patients with intraocular gas still persistent up to 30 days after vitrectomy. Anesthesiology 2002; 97:1305–1308.

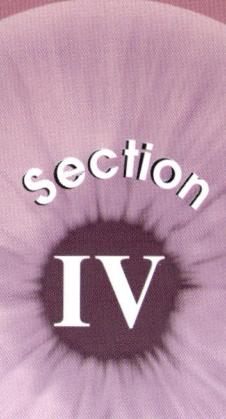

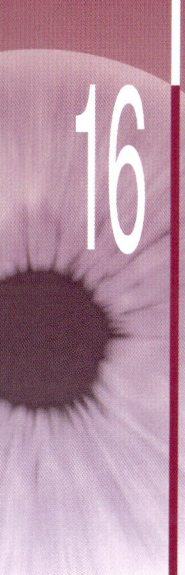

16

PREVENTION AND REHABILITATION OF OCULAR TRAUMA

INTRODUCTION

The eyes occupy 0.1% of the total and 0.27% of the anterior body surface, however, the significance of their injury is magnified as vision is the most important sense. Loss of vision is likely to lead to loss of career, major lifestyle changes and disfigurement.

Ocular trauma remains a preventable cause of visual morbidity globally. Worldwide, more than half a million blinding injuries occur every year. Approximately half of all patients who present to an eye casualty department do so because of ocular trauma. There is a bi-modal age distribution of severe ocular trauma, with a large preponderance of injuries affecting young males as a result of their spending more time outdoors, their employment in higher risk jobs, alcohol use, and participation in adventurous sports and hobbies. Reason for the dip in incidence beyond the age of 30, is the increased maturity and awareness levels from previous experiences.

PREVENTION OF OCULAR TRAUMA

Prevention of ocular injuries can be discussed under the following heads:

- Prevention of occupational eye injuries
- Prevention of eye injuries in motor vehicle accidents
- Prevention of eye injuries in sports and recreational activities
- Prevention of eye injuries in domestic setting
- Prevention of eye injuries in fireworks
- Prevention of ocular war injuries
- Prevention of pediatric ocular trauma
- Prevention of geriatric ocular trauma

PREVENTION OF OCCUPATIONAL EYE INJURIES

Occupational eye injuries account for nearly one-third of all eye injuries seen in an emergency eye department.

Common occupational injuries include superficial corneal foreign body, welder's arc injury, chemical injury, corneal abrasion, ruptured globe, penetrating injury (Fig. 16.1), intraocular foreign body, laceration to eyebrow, electric shock injuries. The majority of these are minor injuries, like superficial corneal and conjunctival foreign bodies.

Activities causing injury include grinding, hammering, cutting metal, welding and drilling.

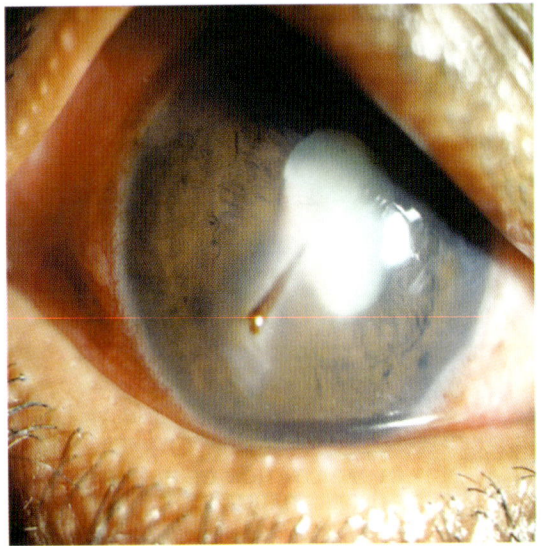

Fig. 16.1 *Penetrating injury by a thorn in a farmer while working in the field causing traumatic cataract*

Eyewear protection, safety training and compliance within the workplace are not universal. A significant proportion of eye injuries still occurs despite reported use of protective equipment, like safety glasses, goggles and welding helmets. This may be due to false reporting, improper usage, the wrong type or poorly designed personal protective equipment (PPE) for the job. Also failure is usually attributed to foreign matter passing laterally around the eyeshield. *Common reasons for non-compliance* are ill-fitting protective eyewear, habit, poor vision due to fogging from sweat and above all non-availability of eyewear. Language barrier between workers and their employers could be an important factor in preventing effective safety training and communication, resulting in a low prevalence of protective eyewear use. Lack of supervision as well as loose legislative efforts are all important factors that contribute to the low prevalence of using protective eyewear as well. In addition to the impact on affected individuals, including risk of causing blindness, there are profound social implications regarding the loss of productivity by young men, unnecessary loss of workdays and socioeconomic costs.

Perhaps, better education on workplace, safety measures and effective preventive strategies for both employers and their employees need to be considered, as well as stricter legal action taken against the non-compliers. There is a need to review the design of eye safety wear, and to improve the comfort and visibility, ergonomics, resistance and durability, in order to increase compliance and maximize protection.

PREVENTION OF EYE INJURIES IN MOTOR VEHICLE ACCIDENTS

Motor vehicle accidents are responsible for a considerable number of eye injuries. Most common are eyelid injuries (Fig. 16.2). Seat belt use is found to be associated with a two-fold reduction in eye injury risk. Penetrating eye injuries from road traffic accidents are shown to decrease considerably after seat belt legislation and the introduction of laminated windscreens. Though frontal air bag deployment has been found to be associated with a two-fold increased risk of eye injury, its protection against life-threatening injuries justifies its use since fewer severe injuries have been found to occur among occupants exposed to air bag deployment. There is increased risk of corneal abrasions for occupants exposed to air bag deployment. Air bag deployment has been found to be associated with traumatic maculopathy. Nevertheless, the air bag seems to have decreased the risk of severe eye injuries. Wearing standard prescription glasses should be discouraged in the front seat of air bag-equipped cars because the fracture of the glass

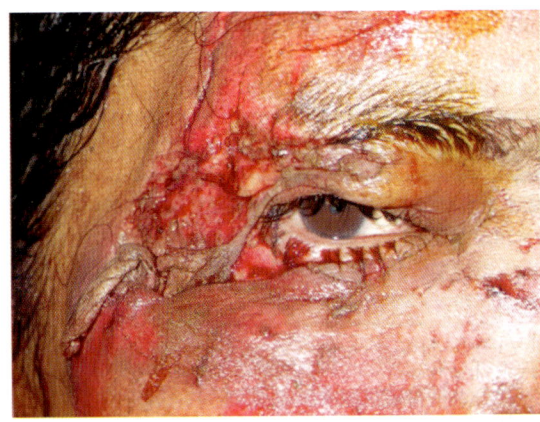

Fig. 16.2 *Laceration of both the upper and lower lids in a patient who met with a motor vehicle accident*

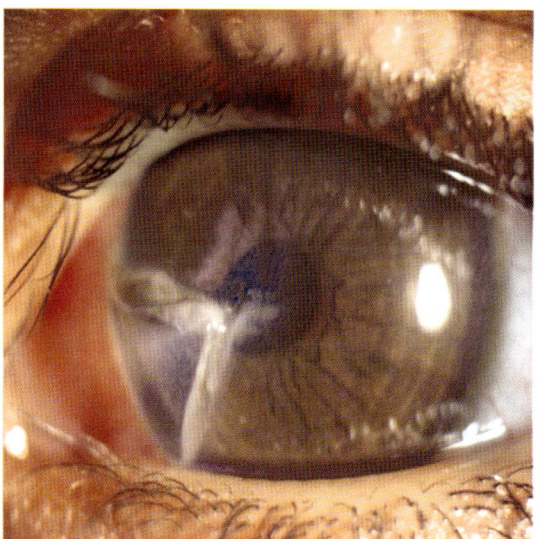

Fig. 16.3 *Corneal laceration caused by fracture of a spectacle glass worn by the patient sitting in the front seat of an air-bag equipped car*

may be responsible for eye injury (Fig. 16.3). The risk of eye injury is highest for frontal collisions, with the most common injury mechanism being the windshield, followed by the frontal air bag, steering wheel, and flying glass.

These days an increasing proportion of the population is undergoing laser refractive surgery. Studies indicate that such surgical procedures weaken the cornea and make it more susceptible to injury for years after the procedure, especially, to injury associated with air bag deployment.

PREVENTION OF EYE INJURIES IN SPORTS AND RECREATIONAL ACTIVITIES

Risk factors in sports

Sports and recreational activities are becoming increasingly popular. About 90% of sports-related ocular injuries are considered preventable. Basketball, water sports, baseball, and racquet sports account for most injuries. When considering the potential for eye injury, it may be more appropriate to categorize sports as low risk, high risk, and very high risk.

Low risk indicates no use of a ball, bat, stick, or racquet, and no body contact. Examples include track/field, swimming, gymnastics, and cycling.

High-risk sports involve the use of a ball, bat, stick, or racquet, and/or body contact. Examples of high-risk sports include baseball, hockey, cricket (Fig. 16.4), football, basketball, racquet sports, tennis, fencing, golf, and water polo.

Very-high-risk sports, such as boxing, wrestling, and contact martial arts, are those in which eye protectors typically are not worn.

Profile of sports injuries

If an object is smaller than the orbit, it causes injury to the eyeball. An object larger than the orbit transmits force to the orbital walls, resulting in fractures of thin or even thick bones. One of the most common injuries is corneal abrasion. Finger and nail scratches to the eyes in contact sports cause pain, tearing and irritation. Blunt trauma could cause hyphema, vitreous haemorrhage, retinal tears and detachment, choroidal rupture, macular oedema, globe rupture, retrobulbar haemorrhage and traumatic optic neuropathy.

Protocol for prevention of sports injuries

In order to prevent these injuries, programmed protocol needs to be followed by sports bodies as under:

1. Pre-participation examination

A complete eye examination should be part of any sports activity. With each athlete, physicians should obtain an ocular history, paying special

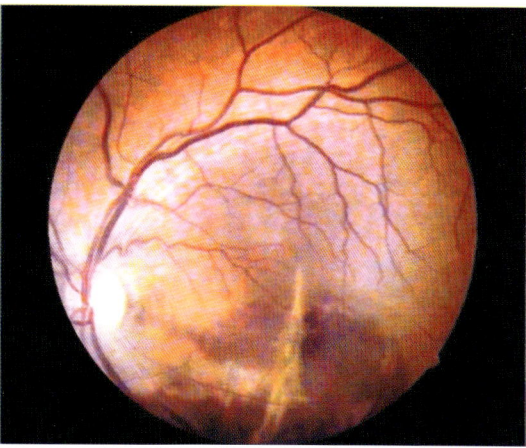

Fig. 16.4 *Choroidal rupture involving the fovea following blunt trauma with a cricket ball*

attention to prior conditions, such as a high degree of myopia, surgical aphakia, retinal detachment, eye surgery, and eye injury or infection. Athletes with any of these conditions may be at increased risk for sports related eye injury. In addition, it is important to assess athletes who have a strong family history of retinal detachment, retinal tears, and diabetic retinopathy. Athletes with such risk factors should be evaluated by an eye care professional before engaging in any high-risk or very-high-risk sport.

2. Protective devices

Eye protection has reduced the number and severity of eye injuries. A protective device should dissipate a potentially harmful force over a larger area. Eye protectors should be such that it can shift impact from the eyes and face to the skull without causing intracranial injury. It may be necessary to integrate helmets with eye and face protectors.

Protective eyewear often is made of polycarbonate, a highly impact-resistant plastic capable of absorbing ultraviolet light. Because this plastic is eight times stronger than other materials, it is preferred for use in protective glasses. Polycarbonate lenses are available as prescription and nonprescription lenses. Contact lenses offer no eye protection, and eyeglasses provide inadequate protection. Regular eyeglasses have only 4 to 5% the impact resistance of polycarbonate of comparable thickness.

Recommendations for protective eyewear include:

- 2 mm polycarbonate lenses in normal streetwear frames (for athletes who need corrective lenses and are involved in low-risk sports).
- Sports frames with a 3 mm polycarbonate lens (for athletes participating in moderate- to high-risk sports). Eye protection should be used by athletes who wear contact lenses and by those who do not need corrective lenses. The athlete with refractive errors should wear prescription polycarbonate lenses.
- A sturdy sports frame meeting impact-resistance standards is required.
- Face masks attached to a helmet should be used in sports such as hockey, cricket, football and baseball.

3. Functionally one-eyed athletes

An athlete is considered monocular when the best corrected visual acuity in the weaker eye is less than 20/40. Such athletes must wear eye protector beneath a face mask in sports that require facial protection (i.e. hockey and football). The athlete should be instructed to wear protective lenses at all times in order to avoid nonsports-related trauma.

Monocular athletes should wear polycarbonate lenses and frames while playing basketball. In hockey, a helmet with a full-face cage, made of either wire or polycarbonate, and sports goggles are needed. While playing football, the monocular athlete should wear a helmet with a face mask, a polycarbonate shield, and sports goggles. Monocular baseball players should wear sports goggles at all times. While batting or running bases, the appropriate helmet with a polycarbonate face guard and sports goggles should be worn. Boxing, wrestling, and full-contact martial arts are contraindicated in monocular athletes because no adequate eye protection is available. The functionally monocular athlete should be evaluated by an ophthalmologist before being admitted to participation in a particular sport.

4. Return to play

Several guidelines for returning to play after an injury should be followed. In patients with significant ocular injury, a full examination and clearance by an ophthalmologist are required. The injured eye should feel comfortable and have adequate retrieval of vision. Eye protectors must be worn. During the game, immediate return to play depends on the athlete's symptoms and the nature of the injury as determined by the team physician. Athletes should never be allowed to use topical anaesthetics to prolong play.

PREVENTION OF EYE INJURIES IN DOMESTIC SETTING

Eye injuries occur in the domestic setting (at home) as well. Women and children commonly fall prey to domestic violence. In addition, children may get themselves injured by innocuously appearing sharp household articles

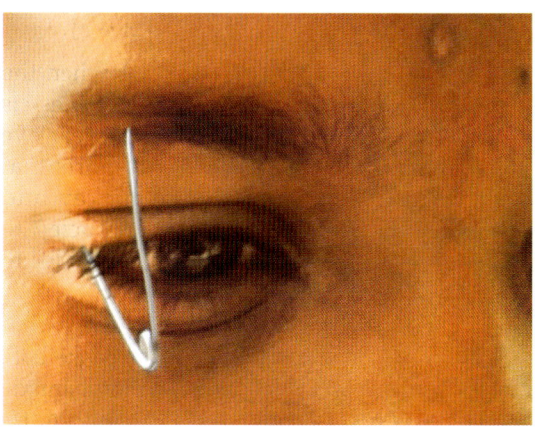

Fig. 16.5 *Retained safety pin in the superior fornix of a young girl*

(Fig. 16.5). In the circumstances of financial constraints most of the household odd jobs are being carried out by the family members. 'Do it yourself' (DIY), car repairs and gardening have been shown to be a common cause of eye injury especially amongst the males of the family. Safety goggles should be worn while using hammers and lawnmowers in gardens. All product packaging should have ocular safety precautions mentioned on them. The local hire shops should rent out eye goggles as well when hiring out commonly used household equipment. Domestic accidents involving chemicals are perhaps hard to prevent, though patients can be advised regarding the correct usage of household consumer items and in the event of injury, they should immediately irrigate themselves.

PREVENTION OF EYE INJURIES IN FIREWORK

Eye injuries caused by **fireworks** are often severe and can cause permanently reduced visual acuity or blindness. Most are unintentional injuries which usually occur at home during Diwali and Dusshera festivals. Persons injured by fireworks are predominantly males. Most injuries are caused by cones and bottle rockets. Bottle rockets account for maximum number of the injuries to bystanders.

Eye injuries resulting from bottle rockets are due to product misuse [e.g. the intentional aiming of the device at others ("bottle rocket wars") and throwing the device after it has been lit but before ignition], device malfunction (especially immediate explosion after ignition), erratic flight characteristics even when used according to manufacturers' instructions, and due to device which ricochets off hard surfaces (e.g. a car or the street). Because of the risks for injury associated with bottle rockets and other firework, it is recommended that persons attending public fireworks displays should wear eye protections and operators firing crackers should not use bottle rockets in public interest. Young children should never indulge in fireworks, older children should be supervised when using fireworks, fireworks should be used only outdoors, a source of water should always be made available nearby in order to do use fire and malfunctioning fireworks. Instructions should be read and followed carefully and malfunctioning fireworks should not be reignited.

PREVENTION OF OCULAR WAR INJURIES

In peacetime where unilateral injuries are the rule, ocular war injuries are bilateral in 15–25% of cases. Ocular blast injuries can be primary, from the blast wave itself; secondary, from fragments carried by the blast wind; tertiary; due to structural collapse or being thrown against a fixed object; or quaternary, from burns and indirect injuries.

Ocular injuries from terrorist bombings occur from missile fragments and small fragments of glass, cement, mortar and other debris associated with the blast that cause minimal damage if they impact on the clothes or skin, but significant morbidity, if they hit the eye. A combination of further urbanization of warfare and increased weapon explosive power with relatively poor ocular protection in relation to the rest of the body leads to an increased incidence of eye injuries from war crimes.

Ballistic eye protection significantly reduces the incidence of eye injuries and should be encouraged from an early stage in military training. Eye protection reduces the number of eye injuries in warfare, particularly secondary blast injuries. Compliance is less as combatants often complain that eye protection degrades their vision due to misting, a poor field of view and easy scratching. However, despite all these enforced use of eye protection is advocated.

PREVENTION OF PAEDIATRIC OCULAR TRAUMA

Worldwide, the incidence of severe visual impairment or blindness caused by **ocular trauma in children** varies from 2 to 14% in different studies. Children are more susceptible to eye injuries because of their immature motor skills, limited common sense and natural curiosity. The causes of eye injuries, therefore, are highly related to physical and psychosocial development.

Paediatric ocular trauma occurs twice as often in boys as in girls, which is similar to other studies. The male–female ratio of ocular trauma is higher in the older age group and lower in the younger age group. This is presumably due to the high physical contact and aggressive nature of play among young boys. Additionally, females are quiet and move gently. This value probably reflects the decreased incidence of ocular trauma in older girls. Closed globe injury is the major type of injury in children. The second most common injury is burns and penetrating injury. Open globe injuries are a leading cause of non-congenital unilateral blindness in children. The most common cause of ocular injury in children under the age of 5 years was a fall against a wall or furniture (Fig. 16.6); many of these patients are either alone or without adult supervision at the time of the event.

This should remind us that children, and infants in particular, should be supervised at all times. A safe environment should be maintained for children. Children of kindergarten age (4–6 years) like to imitate adult behavior without the awareness of possible risks: Pencils, chopsticks, toothpicks, knives and scissors should be regarded as dangerous, and kept away from children. Children engaged in playing sports frequently experience ocular trauma due to body contact. School-aged children who are more physically active tend to take more risks to gain acceptance by their peers. Self-protection should be taught to children to prevent possible ocular injuries. For example, children should be told to avoid dangerous games, such as throwing objects, playing with guns or lighting firework. Also, safety goggles should be offered to children who engage in sports with possible body contact or when using sharp utensils.

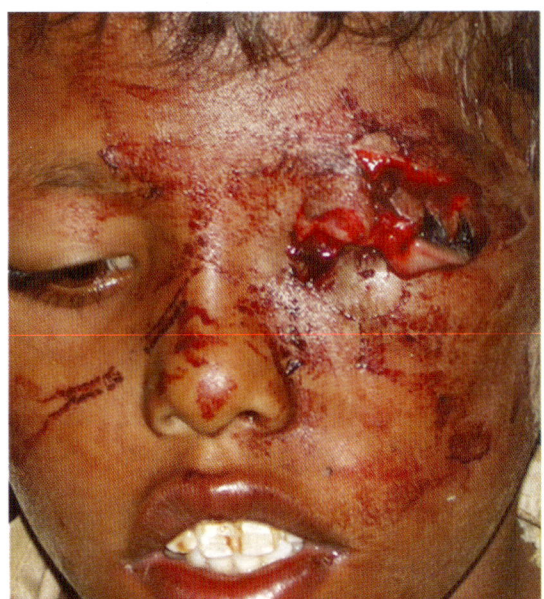

Fig. 16.6 *Laceration of the left upper lid and eyebrow in a child of 5 years following history of fall from height*

PREVENTION OF GERIATRIC OCULAR TRAUMA

The prognosis of open globe injuries is very poor in **geriatric patients**. The most frequent mechanism of trauma is globe rupture due to falls. Age-related structural changes and previous history of surgeries contribute to easy development of a rupture. Systemic hypertension, atherosclerotic diseases and dementia, which are common in the elderly population, also increase fall-related trauma. The prognosis is poor in trauma related to falls since blindness can develop in both eyes simultaneously. Additionally, poor final visual acuity after trauma further increases not only the risk of falls in geriatric patients but also the risk of trauma in the other eye and even the risk of multiorgan trauma. During the treatment process, limited recovery capacity, ocular pathology in patients and low functional capacity in this age group exert negative effects on the prognosis. The enucleation rate is low despite poor final visual acuity in the geriatric age group. This can be explained by the fact that geriatric patients have lower aesthetic expectations than young patients, the risk of sympathetic ophthalmia is lower in the geriatric age group than in the young age group because of shorter life expectancy, and the presence of systemic diseases restricts the performance of additional surgical intervention. Additionally, geriatric patients with normal fellow eye usually do not accept to undergo further surgical interventions required after primary repair and do not receive sufficient rehabilitation because of their satisfaction with the outcome.

REHABILITATION OF PATIENTS WITH OCULAR TRAUMA

Ocular trauma is mostly unilateral but at times bilateral. It is an important cause of monocular visual impairment, leading to difficulty in the assessment of depth perception. Thus, individuals engaged in certain technical profession like surgeons, technicians, engineers, shooters, painters, sculptors, etc. after suffering from injury and thereby monocular visual impairment may have difficulty in pursuing their careers because of lack of stereoscopic vision. Similarly, bilateral trauma leading to bilateral visual impairment has a much more devastating impact on patient's life. Often patients are apprehensive and depressed about their future since loss of vision leads not only to disability but makes them financially and physically dependent on the society.

Therefore, after management of acute condition of the eye, the role of ophthalmologist does not end here. He has to collaborate with his professional colleagues from rehabilitation medicine to work on the patient at the following levels:

• Psychological rehabilitation
• Visual rehabilitation
• Occupational rehabilitation

PSYCHOLOGICAL REHABILITATION

Psychological strengthening is largely carried out by reassurance therapy mainly by the ophthalmologist and partly by clinical psychologist. Ophthalmologist has an important role to play by educating the patient and his relatives about the visual prognosis on the basis of the Ocular Trauma Score. Although, factual information may be given regarding what the patient can do and what he cannot do, but all positive points should be stressed and negative statements must be avoided.

Ocular trauma patients are often particularly stressed and should be counselled to make them as comfortable and relaxed as possible. The key to rehabilitation of almost all people with visual impairment, whether monocular or binocular, is not to let them give up. Patients should be strongly encouraged not to stop performing activities they have a reasonable chance of making adaptations for. The old adage "practice makes a man perfect" definitely applies to the visual system: There are eye surgeons and jewelers who are monocular and golfers who are bilaterally blind.

Reassurance therapy. Lack of confidence can multiply the functional impact of vision loss. Reassurance therapy should therefore be a part of every ophthalmologist's therapeutic armamentarium by providing a credible and acceptable prognosis. A physician should be as specific as possible regarding what the patient can and cannot do. Although he should stress all positive aspects and not volunteer negative and threatening facts but at the same time he should be realistic and avoid raising the patient's expectations so high that they exceed the physician's ability to deliver. He should banish all unwarranted fears as patients usually imagine that problems are worse than they actually are. He should be aware of the power of placebo and refer the patient to a practitioner who has experience in dealing with patients of vision loss.

VISUAL REHABILITATION

Visual rehabilitation should be resumed simultaneously. It consists of utilization of residual vision in a best possible manner so that confidence is built up for finding solutions to the various difficulties of life. Constant efforts in this direction can achieve results even when the fovea is irreversibly damaged. The need of the hour is to develop vision so that visual impairment does not come in the way of the patient for living a life king sized. Rehabilitation training teaches patients how best to use residual vision and offers practical adaptations for activities of daily living. The visual rehabilitation is done by referring the patient to a centre equipped with a variety of low vision aids (LVA). One has to choose the most suitable LVA for the patient depending upon the extent of impairment and based upon his professional requirement (Table 16.1).

Prescription of low vision aids (LVA)

Assistive devices like reading aids (bifocals), high power magnifiers, video-magnifiers, talking books and vision substitution which includes Braille or using a computer with voice synthesis may decrease the disorder related disability. Changes in human and physical environment may increase participation regardless of reduced abilities.

Guidelines for prescribing LVAs

The practitioner should keep following points in mind while prescribing an LVA:

1. The aim should be to provide maximum vision without compromising with the mobility of the patient.
2. It should be borne in mind that as the magnification increases, both the working distance and field of vision decreases.
3. Preferably the aid chosen should be simple, light weight, portable and flexible. It is better to avoid complicated and cumbersome devices. As far as possible, the conventional spectacles with a high addition should be the first choice.
4. The patients visual status, mental status, needs and motivation should be given due consideration while prescribing a LVA. Therefore, the aid needed may vary from person to person even though the cause of low vision may be the same.

5. All the devices with similar magnification should be tried before prescribing a particular LVA.
6. Both eyes should be corrected, if the difference in magnification is insignificant. However, if a complicated and cumbersome device is needed, only one eye may be used to avoid further complicating the situation.
7. A single eyed person with markedly low vision may accept a telescope or high addition.
8. In old patients where keeping the print at a fixed focus may be difficult, it may be worth while to try without magnifier.
9. In children persuasion and understanding is of paramount importance. Therefore, it may be worthwhile to defer prescription of the LVA till the child is old enough and understands their value.

Dispensing an LVA

A. *Magnification trial.* After a meticulously performed work-up the magnification required should be calculated by the practitioner, taking into consideration the influence of scotometry, contrast and glare data. The power of reading correction should be adjusted until the patient can read the target size words and text.

B. *Prescription of appropriate device.* Various LVAs of the calculated power should then be tried systematically in sequence: Convex lens first as a spectacle (either monocular or binocular with converging prism), second as a hand magnifier and third as a stand magnifier. The complex telescopes, microscopic doublet and

S.No.	Vision status	Disability assessment	Low vision device for reading
		Table 16.1 Status of vision, disability and requirement of possible LVA	
1.	Near normal (6/9 to 6/18)	Patient can function fairly normally. Normal performance using shorter reading distance	Stronger Bifocals (3–5D), low power magnifier (5D)
2.	Low vision (6/24 to 6/60)	Near normal performance with magnifiers	Half eye glasses (6–10D) with incorporated prisms for binocularity
3.	Severe low vision (5/60 to 3/60)	Legally blind, slower performance than normal with LVA	High power reading lens (10–20D), video magnifier
4.	Profound low vision (2/60 to 1/60)	Legally blind, reading more strenuous with LVA	Still high power magnifiers (20–40D) video magnifiers, talking books, Braille
5.	Blindness < 1–60	Reading not possible	Talking books, Braille

electronic system should be reserved only for desperate cases.

The major consideration in the choice between a telescope and hand magnifier is the work distance. Other considerations are weight of the spectacles, cosmesis, whether both hands are needed to be free during use, whether or not the hand held magnifier will be steady and the field of view it enhances. In general, a telescope has a larger field of view than a hand magnifier of equivalent power, since they are closer to the eyes.

The user must finally determine what type of visual aid is best for him or her. Every person's adaptability to a particular degree of visual impairment is different, so are his or her needs.

C. *Training to use appropriate LVA.* Once the aid to be dispensed is finalized in view of the guidelines for prescribing an LVA, the patient should be taught how to handle the aid and how to hold the printed material. A common complaint with LVA is that it works much better in the doctor's clinic than at the patient's home. The possible explanation is that the lighting is much better in the doctor's clinic. So, along with the prescription of the visual aid, proper guidance should be given about optimal lighting arrangements as well.

a. *Patients should be trained to*:
- Take care of the device
- Keep it clean
- Decide when to use, where to use, for which activities to use and to explain to others why he or she cannot work without it.

b. *Counselling and motivation* are very important to encourage the patient to use LVA.

c. *Periodic follow-up* is important to assess the user's performance with the prescribed visual aid. Periodic follow-up visits should be scheduled to assess the amount of progress made.

OCCUPATIONAL REHABILITATION

It is the job of occupational therapists along with the orientation and mobility specialists. Their aim is to reduce the functional effect of impairment so that the patient is least dependent on his family/society and to maintain constructive pursuits of the patient so that he continues to be useful to the community and finally he has a life full of satisfaction, contentment and fulfilment.

CONCLUSION

The fact that despite best of the treatment the final visual outcome in a patient of trauma remains unpredictable. Therefore, it is imperative to:

Promote preventive eye care programmes for increasing awareness of protection of eyes amongst all high-risk professionals and automobile drivers.

Use of protective eyewear should be highlighted and legislation for the same by the government agencies needs to be instituted.

Public health education aimed at increasing consciousness among parents, guardians and school teachers regarding the need for supervision of children, and institution of precautionary programmes, especially for vulnerable groups, are urgently needed in order to reduce ocular morbidity due to ocular trauma.

BIBLIOGRAPHY

1. Bhogal G, Tomlins PJ, Murray PI. Penetrating ocular injuries at home. Journal of Public Health 2006;29(1):72–74.
2. Henderson D. Ocular trauma: one in the eye for safety glasses. Archives of Emergency Medicine 1991;8:201–204.
3. Jyh-Haur W, Gangadhara S. Eye Injuries in Singapore – Don't Risk It. Do More. A Prospective Study. Ann Acad Med Singapore 2006;35:706–718.
4. McGwin G Jr, Owsley C. Risk factors for motor vehicle collision-related eye injuries. Arch. Ophthalmol. 2005;123,89–95.
5. Ngo CS, Leo SW. Industrial accident-related ocular emergencies in a tertiary hospital in Singapore. Singapore Med J 2008;49(4):280–285.
6. Thompson GJ, Mollan SP. Occupational eye injuries: A continuing problem. Occupational Medicine 2009;59:123–125.
7. Vats S, Murthy GVS, Chandra M, Gupta SK, Vashist P, Gogoi M. Epidemiological study of ocular trauma in an urban slum population in Delhi, India. Indian J Ophthalmol 2008;56: 313–316.

17

MEDICOLEGAL ASPECTS AND COMPENSATION IN OCULAR TRAUMA

MEDICOLEGAL ASPECTS IN OCULAR TRAUMA

An injury refers to the damage to a person or a tissue/organ caused by transfer of energy: mechanical, thermal, chemical, electrical or radiant. Basic nature of mechanical injuries may be accidental, suicidal or homicidal. The eyeball is fairly delicate organ so it is protected by bony orbit and various physiological reflexes, such as blinking reflex and lacrimation reflex. However, since the eyes are delicate organs, traumatic injuries may lead to even blindness. Ocular trauma is a major cause of visual impairment and morbidity worldwide. In India, there are more than 50 million blind people and this number increases by about 3.8 million per year. Amongst the total number of blind cases, 1.2% are contributed by injuries which are largely preventable. Since the ocular injury may be accidental, suicidal, or homicidal, a lot of questions can arise from the legal point of view. Since visual loss is included as a 2nd clause in the Grievous hurt (Sec. 320 IPC), so ocular injuries are always associated with legal problems.

Undoubtedly, primary duty of a doctor is to provide patient care; however, medicolegal aspects associated with all cases of trauma must get an adequate care along with the execution of treatment. Medicolegal aspects of ocular trauma can be considered under two main headings:
- Medicolegal negligence, and
- Professional negligence.

MEDICOLEGAL NEGLIGENCE

DEFINITION

Medicolegal negligence on the part of attending/treating doctor is defined as failure to carry out

246

the medicolegal duties in an accepted way. If the doctor fails to deliver his medicolegal duties, a case of negligence can also be filed against him and the case may end in the civil or the criminal court.

MEDICOLEGAL DUTIES IN OCULAR TRAUMA

Medicolegal duties in case of ocular trauma include:
- Proper procedure of examination and recording of data,
- Writing accident-cum-wound certificate,
- Written and informed consent, and
- Police information.

1. Proper procedure of examination and recording of data

Whenever a case of injury comes to a doctor, he should know how to examine the patient and record all the findings, and treat him so that whenever he may have to go to the court he can give his opinion as an expert witness.

If any case of ocular trauma reports to the casualty medical officer, he should take consent for examination. During examination, he must note the particulars of the patient and also the name and other details of police officer, if accompanied. He should take short history noting, how he sustained the injuries, date and time of assault, etc. He should carry out the general physical examination and carefully note all the injuries, their type, location, direction, dimensions, presence and absence of foreign body, bleeding or not and also mention about their nature. Preferably he should draw a simple sketch of the injury for future reference.

Photo documentation in ocular trauma

Ocular photographs are very much useful not only for medicolegal purposes but also for clinical records, patient education, teaching and research, interoffice diagnostic opinions and community screening. Ocular photographs are the best evidence to be used in medicolegal cases and for compensatory purposes along with documentation and counselling. The new aspect to be highlighted is to photograph every case of an ocular trauma for the safety of an ophthalmologist and to explain the grave prognosis to the family. This will avoid unnecessary aggravation and harassment to the ophthalmologist in different criminal, medicolegal, and compensatory cases.

2. Writing accident-cum-wound certificate

All the findings must be noted in Medico-Legal Report (MLR) and it should be prepared in triplicate. Original copy of the MLR should be kept under safe custody by the attending doctor, second copy should be submitted to the police as a confidential report and third copy should be kept by hospital in the patient case file. Always take the opinion from the expert of that field (ophthalmologist), and make necessary investigations and treatment, failing to which, a doctor may be charged for negligence.

3. Written and informed consent

Consent is defined as the concurrence of 'will' and its chief essential constituent is the consciousness or knowledge of the act consented to. The Indian Contract Act, Section 13, states "two or more persons are said to consent when they agree upon the same thing in the same sense". The doctors should take consent before each and every examination and institution of treatment. If he fails to do so and if he treats or operates the patient and if the patient suffers any damage than the doctor is liable for the damages and can be prosecuted for his act legally. Consent is to be obtained from conscious, mentally sound adults, or from the parent of a child who is less than 12 years of age. For invasive and diagnostic procedures, general anaesthesia, surgical operations and medicolegal examinations, the age of consent is >18 years.

Consent is not must under following situations:
- *Sections 87 and 88 of IPC* are regarding the exemption of liability when the harm is caused by an act done in good faith and for the benefit of the consenting individual.
- *Section 89 of IPC* deals with cases where the act is done in good faith and for the benefit of child or insane person, by consent of guardian or person empowered to give consent on behalf of the child or the insane.
- *Section 90 of IPC* explains that if the consent is obtained by coercion (under fear of injury),

undue influence, fraud, misrepresentation or misconception of facts, the consent gets vitiated.

- *Section 92 of IPC* explains that if the patient is in coma and needs emergency treatment, consent is not necessary.
- A medicolegal case referred by a court of law for examination also doesn't need consent.

4. Police information

A government doctor must give information to the nearest police station, if any case of injury comes to the casuality, irrespective of its manner and nature of the injury. A private doctor can abstain from such intimation, if the patient does not give consent for the same.

Note. If a doctor takes proper consent, intimates the police, makes an MLR, notes all injuries, investigates the patient and starts treatment, then his medicolegal duties are considered satisfactory. If he fails to perform these medicolegal duties, a negligence suit may be filed against him in a court of law, which may end in civil or criminal court.

PROFESSIONAL NEGLIGENCE

DEFINITION

Professional negligence is the absence of reasonable care and skill or willful negligence of a medical practitioner in the treatment of a patient which causes bodily injury or death of the patient. In simple word, "doing something that one is not supposed to do (act of commission) and failing to do something that one is supposed to do (act of omission)".

TYPES AND CAUSES OF PROFESSIONAL NEGLIGENCE

Types. There are two types of negligence:
- *Civil negligence*: It does not come under the purview of CrPC and IPC.
- *Criminal negligence*: Sec. 304 A deals with criminal negligence.

Causes: Negligence may be either due to lack of knowledge and skill or failure to provide due care during a procedure. Every medical practitioner should have basic reasonable knowledge;

however, it doesn't mean that he should possess the highest degree of skill and knowledge. For example, an MCh doctor is expected of a higher level of skill than an MS doctor, who in turn has a higher level of skill than the MBBS doctor. For the same level of negligence, an MCh doctor may be held responsible, but not an MBBS doctor. No doctor is expected to possess all currently available medical knowledge, and need not apply all known diagnostic and therapeutic techniques.

ELEMENTS OF NEGLIGENCE

There are four major elements in professional negligence:
- Duty of care,
- Failure to exercise duty of care (dereliction),
- Damage to patient on account of dereliction, and
- Direct causation.

1. Duty of care

A doctor begins to owe a duty towards a patient as soon as he agrees to treat him and secondly when he is on emergency duty. A doctor to be charged with negligence must be under a 'duty of care' to the person complaining of negligence. *Doctor cannot be charged for negligence, if he was not under duty of care,* even though there is damage to the complaining party.

Duty of care doesn't exist under following situations:
- While attending an injured person on road-side following an accident, and
- In medicolegal examination for issuing medical certificate for disability and drunkenness.

Doctor cannot refuse to treat a patient who is in emergency. If the patient is in emergency, the doctor must treat him; otherwise charges of criminal negligence may be brought against him, especially if the patient dies.

2. Dereliction of duty

Doctor can be charged for professional negligence, once the presence of duty has been established, and there has to be dereliction of duty on the part of the doctor, i.e. the doctor should have been negligent in performing his duties towards the patient. The dereliction of duty is defined as failure of a doctor to do his duty that is owed to his patient. Such breach of duty may be:

- *Act of commission*, for example, performing any surgery in the normal eye in place of affected or diseased eye, or
- *Act of omission*, for example, failure to give anti-tetanus prophylaxis when it is indicated.

3. Damage to patient on account of dereliction

Damage to patient refers to the injury or disability suffered by the patient due to dereliction of duty, for example, if enucleation of an eye is to be done for a retained intraocular foreign body, which was not diagnosed and treated in the initial stage. Patient cannot sue the doctor for compensation, if no damage has occurred even if he was negligent. Further, it should be proved that the damage has occurred as a result of dereliction.

4. Direct causation

Another element requires that the damage, alleged to have resulted, should bear a direct 'cause and effect' relationship to the negligence of the doctor and not from any other cause. For example, if a patient comes to a doctor with lacerated wound over the right eye, the doctor treats him (*duty is established*), however, the doctor fails to stitch the wound (*dereliction occurs*). Afterwards the patient goes to a quack who applies a cow-dung over the wound and patient develops infection (*damage occurs*), and the patient sues the first doctor for not stitching the wound. However, he cannot succeed because, although there was duty, dereliction, and even damage, but damage was not a direct cause of doctor's dereliction.

PREVENTIVE MEASURES AGAINST MEDICAL NEGLIGENCE

The adage 'a stitch in time saves nine' will definitely help prevent litigation in respect of medical negligence against medical practitioner. Factors likely to prevent initiation of negligence against doctors are listed below:

1. Restrain from criticism of fellow doctors

One of the most common cause of negligence arises out of criticism from another doctor, without knowing the full facts. Sometimes patients go from one doctor to another for asking second opinion. In most of such cases, patients wish to have some psychological reassurance. A casual bad remark by another doctor can create problems by shaking the patient's confidence in the doctor whom he has originally consulted.

2. Creating an environment that engenders trust

At the very top of the list of preventive measures is engendering trust, i.e. trust in the doctors, trust in their staff and trust in their recommendations. Following measures are useful for building a relation of trust between the patient and the doctor:

- Doctors should have a valid insight regarding their own abilities and limitations.
- Doctors and their staff should listen, hear and treat their patients respectfully.
- Doctors and their staff should sincerely care for the patients.
- Clear and adequate communication between patients, staff, and doctors.
- Encouraging patients to maintain their own medical records.
- Encouraging patients to bring written lists of their concerns, medication, and issues they wish to discuss.
- Giving written instructions to patients regarding recommended treatment.

3. Maintaining good medical records

Record keeping must be accurate, perfect and safe because the surgeon may forgot the facts in the due course, but the records will remain as such and can be effectively utilized in a court of law. The patients may die, but the record will never die, and will speak in its own. Keep accurate and complete records. An accurate case record should contain history, present illness, physical examination, investigations, impression about the case, treatment adopted, any cross consultations and any refusal from the side of patient for any investigations and treatment.

4. Sending letters to patients summarizing the results of the patient visit

Sending letters to patients summarizing the results of the patient visit with copies of letters to the referring/treating consultants. The actions especially by doctors and their staff that create an environment in which patients feel cared, heard and respected are essential.

5. Employ qualified staff and associate with good partners

Doctors will be responsible for the act of commission or omission of his assistants, non-technical staff, and partners in the course of treating a patient. So it is emparative to employ qualified and efficient staff.

6. Update the knowledge

Doctor must be exposed to the latest developments in the concerned field by attending local, national and international conferences and consulting the latest journals.

7. Valid consent

Consent must be obtained before starting an examination, diagnostic or investigative procedure or treatment. For the consent to be valid it must be informed, with patient being informed of relevant facts regarding procedure and its complications and consequences.

8. Ensure reasonable skill and care

Doctor should use reasonable skill and care in both diagnosis and treatment. When in doubt, it is always better to take a second opinion. A doctor must ensure that all the instruments used by him are maintained well and sterilized properly.

9. Guard against therapeutic hazards

Before starting treatment, doctor should enquire about the past history of any adverse drug reactions. All the facilities to manage a case of drug reaction must be available.

DEFENCES AGAINST NEGLIGENCE

Defences against negligence are as below:
1. No duty owed to the plaintiff.
2. Duty discharged according to prevailing standards.
3. Therapeutic misadventure.
4. Error of judgement.
5. Contributory negligence.
6. Res judicata (Sec 300 CrPC): If a question of negligence against a doctor has already been decided by a court, the patient will not be allowed to contest the same in another proceeding between himself and a doctor.
7. Limitation. As per Sec 24-A of CPA 1986, a suit for damages for negligence against a doctor should be filed within 2 years from the date of alleged negligence, whereas the limitation period for filing a case is maximum up to 3 years under the Limitation Act.

COMPENSATION IN OCULAR INJURIES

GENERAL CONSIDERATION

INTRODUCTION

Eyes are very important organ for every human being. Injuries to the eyes are not uncommon and can be very distressing to the individual. The distress may vary from the mild conjunctival irritation to the loss of eye sight. Cause of an eye injury can vary from the smallest dust particle entering the eye to the ocular damage resulting from roadside accident or an accident at work place. Ocular injuries may also result from an assault by blow, or a blunt or sharp instrument as well or due to medical negligence in operative procedures of eye. During roadside accident, injury to the eye can occur due to the broken pieces of glass of windshield or due to the air bag compressing the chest and causing injury to the eye.

COMPENSATION: PURPOSE, TYPE, ASSESSMENT AND CATEGORIES

Purpose of awarding damages in a tort action is to ensure that a person who has suffered damage (injury/harm) is made 'whole' or is returned to the previous condition that existed before the injury.

Two types of compensatory damages have generally been recognized:

- General damages—awarded for non-economic losses, and
- Special damages—awarded for past and future medical, surgical, hospital and other related costs, past and future loss of income and expenses for cremation.

Assessment of compensation. Damages are assessed by the court based on parameters like loss of earning capacity, medical and surgical cost and/or reduction of quality of life.

Categories of damage. Potential damages (financial compensation) in negligence suits fall into three categories:

- Economic or the monetary costs of an injury (medical bills and/or loss of income),
- Non-economic (e.g. pain and sufferings, loss of ability to have sex), and
- Punitive or damages to punish a defendant for wilful and want on conduct.

CIVIL MATTERS RELATED TO COMPENSATION

1. *When a doctor has treated the case as a second expert.* When either the patient is referred by the first ophthalmologist for opinion and/or further treatment or the patient has gone of his own to the second expert for treatment and if the case goes in the court under CPA, then the first and/or second doctor treating the case may be called in the court as witness or to provide opinion.

2. *When the patient is referred or comes himself for examination and a certificate for compensation purposes is required.* If there is loss of vision causing disability or blindness or disfiguration a certificate for compensation may be required in following situations:

- *Under Employees Compensation Act*, the treating doctor has to certify the extent of damage to the concerned authority or the court. When there are damages during working in the organization.
- *For insurance and re-imbursement.* In insurance cases, the doctor has to certify the extent of damage to the insurance company or the court.

- *Under Consumer Protection Act (CPA).* When a doctor has treated the patient as second expert doctor and the court requires the extent of damages to calculate the loss and compensation.
- *As a certifying expert after examination of a case.* The court may send a case for examination and certification of the condition of the patient.

CRIMINAL MATTERS IN RELATION TO COMPENSATION

1. *Accidental trauma.* When trauma is caused in a vehicle accident case, doctor may be required to give certificate to the court or insurance company indicating the amount of loss of function. Record of such cases has to be kept for a minimum of 3 years.

2. *Trauma by assault.* Patient may give history of an assault and when it is taken on record, or when patient is referred by police or court, the doctor has to note the injuries in detail, in a separate register called medicolegal examination (MLE) register. It has to be noted whether injury is simple or grievous in nature. The amount of loss of function (vision) is also to be noted.

3. *Trauma while working.* When a worker is referred for the ocular injury sustained while working, one has to keep record of the injury and percentage of loss of function or percentage of eye injury.

LAWS (STATUES) AND PROVISIONS FOR COMPENSATION IN INDIA

The law in our country provides adequate compensation for each ocular injury under various sections. Some of the common situations for compensation in ocular injuries include:

- Compensation for ocular injuries due to an assault
- Compensation for ocular injuries at work place
- Compensation in Motor Vehicle Act
- Compensation for medical negligence in ocular injuries

COMPENSATION FOR OCULAR INJURIES DUE TO AN ASSAULT

According to section 319 IPC, hurt means bodily pain, disease or infirmity caused to any person. Grievous hurt, covered under Section 320 IPC, is a hurt of more serious nature. Clause 2 of section 320 IPC for grievous hurt for eyes pertains to the permanent privation of sight of either eye which could even include partial loss of sight. Operative interferences are not taken in account.

Compensation for various simple and grievous injuries is covered under sections 323 to 326 of IPC depending upon the weapon and intention of infliction of the injury.

- *Under section 323 IPC*, a punishment for voluntarily causing the hurt is punishable with imprisonment up to 1 year and/or fine of ₹ 1000.
- *Under section 324 IPC*, voluntarily causing the hurt by a dangerous weapon is punishable with imprisonment up to 3 years and/or fine of any amount.
- *Under section 325 IPC*, a punishment for voluntarily causing the grievous hurt is punishable with imprisonment up to 7 years and/or fine of any amount.
- *Under section 326 IPC*, voluntarily causing grievous hurt by dangerous weapon is punishable with imprisonment for the life or imprisonment which may extend up to 10 years and/or fine of any amount.

COMPENSATION FOR OCULAR INJURIES AT WORK PLACE

Workmen's Compensation Act 1923 is one of the earliest labour law legislation enacted in India. This act provides compensation for the various injuries to the employees at the workplace. The 'Workmen's Compensation Act' which came into force with effect from 1.7.1924 has been amended several times. It has been enacted to provide for payment by certain classes of employers to their workmen as compensation for the injuries inflicted by an accident occurring during the discharge of their duties.

In 1929, an amendment removed restriction on compensation in building trades. In 1931, the categories of workmen covered by the act were increased, scales of compensation were raised and the waiting period reduced. In 1946, the wage limit of a worker covered by the act was increased from ₹ 300 to 400/–.

The 'Workmen's Compensation Act of 1946' should be further revised and provision should be made for temporary workers also.

Definitions under Workmen's Compensation Act

- *A workman* is defined as any person whose employment is not of a casual nature.
- *Total disablement* means a disablement, temporary or permanent, which incapacitates a workman for all the work which he was capable of doing at the time of accident.
- *Partial disablement* means one of temporary nature which reduces the earning capacity of a workman for the profession he has been following at the time of accident. It is called permanent when it reduces the earning capacity in any profession even employed elsewhere.

Compensation under Workmen's Compensation Act

Employer is liable for compensation when the personal injury is caused to a workman by accident arising out of and in course of employment.

Employer is not liable for compensation when:
- Injury does not disable workmen totally or partially
- Disablement is for less than 3 days
- Injured workman was under the influence of drink or drugs
- Injured workman ignored safety rules
- Injured workmen disregards safety devices

Note. No claim for compensation can be entertained unless notice has been given as soon as practicable after the accident, but within 2 years of occurrence of death, disability or accident.

Compensation in corneal opacities. Industrial trauma causing corneal opacities can be of a multiple nature. A simple tiny corneal foreign body may become infected giving rise to a sloughing corneal ulcer and a thick corneal leucoma. Panophthalmitis and loss of eye has also been noted in some cases. The cases of leucomas must be submitted to keratoplasty before the compensation is decided.

Compensation is payable by the employer and the amount payable depends upon the gravity of injury. Amount of compensation in case of permanent total disablement is equal to [60% of monthly salary of the injured worker] × [relevant factor] or ₹ 90,000 whichever is more.

Younger the person, higher is the relevant factor. For example, relevant factor for 16 years worker is 228.54; for 25 years old 216.91; for 50 years old 153.09; for > 65 years 99.37, and so on.

PRE-RECRUITMENT MEDICAL EXAMINATION

This is a very important factor, if we are not going to be caught unaware when an accident occurs. The medical examination should be by an industrial medical officer or a board of specialists.

Haphazard record of vision may give rise to a lot of difficulties later on. Several cases have been discovered on a routine check-up of records where vision has been recorded as, both eyes equal to 6/6. Probably, in such cases, vision was recorded by a general duty doctor with both eyes together. After an accident, the workman can claim that each eye was normal before accident. One eye, however, may have been blind at the time of employment.

Colour vision must be recorded in all cases, whether good colour vision is essential for the job or not. A workman not requiring good colour vision at the time of recruitment may be transferred later to a job where good colour vision is essential. Leaving aside railway jobs and crane operators in whom good colour vision is essential, ordinary workers, like electricians, also require good colour vision. The colour of wires red, blue and green if mistaken may lead to serious accident and death. In all such cases, heavy compensation may have to be paid just because proper medical examination was not undertaken earlier.

Malingering

Many people pose a problem to the industrial ophthalmologist by malingering. A few examples are given below.

1. *Mr AK was exposed to hot coal tar gases and developed severe conjunctivitis* in both eyes. It settled down in two days after which period a thin nebula was discovered on the left cornea reducing his vision to 6/36 with best correction. His pre-recruitment records showed "vision both eyes equal to 6/6". Even six months after the accident, the nebula was as before and must have been there before the accident. The latter fact, however, could not be proved and a partial disability compensation had to be paid.

2. *Two years after a hot metal burn on face and hands* Mr JPC claimed that his reduced eye-sight was due to the accident at workplace. On examination, he was found to have myopic astigmatism which could be corrected to 6/6. No compensation was paid inspite of the loud protests by the worker and the workers' Union.

3. *Mr CP, after a head injury at workplace was alright for 6 months.* Then he reported loss of sight in the left eye. A simple fogging test proved him to be faking blindness.

COMPENSATION IN MOTOR VEHICLE ACT

Ocular injuries accidents occur by way of splinters entering into the eye or by other modes. Ocular injuries can lead to either blindness or low vision. Blindness has been defined as:

- Total absence of sight; or
- Visual acuity not exceeding 6/60 or 20/200 (Snellen) in the better eye with best correcting lenses; or
- Limitation of field of vision subtending an angle of 20 degrees or worse.

Low vision. A person with impairment of vision from less than 6/18 to 6/60 with best correction in the better eye or impairment of field of vision in any one of the following categories:

- Reduction of visual fields less than 50 degrees; or
- Hemianopia with macular involvement; or
- Altitudinal defect involving lower half of field of vision.

CATEGORIES OF VISUAL DISABILITY

While assessing function loss (vision disability) resulting in permanent physical impairment

Table 17.1 *Categories of visual disability*

Category	Better eye (Best corrected vision)	Worse eye (Best corrected vision)	Percentage impairment
Category 0	0 6/9–6/18	6/24–6/36	20 %
Category I	6/18–6/36	6/60–Nil	40%
Category II	6/60–4/60	3/60–Nil	75%
Category III	3/60–1/60	FC at 1 ft–Nil	100%
Category IV	FC at 1 ft	Nil FC at 1 ft	100%

FC = Finger Counting

(disability) following variables need to be taken into consideration:

- Acuity of vision,
- Field of vision (in degrees),
- Hemianopia, and
- Altitudinal defect (in lower field).

Categories of visual disability are depicted in Table 17.1.

Percentage of visual disability is duly calculated and compensation is equally awarded.

One-eyed person. Having visual acuity of 6/6 in one eye and FC at 1 ft. to Nil or field of vision <10° in the other eye. Visual disability without disfigurement in such cases is 30%.

OCULAR INJURIES AND CONSUMER PROTECTION ACT (CPA)

When a patient with injury comes to an ophthalmologist many a times because of fear of CPA, he is in dilemma whether he should take the case or not, particularly when he is a general ophthalmologist. In such cases, when he wants to refer the case, he should give primary treatment and should give a referral letter to the patient and a copy of letter with "received" signature of patient or guardian with date and time should be kept with him.

Defenses against CPA

A doctor should not be afraid of CPA, as the Court expects only that much care and treatment that a "*Prudent doctor*" will give. So in such cases, the doctor should record the injuries in detail with figures or photographs. Defenses against CPA:

- Do necessary investigations and should keep records.
- Should tell relatives the prognosis and take them in confidence.
- Should take informed consent in their vernacular standard language, if surgery is to be done.
- Treat the patient as per the textbook norms.
- Refer the patient to higher centre, if you feel.
- Be transparent and polite with patient and relatives.

COMPENSATION FOR MEDICAL NEGLIGENCE IN OCULAR SURGERY AND EYE CAMP CASES

With the advancement of medical knowledge and recent technical developments, eye diseases which were considered incurable have now become curable. Since the treatment depends upon the latest equipment, which are somehow costly so the amounts spend on the ocular surgery is increasing. Treatment outcome depends on the quality of treatment and the biological response from the patient. As the amount spend on surgery is increasing, the litigations are also increasing as the patients want immediate results and that too without any complication. Of all the surgeries being conducted in ophthalmology, cataract surgery accounts for the major chunk. As these surgeries are being conducted in various charitable hospitals or in private set ups in large scale, the Supreme Court has laid down certain guidelines while performing the surgeries in eye camps. These include:

1. *Operations in the camps should only be performed by qualified, experienced ophthalmic*

surgeons registered with Medical Council of India or any state medical council. The eye camp should not be used as a training ground for postgraduate students, and operative work should not be entrusted to postgraduate students.

2. *Pathologist* should be there to examine urine, blood, sugar, etc. It is preferable to have a dentist to check the teeth for sepsis and a physician for general medical check-up.

3. *All medicines to be used should be of standard quality* duly verified by the doctor in-charge of the eye camp. Purity of the drugs and medicines intended for human use would have to be ensued by prior tests and inspection.

4. *Necessity of maintenance of the highest standards of sterile conditions* at places where ophthalmic surgery or any surgery is conducted cannot be over-emphasized. It is not merely on the formulation of the theoretical standards but really on the professional commitment with which the prescriptions are implemented that the ultimate result rests. The maintenance of sterile, aseptic conditions in hospitals to prevent cross-infections should be ordinary, routine to high standard.

Note. If the above guidelines are not followed the treating doctor are liable to be sued for compensation for the medical negligence.

BIBLIOGRAPHY

1. Aggarwal A. Textbook of Forensic Medicine and Toxicology. 1st ed. p 51–52.
2. Aggarwal A. Textbook of Forensic Medicine and Toxicology. 1st edition. Avichal Publishing Company, New Delhi. p 36.
3. Biswas G. Review of Forensic Medicine and Toxicology. 2nd edition. p 13–14.
4. Categories of Visual Impairment in India. [Internet] [Updated 18 March 2015]. http://www.medindia.net/health_statistics/general/visualimpairment.asp
5. M Rangnath. AS Mittal and Ors Vs State of UP and Ors on 12 May, 1989: 1989 AIR 1570, 1989 SCR (3) 241. http://indiankanoon.org/doc/338680/
6. Misra S, Nandwani R, Gogri P, Misra N. Clinical profile and visual outcome of ocular injuries in a rural area of western India. AMJ 2013, 6, 11, 560–564.
7. Raju KV. Medicolegal aspects of ocular trauma. Kerala Journal of Ophthalmology. Vol. XXII, No. 3, Sept. 2010, p 277–278.
8. Reddy KSN. The Essentials of Forensic Medicine and Toxicology. 32nd ed. p 278-280.
9. Reddy KSN. The Esssentials of Forensic Medicine and Toxicology. 33rd edition. p 34.
10. Subrahmanyam BV. Law in relation to medical men. In: Modi's Medical Jurisprudence and toxicology, 22 ed, 2001. Butterworths India, New Delhi. 683–740.
11. Vij K. Textbook of Forensic Medicine and Toxicology. Principles and Practice. 6th edition. Elsevier, New Delhi. p348–349, 356.

Index